A Practical Guide to Beauty Therapy

for NVQ Levels 1 and 2

Janet Simms
Chief Examiner for C&G

Stanley Thornes (Publishers) Ltd

First published in 1993 by:
Stanley Thornes (Publishers) Ltd
Ellenborough House
Wellington Street
CHELTENHAM GL50 1YD
England

Reprinted 1993
Reprinted 1994 (twice)
Reprinted 1995

A catalogue record for this book is available from the British Library.

ISBN 0 7487 1508 8

Typeset by Tech-Set, Gateshead, Tyne & Wear
Printed and bound in Great Britain by Scotprint, Musselburgh

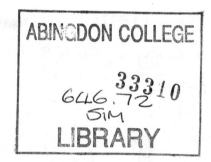

Contents

Introduction

There has never been a more exciting and challenging time for vocational education than the present, and the publication of A Practical Guide to Beauty Therapy (NVQ Levels 1 and 2) will provide a reference text for the first students and tutors involved with the new NVQ qualifications. The book has been developed concurrently with the design of the Levels 1 and 2 awards and faithful regard has been paid to providing the underpinning knowledge required for successful completion of each unit.

Whilst accepting the need to identify specific subject areas for the purposes of assessment, the contents of some units have been integrated with other chapters to provide relevance and increase understanding.

The study matrix will guide students through this integrated approach.

Each chapter includes activities to help students develop practical learning skills and increase their knowledge of current working practice.

The self-checks provide opportunity for testing knowledge and understanding at an appropriate stage of each chapter. This will help prepare students for the oral and written testing which will form the basis of their assessment for Levels 1 and 2 awards in Beauty Therapy.

Acknowledgements

Cover photograph courtesy of Mary Cohr Cosmetics, visagiste Michel Limongi.

I would like to give special thanks to my husband Iain, my boys Adam and David and my family and friends who have supported and encouraged me with this book. Also, in recognition of their technical and professional contribution, usually knowingly (but not always!): Pam Ledgard, June Hunt, my friends and colleagues at City College Manchester, Alan Glen, Kate Jenkins (Inverness U.K. Ltd.), Bryn Williams (Sterling Supplies Ltd.) and Raymond Langford-Jones (City and Guilds).

Study matrix for NVQ units

Chapter	A01	A02	A03	B04	B05	B06	B07	B08	B09	B10	B11	B12	B13	B14	B15	B16	B17	B18	B19
1	•	•	•			•	•		•	•	•	•	•	•	•		•	•	•
2	•	•	•	•	•	•	•									•	•	•	•
3	•	•	•	•	•	•	•	•								•	•	•	•
4	•	•	•		•		•		•	•	•			•	•	•			
5	•	•	•	•	•		•		•	•						•			
6	•	•	•	•	•		•			•						•			
7	•	•	•	•	•		•				•					•			
8	•	•	•		•		•					•	•			•			
9	•	•	•	•	•		•					•	•			•			
10	•	•	•	•			•						•			•			
11	•	•	•	•	•		•					•				•			
12	•	•	•	•			•							•		•			
13	•	•	•	•			•								•	•			

Key to chapters

1 Health, hygiene and safety in the salon
2 Reception
3 Selling products and services
4 Examining the face and neck
5 Facial massage and skin care
6 Make-up
7 Lash and brow treatments
8 Examining the hands and nails
9 Manicure and hand treatments
10 Nail technology
11 Pedicure
12 Wax depilation
13 Ear piercing

Key to units

A01 Maintain employment standards
A02 Support a healthy, safe and secure salon environment
A03 Liaise with clients and colleagues in a salon environment
B04 Undertake salon reception duties
B05 Providing a service to the customer
B06 Processing the sale
B07 Achieving a sale
B08 Dealing with returned goods and complaints
B09 Provide facial massage and skin care
B10 Apply and instruct on make-up
B11 Provide lash and brow treatments
B12 Provide and advise on nail care
B13 Provide artificial nail structures
B14 Provide wax depilation
B15 Pierce ears
B16 Marketing cosmetics and perfumes
B17 Handling stock
B18 Displaying and merchandising stock
B19 Maintaining stock records

Chapter 1

Health, hygiene and safety in the salon

After working through this chapter you will be able to:

- ▶ understand the importance of health and safety in the salon
- ▶ explain the influence of legislation on working practices
- ▶ identify potential hazards in the salon
- ▶ carry out emergency procedures
- ▶ describe professional standards of hygiene and appearance
- ▶ understand the basis of effective working relationships
- ▶ carry out security procedures.

Employment standards

The law demands that every place of work is a healthy and safe place to be, not only for the people who work there but also for clients and other visitors. Failure to comply with the law has serious consequences and can be very expensive for the salon in the event of the following:

- claims made by injured staff
- claims made by injured clients
- prosecution and fines
- closure of the business
- loss of trade through bad publicity
- loss of staff through damaged reputation.

Would you want to work for a salon which neglected the health and safety of its clients and staff?

Health and Safety at Work Act 1974

The *employer* must:

- safeguard as far as possible the health, safety and welfare of themselves, their employees, contractor's employees and members of the public
- keep all equipment up to standard
- ensure the environment is free from toxic fumes

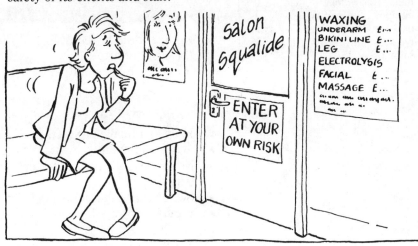

> *Remember*
> Under the Health and Safety at Work Act, everyone working in the salon is obliged always to work safely and to have consideration for their fellow workers.

- have safety equipment checked regularly
- make sure all staff know the safety procedures and provide safety information and training
- ensure safe systems of work.

The *employees* must:
- take reasonable care to avoid injury to themselves and others
- co-operate with others
- not interfere with or misuse anything provided to protect their health and safety.

Fire Precautions Act 1971

- All premises must have fire fighting equipment in good working order.
- The equipment must be readily available and suitable for the types of fire that are likely to occur.

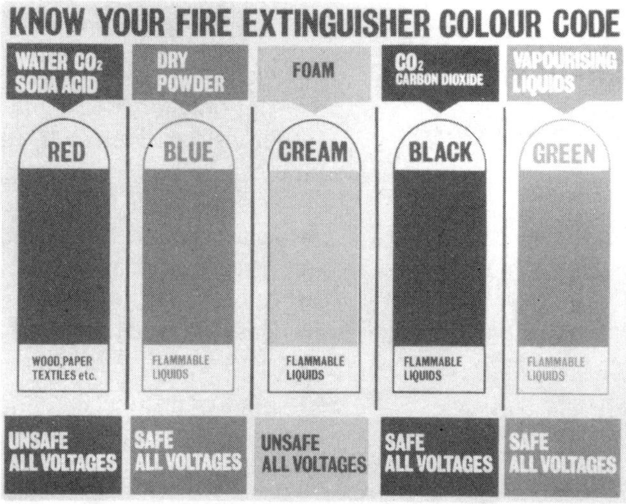
KNOW YOUR FIRE EXTINGUISHER COLOUR CODE
WATER CO2 SODA ACID
DRY POWDER
FOAM
CO2 CARBON DIOXIDE
VAPOURISING LIQUIDS
RED
BLUE
CREAM
BLACK
GREEN
WOOD,PAPER TEXTILES etc.
FLAMMABLE LIQUIDS
FLAMMABLE LIQUIDS
FLAMMABLE LIQUIDS
FLAMMABLE LIQUIDS
UNSAFE ALL VOLTAGES
SAFE ALL VOLTAGES
UNSAFE ALL VOLTAGES
SAFE ALL VOLTAGES
SAFE ALL VOLTAGES

> *Remember*
> Water or foam extinguishers are not suitable for a fire in the salon, which would usually involve flammable products or electrical equipment. A carbon dioxide gas or dry powder extinguisher is the type normally recommended for salon use.

- Doors should be left unlocked so that a quick exit can be made in the event of fire.
- Room contents should not obstruct the exits.

What you must do

- Keep flammable products away from heat.
- Avoid overloading electrical circuits.
- Never leave the flex of an electric heater trailing where it could be tripped over.
- Switch off and disconnect electrical appliances after use.
- Provide ashtrays for clients who smoke (ideally smoking should not be allowed in the salon).
- Never smoke in the stock room.
- Avoid placing towels over electric or gas heaters.

> *Remember*
> If you have time, shut windows and doors and turn off electric and gas appliances. Sound the alarm if there is one.

Fighting fire

Your priority is to remove clients to safety. If the fire is small, use an extinguisher or glass fibre blanket to smother the fire. If the fire is too big to tackle, leave the premises quickly, closing doors behind you.

Calling the Emergency Services

Dial 999. Try not to panic: speak clearly and not too fast. Tell the operator you want the Fire Service and give them your telephone number. Wait for the Fire Service to come on the line. Give them the full address of the emergency and other relevant details of the fire. Listen carefully to any questions you are asked and answer them calmly. After the call, replace the receiver and wait in a safe place for the fire service to arrive.

> Remember
> It is very important that you understand the safety procedures in your salon. Make sure you know where the fire-fighting equipment is kept and how to use it. Find out where the escape routes are and how to operate the fire alarm if there is one.

The fire service provide advice on all aspects of fire safety, including evacuation procedures for a salon and the choice and positioning of fire extinguishers. They also carry out periodic checks on safety equipment.

The salon should have regular fire practices to prepare staff for a real emergency.

Electricity at Work Regulations 1990

Every electrical appliance at work must be tested at least once a year by a qualified electrician. A written record must be kept of these tests and be available for inspection by the Health and Safety authority.

What you must do

When using an electrical appliance or piece of equipment, always check that:

- cables and flexes are in good condition with no signs of fraying or worn insulation. They should not be trailing where they could cause someone to trip
- the plug is intact. If it is cracked or broken then it must be replaced
- there are no loose connections. Leads should feel firmly attached and switches secure
- the appliance is on a level and stable base
- there is no water in the immediate area
- the appliance is switched off and disconnected from the mains after use
- the appliance is left clean and stored properly
- cables and flexes are wound up and secured to avoid them becoming damaged in between uses.

> Remember
> Do not touch equipment, plugs, sockets or flexes with hands which are damp or wet. This could give you an electric shock, which at best is unpleasant, at worst is fatal.

> Remember
> If you spot an electrical fault or potential electrical hazard in the salon, report it to your manager. Never use equipment or an appliance which you know is unsafe.

You should know how to wire a plug:

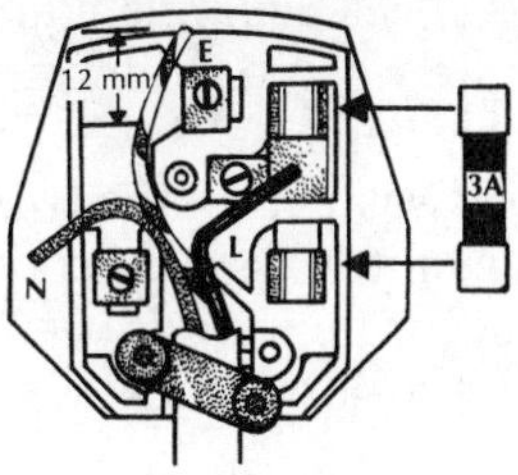

1 Cut away the outer cable, unscrew the cable grip and insert the cable

N = Neutral = Blue
E = Earth = Green/Yellow
L = Live = Brown

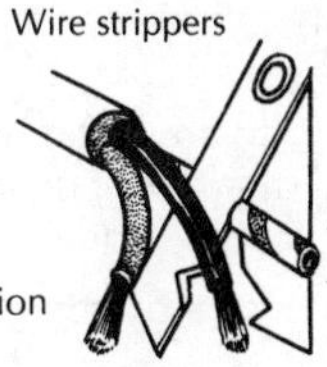

2 Cut away the insulation using wire strippers

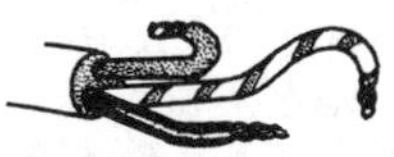

3 Twist the copper strands together

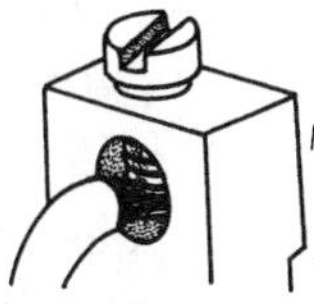

4 Insert each wire into the correct pin

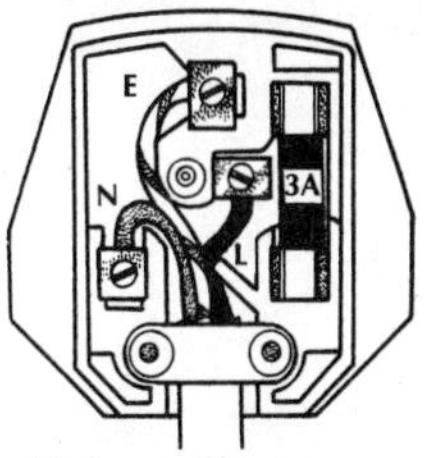

5 Tighten all the screws and the cable grip. Attach the plastic back

The Employer's Liability (Compulsory Insurance) Act 1969

The law requires that employers have everyone on their payroll covered by this insurance and that a current certificate of insurance is displayed at the place of work. The insurance provides cover for claims that might arise when an employee suffers injuries or illness as the result of negligence by either the employer or another employee. Employees who are injured as a result of their own negligence are not covered by the act.

> Remember
> Accidents can happen not just when you are treating clients, but also when taking breaks, returning equipment to store, dealing with stock, cleaning up or even just moving around the salon.

What you must do

- Keep alert and, as soon as you spot a potential danger, either do something about it or report it to someone who can.
- Be conscientious in all aspects of your work. Protect yourself and those around you.

Public Liability Insurance

Public liability insurance is not statutory, but is taken out by employers to cover them for claims made by members of the public as a result of injury or damage to personal property caused by the employer or employee at work.

A special *Professional Indemnity* insurance extends this liability to cover named employees against claims, by clients, of personal injury resulting directly from a treatment.

> Remember
> Injuries which are proven to be caused by professional negligence can result in very expensive fines and claims for compensation.
>
> All employees who give treatments should be covered by Professional Indemnity Insurance. This is particularly important in respect of 'higher risk' treatments such as ear piercing, wax depilation and electrical depilation.

What you must do

- Avoid working on clients if you have a contagious disease or infectious illness.
- Keep your working area clean and tidy.
- Maintain high standards of hygiene in all aspects of your work.
- Always check that the client is suitable for treatment, with no contra-indications.
- Explain treatments clearly to the client beforehand.
- Take all necessary safety precautions before and during the treatment.
- Use correct techniques and never skimp on treatments.
- Adapt treatments appropriately to suit individual clients.
- Always check equipment and machines before use.
- Take care when handling and disposing of substances (COSHH, See table opposite).
- Remove waste from the treatment area as soon as possible and dispose of it in a sealed container.
- Keep accurate records of treatments given and note any abnormal reactions or problems.

> Remember
> If you spot a potential danger in the salon, do something about it! Don't leave it to someone else.

COSHH: The Control of Substances Hazardous to Health Act 1989

This law requires employers to control people's exposure to hazardous substances in the workplace. Some of the products used in the salon are safe in normal use but become hazardous under certain conditions. You need to know the potential hazards in your salon and carry out the necessary safety precautions.

Handling and disposal of hazardous substances

Product type	Health Hazard	Use/handling	Storage	Disposal	Caution
Aerosols: spray cleaners, nail dry sprays	*Flammable:* contents are under pressure and can cause an explosion or fire	Use in well ventilated area. Do not smoke while using. Keep away from eyes. Do not inhale. Do not spray near naked flame or on hot surfaces. Keep cans cool	Cool dry place away from sunlight	Do not pierce or burn aerosol container	In case of fire, evacuate, quickly, areas known to contain aerosols and let fire service know of their location
Cuticle remover	*Caustic*: can burn the skin	Keep away from eyes. Follow the instruction for use. Do not use on damaged or sensitive skin	Cool dry place	Wear gloves. Mop up spills with damp cloth. Rinse well	Rinse out from eyes immediately with plenty of cold water and seek medical advice. Rinse well off skin and seek medical advice if skin irritation persists
Acetone, astringent, equipment cleaner, nail enamel thinners, nail enamel remover, solvents, some sterilising agents, surgical spirit, witch hazel	*Flammable:* vapours catch fire if exposed to flame or ignited by other means	Do not smoke when dispensing. Ensure bottles are clearly labelled. Use only in a well ventilated room. Avoid excessive inhalation	Cool place. Keep sealed. Do not store large quantities together. Always read product labels and follow the advice given	Seek advice from your local Environmental Health Officer. Do not flush down toilet or pour into drains	As above. Move to fresh air immediately if feeling nauseous. Seek medical advice if nausea persists
Equipment cleaner, some sterilising agents, most nail technology products, brush cleaner, nail glue, eyelash tint	*Sensitising:* risk of causing acute allergic reaction	Avoid contact with the skin	Cool, dry place	Small quantities can be disposed of normally. For advice on disposing of large quantities, contact the local Environmental Health Officer	As above. Move to fresh air if feeling nauseous and seek medical advice if it persists
Skin bleach	May cause skin irritation	Use in well ventilated area. Wear protective gloves. Avoid inhaling dry powder or contact with eyes and face. Do not use on damaged or sensitive skin	Cool dry place away from sunlight and other sources of heat. Reseal container after use	Do not incinerate. Use water to dilute and mop up spillages. Dispose of dry powder by washing it down the drain with plenty of water	As above. If dry powder is inhaled, move to fresh air. If coughing, choking or breathless-ness persists for longer than 10–15 minutes, seek medical advice
Hydrogen peroxide	Irritant to skin and eyes	Always wear protective gloves. Avoid contact with eyes and face. Do not use on damaged or sensitive skin. Always use non-metallic equipment	Cool dry place, away from sunlight and other sources of heat. Store in container supplied and replace cap immediately after use	Flush down the drain with plenty of water. Do not incinerate or store with easily combustible materials, e.g. paper	Rinse away from eyes with plent of water and seek medical advice. Rinse the skin well and seek medical attention if irritation persists
Gluteraldehyde solution	Can cause allergic reaction by contact or following excessive exposure to vaporised fluid	Avoid breathing in vapour. Keep off the skin. Wear rubber gloves when handling. Utensils which have been treated should be rinsed with water before using on the skin	Cool, dry place. Keep in a closed, covered container	Rinse away down the drain with plenty of water. Empty containers should be rinsed thoroughly with water and treated as household waste	Rinse eyes continuously for 10–15 minutes. Wash skin and seek medical advice if irritation persists. If headaches and chest discomfort occur, move to fresh air and get medical advice if symptoms persist
Fine powders; acrylic nail powder, bleaches, loose powder cosmetics, talcum powder, clay mask powders	Irritation caused by inhalation of fine particles	Take care to control powders when using and mixing them. Avoid creating dust when using them. Do not inhale, even in small quantities. Wear a face mask when dispensing large quantities of powder	Cool, dry place in a closed container	Treat as domestic waste unless otherwise instructed by the manufacturer	Rinse eyes with plenty of water. Wash skin to remove particles inhaled, move to fresh air. If irritation or coughing persists, seek medical advice

What you must do

- Understand how COSHH affects you and your work.
- Put the theory into practice!

Hazard warning symbols - Classification, Packaging and Labelling of Dangerous Substances Regulations 1984.

Safety signs are the subject of EC legislation

Controlling the salon environment

The employer has basic legal duties regarding the health and welfare of employees at work. These are covered in broad terms by the Health and Safety at Work Act 1974. More detailed and specific requirements are covered by the Offices, Shops and Railways Premises Act 1963.

The main requirements for which the employer is legally responsible are summarised below.

> Remember
>
> When handling breakages, spillages and waste:
> - clear away immediately
> - wrap glass before placing in waste bin
> - wipe up spillages immediately
> - dispose of waste in covered bins
> - remove waste daily
> - dispose of contaminated needles in yellow 'Sharps' boxes.

Clean premises

The premises, furnishings and fittings should be kept clean. Floors and stairs should be cleaned at least once a week. Dirt and refuse should not be allowed to accumulate.

The Local Government (Miscellaneous Provisions Act) 1982 empowers local authorities to register businesses which practise beauty therapy treatments, in particular electrical epilation, wax depilation and ear piercing, which carry a higher risk of cross-infection and skin damage. The act states that:

- a person may not carry out their practice unless registered by the local authority
- premises have to be registered to carry out treatments.

A certificate of registration is awarded by the local authority, who may charge reasonable fees at their discretion for registration purposes, and they may make bye-laws for securing:

- the cleanliness of the premises and fittings
- the cleanliness of persons registered and their assistants
- the cleansing and sterilisation of instruments, materials and equipment used.

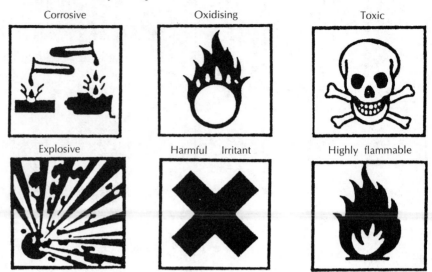

Local Environmental Officers have the authority to fine or cancel the registration of businesses which do not maintain appropriate standards of hygiene.

Adequate heating

The working temperature should be 16 °C (60-80 °F) after the first hour. Thermostatically controlled heating systems keep the salon at a comfortable temperature. They have a device which switches off the heat when the required temperature has been reached and then turns it on again as the temperature begins to fall. The heating method should not give out dangerous or offensive fumes.

Fresh or purified air

There should be enough ventilation to keep the air fresh and to prevent build up of fumes. Extractor fans and open windows help to remove the pungent smells produced by solvent-based manicure preparations and some nail technology products. Too much exposure to these fumes can cause nausea and headaches. Full air conditioning is ideal for keeping the salon comfortable and fresh. This method draws out stale air and replaces it with clean fresh air heated to the correct temperature.

Stale air makes us feel tired and listless. This is because of the build-up of carbon dioxide in the air. If the salon is warm and air is not circulating, sweat does not evaporate as readily from the skin surface. The body does not cool and we feel very uncomfortable.

What you must do

- Know how to control the heating and ventilation systems in your salon.

Sufficient lighting

The lighting in the salon should be bright enough for everyone to move around safely and see what they are doing, but not so bright as to create glare.

Natural daylight is the best sort of light and has the advantage of showing up 'true' colours. Artificial lighting often distorts colours: a client would be very disappointed to find that the colour of a nail enamel or lipstick looked quite different once they had left the salon, particularly if they had been bought to match up with a special outfit. Warm white fluorescent tubes are nearly as good as daylight for colour matching. The special lighting needed for close work is usually provided by a magnifying anglepoise lamp containing a circular fluorescent tube.

> *Remember*
> Bad lighting can cause eyestrain and headaches.

What you must do

- Always make sure that you have enough light to work safely and accurately.
- Ensure that neither your client nor yourself are dazzled by a bright light.
- Report glaring light bulbs and flickering tubes to your manager so that they can be checked or replaced.

> Remember
> Water is heated up by either gas, oil or electricity, all of which have to be paid for. Heating costs are a major expense for the salon. Wasting hot water is pouring money down the drain!

Adequate sanitary and washing facilities

The salon needs a constant supply of clean hot and cold water. Problems with plumbing and drainage may mean that treatments have to be delayed or even cancelled. This can cause financial loss to the business.

What you must do

- Report blocked sinks immediately. Standing waste water smells unpleasant. Also, bacterial growth increases which may spread disease.
- Do not leave hot water taps running longer than necessary. This is both wasteful and expensive.
- Do not flush solid or semi-solid materials down the sink. They may cause a blockage in the pipes which transport water away from the salon to the drains outside.
- In the event of a pipe bursting, turn off the water at the stopcock. This will stop the supply of water to the salon from outside. It is advisable to turn off the electricity as well as the water. Until you have done this, you should not touch any light switches or electrical appliances. You could get electrocuted.
- If water comes out of the tap discoloured or with a strange smell, report it to your manager who should contact the Local Water Authority for advice.

Other working conditions which an employer is legally bound to provide are:

- adequate space for each employee
- rest and eating facilities.

> Remember
> The plumbing beneath the basin has a waste trap which holds water and stops gases and smells from the drains travelling back up the pipes. If a small object accidentally falls through the plug hole, the waste trap can be investigated to see if it has settled there.

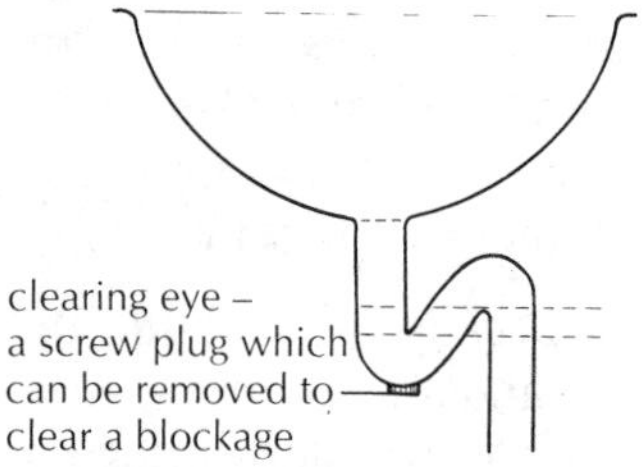
clearing eye – a screw plug which can be removed to clear a blockage

An S-bend siphon trap beneath a wash basin

Employment standards: Multiple choice quiz

There may appear to be more than one right answer. Read the sentence carefully before choosing the best one.

1 During a beauty treatment, the safety of a client is the responsibility of the:
a) employer
b) client
c) manageress
d) employee (you).

2 Bad publicity is expensive for a salon because:
a) advertising has to be paid for
b) clients are put off coming to the salon
c) other salons pinch the clients
d) the staff have to be paid more.

3 Smoking is prohibited in the stock room because of the:
a) unpleasant smell
b) hygiene regulations
c) flammable products
d) salon's image.

4 A fire blanket is used to:
a) cover a person who has been injured in a fire
b) smother a large fire
c) smother a small fire.
d) cover flammable products during a fire.

5 During a fire, doors should be shut to:
a) prevent the fire from spreading
b) prevent the smell from spreading
c) show that the salon is closed
d) stop air getting to the fire.

6 The safety of the salon's electrical equipment is the responsibility of the:
a) electrician
b) employer
c) employee (you)
d) manufacturer.

7 Details of abnormal reactions or problems with treatment should be recorded so that:
a) the client does not have the treatment again
b) accurate information is available for insurance purposes
c) the salon cannot be held responsible for accidents
d) the client cannot be held responsible for accidents.

8 Good ventilation is important in the salon to keep the air:
a) dry
b) warm
c) humid
d) fresh.

9 Poor lighting in the salon can cause:
a) headaches
b) short-sightedness
c) long-sightedness
d) colour blindness.

10 A small object which has fallen down the plug hole can usually be recovered from the:
a) stopcock
b) mains
c) drains
d) waste-trap.

Employment standards: Self-checks

Fill in the missing words: sometimes you may need more than one word to fill the space correctly.

1 Caustic substances can ____ the skin. One example of a caustic manicure preparation is ________________.

2 ________ substances can cause fires. Three examples are ________ ____, ________________ and ________________.

3 __________ sterilising agents such as ________________ may cause an ____________ reaction. Always wear ______ when handling these substances and avoid them contacting the _____ and ______.

4 An aerosol container may ______ if it is burned or ______ after use. Always keep aerosols away from ________ and use in a well ________ __ area.

5 The best conditions for storing beauty products are in a place which is _____, _____ and _____.

Employment standards: Activities

> Remember
> Domestic cleaning products are also covered by COSHH (see page 4).

1 It is very important that you understand the safety procedures in your salon. Make sure you know where the fire fighting equipment is kept and how to use it and, also, where the escape routes are.

2 Have a word with your supervisor or tutor. Find out exactly what the electrician does during the regular checks of electrical appliances. Ask if you can see how the results of the checks are recorded.

3 Have a good look around your salon and see if you can spot any safety hazards. If you can, make a note of them and report them to your supervisor.

4 Find out where and how the products in your salon are stored. Read packaging and containers for specific safety instructions.

5 Find out how to operate the heating and ventilation systems in your salon.

6 Have a good look at a colour chart, for example for lipsticks or nail enamels in reception and in the salon. Take the chart to a window so that the colours can be seen in daylight. Can you see any difference? If you can, think how it will affect the recommendations you make to your clients for choosing cosmetic colours.

7 Check the plug holes in the sinks in your salon. Are they clear or is there a build up of waste? If they are getting blocked, you know what you have to do! If they are not clear, there could be a problem developing further down the system.

8 Think about ways in which you and your colleagues could keep down the plumbing bills.

Salon security

> Remember
> It is a good idea before opening a business to consult the crime prevention officer at the local police station, and also to arrange for a good security firm to inspect the premises and install all necessary safety devices.

> Remember
> It is not only money that attracts burglars: stock also has a 'street' value. It pays to have a good system of stock control. If your salon is burgled, you will find it easier to list what has been stolen and this will help prompt settling of insurance claims.

A salon owner is required, by law, to ensure adequate security of the business premises. This is particularly important for obtaining insurance cover in the case of theft from or damage to the property and, also, for leasing and mortgaging purposes.

It is virtually impossible to make the salon completely burglar-proof, but steps can be taken to make it more difficult to burgle, and minimise the possible damage once the property has been entered:

- fit locks and/or bolts on all doors and windows, including basements and attics
- install a burglar alarm
- check that glass window panels are intact and that they are not loose. Double glazing and/or window bars give extra security.

Strict salon procedures are required to ensure the security of the building both during and outside business hours. There is obviously a greater risk of burglary when the salon is closed. Particular attention must be paid to locking up:

- there should be a minimum number of key-holders, with every key accounted for at all times. The police should be given details of key holders in case they need to contact them when the salon is closed
- a light should be left on all night, preferably at the front of the salon. This may deter a burglar and will help patrolling policemen to keep watch on the premises
- money should not be left in the till overnight. Large sums of money should be banked during the day or deposited in the night safe after banking hours

- the till drawer should be left open at night. A thief would try opening it anyway and cause unnecessary damage
- all entrances, lockable cupboards, doors and windows should be checked and the burglar alarm tested before the premises are left. External doors should be locked while the internal checks are carried out.

The person responsible for opening up the salon usually has jobs to do in preparation for the day's business. This person is normally expected to arrive early, before the rest of the staff, which means they are on their own for a short while. During this period:

- the main entrance should remain locked until the opening time of the salon. Staff can be let in as they arrive, preferably through an alternative staff entrance
- the burglar alarm should be switched off
- the till and lighting for shop window and display areas should be switched on
- post which has arrived should be put in a safe place for collection
- all internal doors and fire exits should be unlocked to satisfy health and safety regulations.

Security during business hours

It is important to establish the identity of anyone entering the premises and their reason for being there. In most cases, visitors will be attending the salon on legitimate business and will have an appointment card or professional identification. Casual callers will go to reception and be attended to there.

> *Remember*
>
> If you are suspicious about someone who you think is not authorised to be in an area of the premises, politely ask for their identity and offer them assistance. If you are still not happy, try to alert your supervisor or another member of staff.
>
> *Do not put yourself in danger.* If the intruder runs away, report the incident immediately to your supervisor who will contact the police.
>
> Check the area for evidence of damage or theft. Write the details down as soon as possible. It will help the police if you can also provide them with an accurate description of the intruder.

Beauty Box Salon

Incident Report Form

NAME OF PERSON MAKING REPORT: CATHERINE ARNOLD

A. DETAILS OF INCIDENT

Date 17.5.93 Time 11:30 (approx.) Location Reception

Details of any witnesses Mrs. C. Jones (Client) 765 - 3987
Sue Ruby (Therapist)

Description of the incident Two girls aged 13-15 came in to the salon enquiring about nail extensions. As I spoke to one of them, the other one moved away and began acting suspiciously around the make-up display. When I offered her assistance she grabbed a couple of items and ran out of the salon followed by her friend. I gave chase but could not catch up with them. Both girls wore blue jeans and a black leather jacket. The girl who I was speaking to was approx. 5'2", slim with short, spikey blonde hair, heavy make-up and pierced ears. Her friend was about the same size. She had long red, curly hair, wore little make-up and was carrying a large black canvas bag.

Signed Cath Arnold. Date of report 17.5.93.

B. ACTION TAKEN (to be filled in by supervisor)

I contacted the Police immediately. They came and took statements from Cath, Sue & Mrs. Jones. I offered Mrs. Jones a complimentary facial for her co-operation.

Signature and name Jenny Wilson JENNIFER WILSON Date 17.5.93.

An example of a completed incident report form

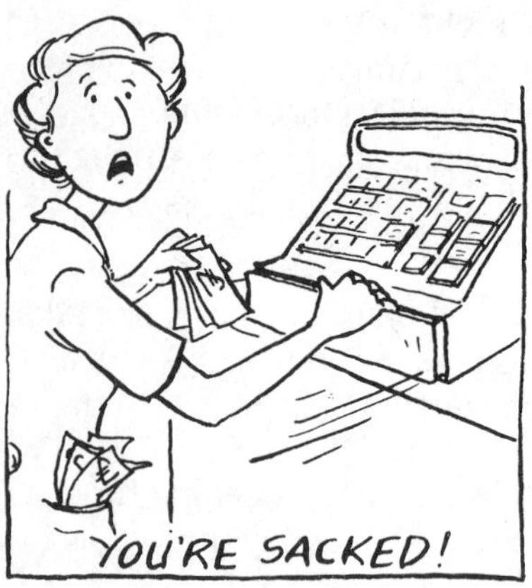
YOU'RE SACKED!

Remember

Every salon has rules regarding the security of money, equipment and stock. Make sure you know these rules and stick to them.

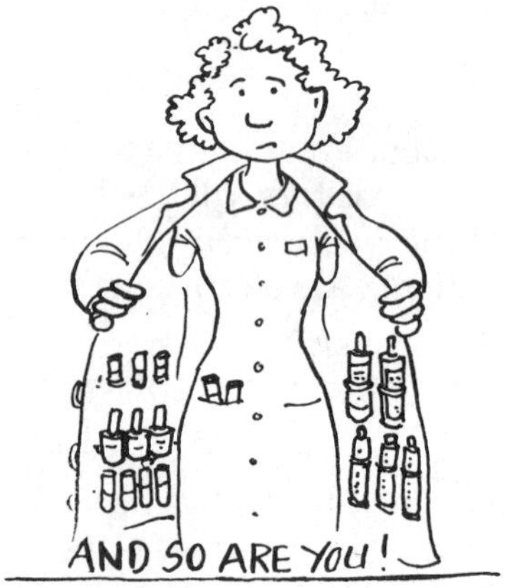
AND SO ARE YOU!

Remember

Do not take salon stock for granted. It does *not* belong to you until you have paid for it. Your salon will have rules regarding employees' own purchases which will probably qualify you for a discounted price. Helping yourself to goods without paying for them is stealing.

Remember

The client may prefer to have very valuable items of jewellery stored in the safe, particularly if her treatments require her to move between different areas of the salon.

Regrettably, theft by burglary is not the only way in which stealing may take place in the salon. Pilfering by staff and clients (politely known as 'shrinkage') is something that the salon owner must protect against. Pilfering by staff could take the form of 'a hand in the till' or stealing from stock. This type of stealing is much less likely to occur in a salon which operates efficient stock control and reception procedures.

Security of money

It is worth the salon investing in an electronic till for recording and storing payment. The till can be kept locked in between uses and, where only one or two named people have the authority to use and have keys for the till, the risk of theft becomes very small.

An electronic till keeps a running total of takings and updated information can be provided instantly for cashing up purposes throughout the day. In this way, discrepancies between the takings and till receipts can be spotted and acted upon quickly.

Ideally, money which is cashed up during the working day should be paid straight into the bank but this is not always possible. The salon should have a safe for the short-term storage of money and valuables.

It is up to the employer which staff are entrusted with the special combination code which opens the safe, but, clearly, confidentiality is essential for providing security.

Security of stock

A good system of stock control monitors the use of consumable and retail products and keeps supplies stored safely in a locked stock room or cupboard.

Usually only one or two people will have keys to the storage areas and they will have responsibility for issuing items to staff and keeping stock records. In this way, general access to stock is limited and the rate of replacement is monitored closely.

Stealing by clients

In the retail industry, stealing by clients is known as shoplifting and refers to the theft of items on display for resale. Shoplifting is not a big problem in beauty salons, but there are obviously risks where items are displayed at reception or in treatment rooms. These risks are reduced if shelves and display stands are kept well lit and stocked up neatly.

Personal property

Staff and clients also need protecting against theft. It is the responsibility of the therapist to ensure that the client's handbag and jewellery are kept safely in the treatment area, preferably where they can be seen by the client, or in a locked cupboard. The client's property should not be visible if the treatment area is left unattended.

It is sensible for staff to keep the amount of money and valuables they take to work to a minimum. This reduces the risk of disappointment and upset caused by loss or theft. In larger businesses particularly, leaving handbags and purses on open display in staff rooms or other shared areas is asking for trouble.

> *Remember*
> Security in the salon relies to a great extent on the day-to-day vigilance of staff. Stay alert and notice what is going on around you! Make your contribution to protecting the business which employs you.

If the salon does not provide secure storage facilities for staff belongings, it is best to confine personal possessions in a small purse or wallet which can be kept safely, nearby, throughout the working day.

An employer would be justified in feeling very angry about losses to the business and personal losses suffered as a result of staff negligence.

Security: Self-checks

1. How might a burglar try to gain entry to the salon outside working hours?
2. What security procedures should be carried out at night before leaving the salon?
3. State three functions of an electronic cash till.
4. How does good stock control contribute to salon security?
5. List the precautions which should be taken at work to ensure the safety of
   a) personal property
   b) the client's property.

Security: Activity

Working with a partner or in a small group, decide how effective the security procedures are in your salon and, where appropriate, make recommendations for improvements.

Consider more than the security just of the building: look at how closely the use of salon stock and towels is monitored and, also, the safety of money and retail stock on display. How adequate are the facilities available for storing property belonging to clients and staff?

Protecting against disease

We spend our lives surrounded by what are commonly known as 'germs'. Some germs are harmless, some are even beneficial, but others present a danger to us because they cause disease.

The germs which cause disease are usually spread by:

- unclean hands
- contaminated tools
- sores and pus
- discharges from nose and mouth
- shared use of items such as towels and cups
- close contact with infected skin cells
- contaminated blood or tissue fluid.

Viruses

Viruses are the tiniest germs, yet they are responsible for an enormous range of human diseases. Viruses can only survive in living cells. The following are examples of viral infections:

- common cold: the virus is spread by coughing and sneezing and is carried through the air as a droplet infection

- cold sore: this virus remains dormant in the mucous membranes of the skin and is triggered off by sunlight or general debility. Cold sores are most likely to spread when they are weeping
- warts: there are several types of wart. Verruca plantaris is a wart which occurs commonly under the feet and is spread by close contact.

Bacteria

Bacteria are tiny single celled organisms. They grow from spores and multiply very quickly. Bacteria are capable of breeding outside the body and can therefore be caught easily through personal contact or by touching a contaminated article.

Some bacteria cause diseases and infect wounds. Bacteria develop from spores which are very reproductive and highly resistant. The following are examples of bacterial infections:

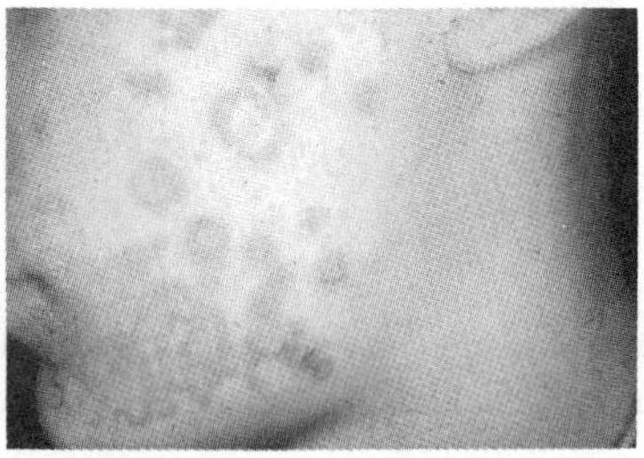

Impetigo

- impetigo: bacteria enter the body through broken skin and cause blisters which weep and crust over. The condition is highly infectious and can be spread easily by dirty tools.
- boils: these can occur when bacteria invade the hair follicle through a surface scratch or by close contact with an infected person.
- whitlow: this can be caused by the bacteria invading the pad of the finger through a break in the skin, which has often been caused by a splinter.

Fungi

Fungi consist of yeasts and moulds. Moulds break down all sorts of materials but rarely cause disease. Yeasts are single cells which can cause disease. Fungal infections are very easily transmitted by personal contact or by touching contaminated articles. The following are examples of fungal infections:

- tinea pedis (athlete's foot): in this condition, the fungus thrives in the warm, moist environment between the toes and, sometimes, under the feet. The condition is picked up easily by direct contact with recently shed infected skin cells.
- tinea unguium (ringworm of the nail): this condition may result from contact with the fungus present on other parts of the body. For example, toenails may become infected during an outbreak of athlete's foot which if touched could then spread to the hands.

Animal parasites

Animal parasites are small insects which cause disease by invading the skin and using human blood or protein as a source of nourishment. Diseases caused by animal parasites usually occur as the result of prolonged contact with an infected person. The following are examples of diseases caused by animal parasites:

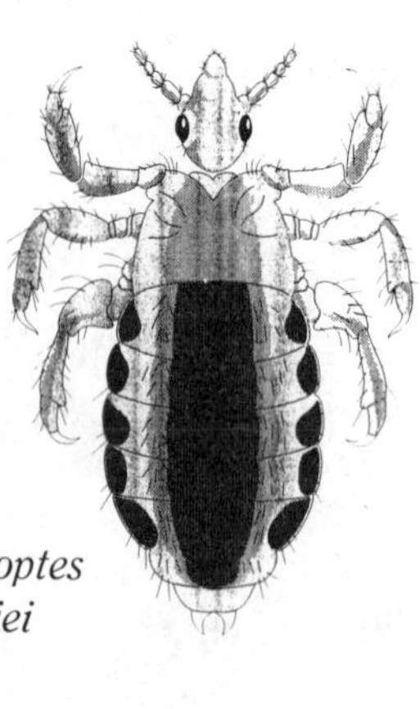

Sarcoptes scabiei

- scabies: tiny mites burrow through the outside layer of epidermis and lay their eggs underneath the skin surface. The condition is very itchy and causes a rash and swelling. Characteristic line formations show where the burrows have been formed.

> Remember
> You have a responsibility to yourself, your clients and your colleagues to always work hygienically and to do everything you can to avoid the spread of infection.

> Remember
> Dirt and bacteria accumulate in cracks. You must not use tools with a damaged edge as they cannot be sterilised effectively.

> Remember
> Waste should not be handled or left exposed. Make sure that the waste resulting from your treatments is placed in a lined container, tied up tightly and disposed of in a large sealed refuse sack with other salon waste.

> Remember
> All work surfaces should be cleaned regularly with hot water and detergent. The treatment table, trolley, sink and stools should be wiped down at the end of each working day with a solution of disinfectant.

- head lice: these are small parasites which puncture the skin and suck blood. They lay eggs on the hair close to the scalp. The hatched eggs are called nits and can be seen as shiny, pearl coloured oval bodies which cling to the hair shaft.

What you must do

- Provide each client with clean towels and gown.
- Carry out an examination before each treatment so that contra-indications are spotted in time.
- Use only tools which have been cleaned and sterilised.
- Keep cutting tools sharp and in good working order.
- Use correct treatment techniques to avoid injuring the client.
- Dispose of waste properly after each treatment.
- Keep your work area clean and tidy.
- Wash your own hands before each treatment, and more often if necessary.
- Maintain high standards of personal hygiene.

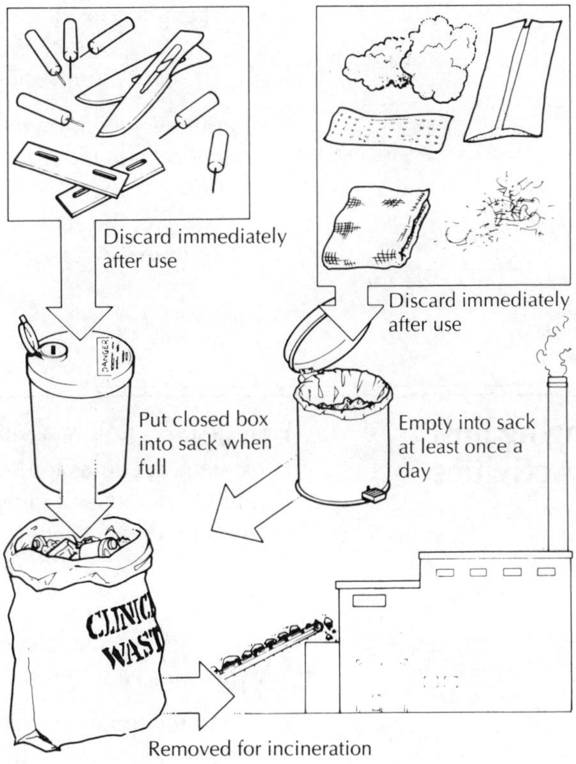

Discard immediately after use
Discard immediately after use
Put closed box into sack when full
Empty into sack at least once a day
CLINIC WAST
Removed for incineration

Waste disposal methods

Protecting against disease: Multiple choice quiz

There may appear to be more than one correct answer. Read the sentence carefully before choosing the best one.

1 Bacteria can breed:
   a) only in living cells
   b) both inside and outside the body
   c) only outside the body
   d) only in infected cells.

2 A cold sore at the side of the mouth may be spread by:
a) kissing an infected person
b) sharing the same toothbrush
c) close contact with an infected person
d) close contact with infected tissue fluid.

3 Viruses survive only in:
a) warmth and moisture
b) living cells
c) contaminated skin
d) unhygienic conditions.

4 Athlete's foot is caused by:
a) a virus
b) an animal parasite
c) a fungus
d) bacteria.

5 Waste should be disposed of in a sealed container in order to:
a) keep the trolley tidy
b) keep the inside of the bin clean
c) prevent germs from spreading
d) present a professional image.

6 Strict hygiene procedures are essential in the salon to:
a) eliminate the risks of cross-infection
b) protect the clients
c) protect the staff
d) eliminate diseases.

Protecting against disease: Activities

1 Is there a cleaning policy in your salon? Do all the staff follow the same procedures for keeping their working areas clean? Is a cleaner paid to do general cleaning or is there a cleaning rota for general jobs? Assume that you work in a salon where a cleaner comes in daily just to clean the floors and toilets.

Working with a partner or in a small group, design a schedule which identifies specific cleaning duties for the staff to maintain their own work areas and the salon in general. Don't forget the staff room !

2 Go to the library and find an illustrated dermatology book. Try to find coloured pictures of the skin infections mentioned here. Look through chapters on bacterial, fungal and viral infections. Discover other skin conditions which you may come across in the salon.

Appearance and personal hygiene

The effort you put in to getting ready for work reflects your pride in the job. Clients will initially judge your professionalism on how you present yourself. You are in an industry where image and appearance are important, so represent your industry well and win the confidence of the client at first sight. It is fine for you to have your own individual look provided that you appreciate that there are professional standards of dress and appearance which must be followed.

> Remember
>
> Each salon has specific rules on dress which reflect their 'house style' or professional image. Always stick to the rules! Do not try changing them without consulting your manager first.

You must allow yourself plenty of time in the morning for getting ready for work. It is not enough to turn yourself out looking nice. You must also be clean and fresh. Intimate personal hygiene consists of scrupulous cleanliness and the wearing of clean, fresh underwear every day and more often if necessary. Standard body care preparations and perfumes are not suitable for the intimate areas of the body due to the sensitivity of the skin and risks of infection. Good personal hygiene helps to keep the body healthy. It also ensures that you do not offend your colleagues and clients with body odours and stale breath.

Here are some general recommendations.

- Your overall should always be clean and well pressed; it will probably be made of cotton, or polycotton which is easier to launder. These fabrics are lightweight and comfortable to wear for working, but make sure your overall is not too tight. It should be loose enough to allow air and moisture to circulate, keeping the body cool and feeling fresh. Do not travel in your overall or wear it anywhere it may pick up undesirable smells.

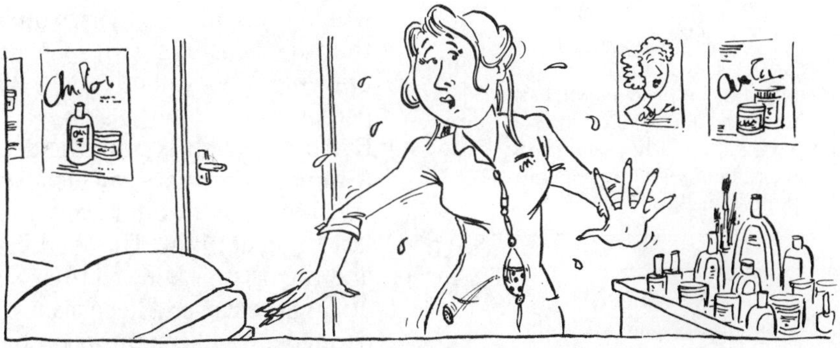

- Keep jewellery to a minimum. Do not wear bracelets, rings or chunky jewellery.
- Have clean, shiny hair in a smart, manageable style. Do not let hair fall over your face: a face which is hidden behind a mass of hair cannot communicate very well. It is also unhygienic when working over the client. Hair care includes regular washing and conditioning so that it never looks greasy, lank and unkempt. There are plenty of shampoos and hair cosmetics to choose from. Regular brushing of the hair helps to remove dust, scurf and parasites which would otherwise build up on the hair.

> Remember
>
> You should not wear jewellery which could scratch clients during treatment. Also, you should avoid 'out dressing' your clients. They could find it rather intimidating!

> Remember
>
> Wash and disinfect combs and brushes regularly to avoid a build up of grease, loosened hair, dust and debris. Infection can occur if the scalp is scratched with dirty hair equipment.

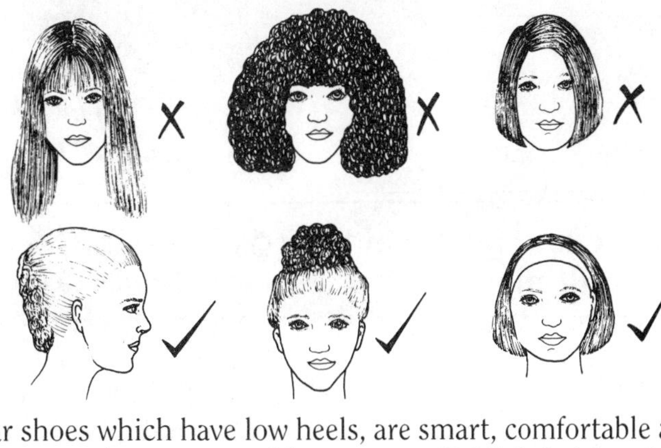

Suitable hair styles for a therapist

- Wear shoes which have low heels, are smart, comfortable and appropriate for wearing with your overall. High fashion shoes have their place, but not usually as part of a uniform. Foot sprays and medicated foot powders help to keep the feet cool and dry. Clean stockings, tights or socks should be worn each day.

Remember
If you work as a manicurist or a nail technician, you may be required to wear nail enamel as part of your professional image. If you work as a therapist, treating the face or body, you must not wear nail enamel. This is for two reasons:
a) Your nails may come in to direct contact with the skin and the client may be allergic to your enamel.
b) Nails which are free from enamel can be seen to be clean. This is particularly reassuring for clients who are due to undergo facial or body therapy.

Remember
A brisk rub with the towel afterwards helps to stimulate the circulation and perk up the body – particularly useful if you have difficulty getting going in the mornings!

Remember
The smells of cigarettes, garlic and curries stay on the breath for some time. Others can smell them long after you've tasted them!

Remember
Sweat evaporates freely from skin which is exposed to the air but not from areas where two surfaces of skin meet or where clothes and shoes fit tightly.

- Wear plain fine tights or stockings which are not pulled or laddered. You should keep a spare pair at work for emergencies.
- Apply make-up before leaving for work and refresh it during the day if necessary. A fresh application of lipstick always brightens up the face.
- Keep your hands and nails well groomed and spotlessly clean, with the skin kept smooth to avoid cracking – breaks in the skin provide a route for bacteria. Use hand cream regularly and wear rubber gloves for cleaning.
- Nails trap dirt underneath. The shorter nails are, the easier they are to keep clean. Use a nail brush as part of your regular cleansing routine. Clean hands are hygienically 'safe', and hands that are well groomed set a good example for the client.
- General body care consists of at least one bath or shower a day to remove the build up of sweat from the skin and to remove loose, dead skin cells. The armpits, feet and genital areas have a lot of sweat glands. They are warm and moist and certain bacteria thrive there. Unfortunately, these bacteria produce the unpleasant smells which everyone recognises but nobody likes to mention! Regular, thorough washing with soap and water is the only way of preventing body odour (BO). Washing removes surface bacteria and perspiration from the skin.
- Bad breath results from the decay of food particles left on the teeth. (Stomach disorders can also be a cause.) It is important to brush teeth thoroughly after every meal as well as in the morning and last thing at night. The toothbrush should be rinsed well after use and the bristles allowed to dry in the air. Be careful what you eat during the day and keep a spare toothbrush at work. Use breath freshener and keep mints on hand just in case.
- Anti-perspirants have a cooling, astringent (tightening) effect which reduces sweating and minimises the build up of bacteria which cause odours. They also usually contain bactericidal ingredients. Under normal circumstances, anti-perspirants stay effective all day, but it is a good idea to keep one at work just in case.
- Deodorants really only mask smells. They have bactericidal properties but they do not deal with the real cause of the problem, which is a build up of sweat. Although they are less effective than anti-perspirants, some people prefer to use deodorants as their skin can be sensitive to the extra ingredients contained in an anti-perspirant.

Appearance and personal hygiene: Multiple choice quiz

1 Long nails are less hygienic than short ones because:
a) they spread infection easily
b) they are more prone to infection
c) they collect more germs beneath them
d) they break and cause germs to enter.

2 The function of a tooth brush is to:
a) make the teeth white
b) remove particles of food from the teeth
c) spread toothpaste over the teeth
d) prevent bad breath.

3 An overall should be loose enough to:
a) disguise figure defects
b) adjust to changes in body shape
c) prevent sweating
d) allow sweat to evaporate.

4 The therapist's hands should be washed before each treatment so that:
a) the hands look clean
b) infection is not spread
c) surface bacteria are removed
d) the client feels safe.

Appearance and personal hygiene: Activities

1 What do you do between getting up in the morning and going to work? Are you ready for work when you leave the house or are you still half asleep when you reach the salon? Be truthful with yourself. If you know there's a problem, think of how you could improve the efficiency of your morning routine. Be warned, it may involve re-scheduling your social life and getting up earlier!

2 How strict is your salon about the appearance of the staff? How important do you think it is to have rules about dress?

Have a small group discussion. Look at yourself and your colleagues. Is there room for improvement? Does everyone present a professional image? Be diplomatic with your comments!

Sterilisation and disinfection

Sterilisation

Sterilisation is the destruction of all living organisms. It is very difficult to maintain sterile conditions. Once sterilised items have been exposed to the air they are no longer sterile. Articles which have been sterilised and stored hygienically are safe to use on the client.

Autoclave

The most effective method of sterilisation is steaming at high pressure in an autoclave. This works on exactly the same principle as a pressure cooker. Steam is produced from a reservoir of water and is contained under pressure at a minimum of 121 °C for 15 minutes. Modern autoclaves have thermochromic indicators which change colour when the required temperature has been reached. Stainless steel and glass items are suitable for sterilisation by this method. A stacking facility is usually provided so that articles can be placed at different levels in the autoclave. Unfortunately, this method is not suitable for some of the items used in salon treatments. The very high temperature required to kill spores destroys certain materials in much the same way that over cooking ruins food.

When autoclaving is not possible, other methods of controlling infection are used which are less effective, and so rely more on recognising infection and avoiding contact with it.

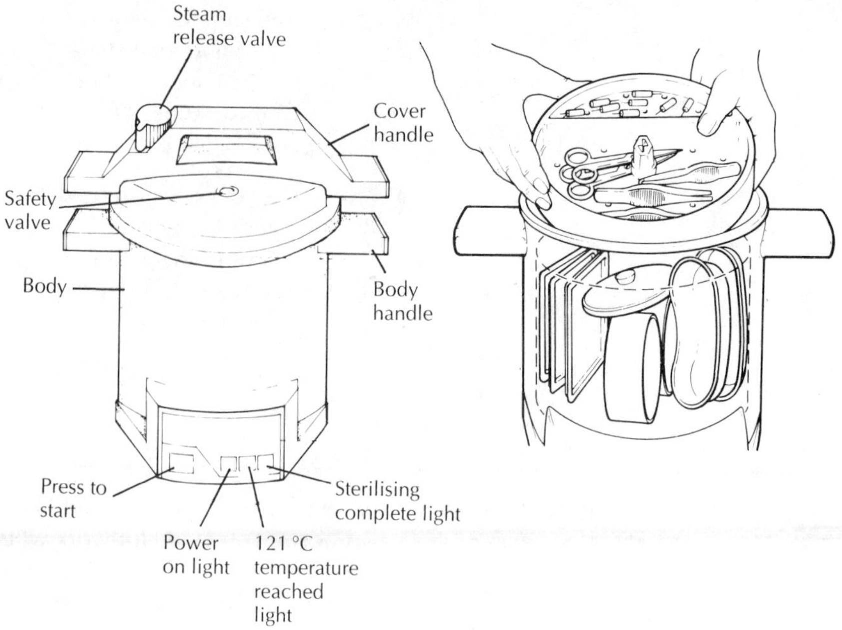

An autoclave

When autoclaving is not possible, other methods of controlling infection are used which are less effective, and so rely more on recognising infection and avoiding contact with it.

Ultraviolet rays

Ultraviolet rays also sterilise but they have a very low rate of penetration. The rays are emitted in a cabinet which may be wall-mounted or kept on a surface. Ultraviolet irradiation sterilises only the surface of objects, so it is suitable only for solid tools such as cuticle nippers. Items have to be turned halfway though the sterilisation process to ensure that all surfaces have been treated.

The generally recommended exposure time is 15 minutes each side. Equipment is often stored in an ultraviolet cabinet until it is required for use.

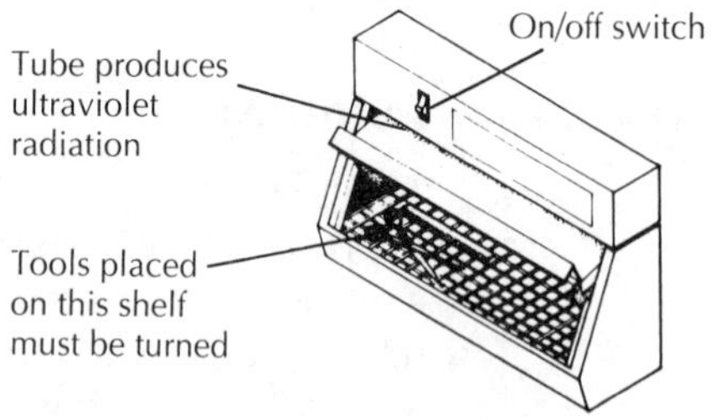

An ultraviolet cabinet

Glass bead sterilisers

Glass bead sterilisers reach a temperature of between 190 and 300 °C (374-572 °F) depending on the model. This temperature has to be maintained for 30-60 minutes. If extra items are put into the steriliser during this period, the temperature of the beads drops and the effects are lost. Timing has to begin again. Glass bead sterilisers can hold only very small items and have limited use in the salon.

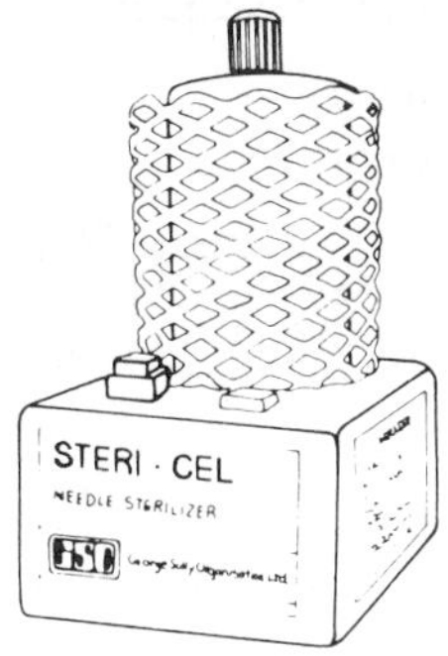

Glass bead steriliser

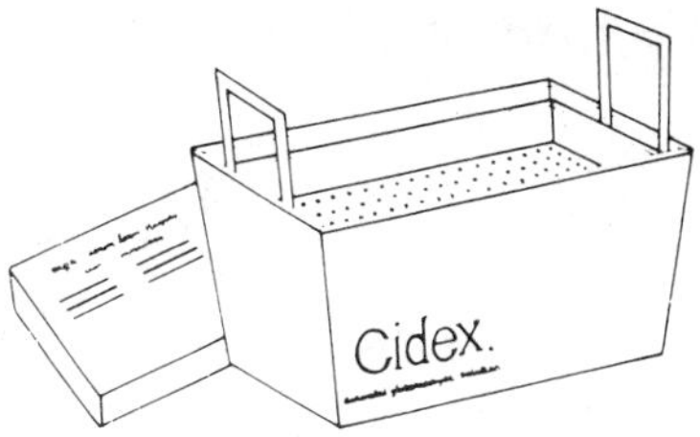

Liquid chemical steriliser

> Remember
> You must be sure that you are carrying out safe and effective hygiene procedures. Always read and follow the manufacturer's instructions carefully when preparing, using and disposing of chemical solutions.

Chemical methods of sterilisation

Concentrated liquid chemical agents are available which have to be diluted for use. Some chemical agents act either as a disinfectant or as a sterilant, depending on the strength of their solution and the time for which items are kept in contact with them. Some liquid chemical sterilisers are very harmful to the skin and great care is needed when handling them (see the table on page 5).

Disinfection

Disinfectants work against bacteria and fungi but just remove contamination; they do not necessarily kill spores. Disinfectants only reduce the number of organisms. Examples of good chemical disinfectants are:

- gluteraldehyde (e.g. Cidex): a 2% solution is used which remains active for 14-18 days, after which time it must be discarded. Gluteraldehyde is a very valuable disinfectant. It is particularly useful for soaking metal instruments and applicators, but must be handled with great care (COSHH)
- alcohol (e.g. 70% isopropopyl alcohol, surgical spirit): alcohol disinfectants have a very effective bactericidal effect. They must be used once only and then discarded
- quartery ammonium compounds (e.g.Cetrimide): these are bacteriostatic cleansing agents. They prevent bacteria from spreading but they are not effective against very resistant organisms. QUATS are inactivated by soap
- hypochlorites (e.g.Milton, Domestos): these products contain sodium or calcium hypochlorite and are effective against most bacteria and some types of spore. They are often used for general cleaning purposes because they are relatively cheap. Some are corrosive and should not be used for soaking metal instruments.

> Remember
> Tools should always be washed in warm soapy water and rinsed well in clean water before disinfecting or sterilising them. This ensures the removal of debris which would act as a barrier. It also prevents contamination of the soaking solution.

Antiseptics

Antiseptics are disinfectants used specifically on the skin and for treating wounds. Ready-for-use swabs impregnated with 70% ispropopyl alcohol are often used for convenience.

> Remember
> The risks of cross-infection will only be eliminated if potential disease is identified, immediate measures taken and tools and equipment are kept scrupulously clean throughout the treatment.

Sterilisation and disinfection: Activity

1 Find out about the cleaning and sterilising methods used in your salon. Make a note of any special instructions on diluting, using and disposing of the chemical disinfectants and sterilising agents used. Make sure you know how to use the sterilising equipment. Find out where the rubber gloves and cleaning materials are kept.

Emergency aid

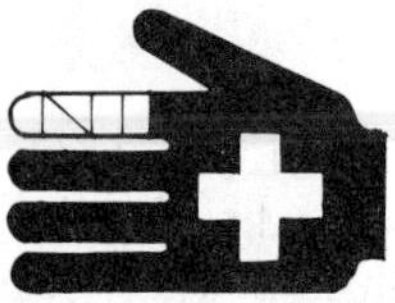

You need a basic knowledge of first aid so that you can assist with minor accidental injuries or unexpected situations which happen from time to time in the salon. More serious injuries, for example those involving acute pain, loss of consciousness or serious bleeding, should be dealt with by a qualified first aider, doctor or nurse.

Remember
It is advisable to keep in the box a card which lists names, addresses and phone numbers of the local health centres and hospitals.

First Aid kit

The Health and Safety regulations require the salon to have a First Aid kit readily available. The contents are specified and are intended to cover most emergency situations:

- a First Aid guidance card
- assorted plasters (preferably waterproof)
- different sizes of sterile dressings
- bandages(including a triangular bandage)
- sterile eye pads
- scissors
- tweezers
- safety pins.

Remember
Contaminated cotton wool and dressings should be disposed of in a plastic bag which has been tied up.

Useful additions to this list are:

- surgical adhesive tape and lint
- antiseptic cleansing products, i.e. liquid and cream
- an eye bath
- gauze
- crepe bandages
- an antihistamine cream
- medical wipes
- cotton wool.

If the salon has a fridge with a freezer compartment it is a good idea to keep an ice pack for injuries which produce swelling.

It is advisable to keep a stock of disposable gloves to wear when dealing with open wounds. These give some protection from hepatitis B and AIDS if an infection is present.

All staff should know what the First Aid box looks like and where it is kept. It is recommended that the box is green with a white cross marked on it and that it is dustproof and free from damp.

Remember
All accidents which occur in the salon must be recorded in an accident register. This is a requirement of the Health and Safety at Work Act.

What you may have to deal with

Problem	Priority	Action
Minor cuts	To stop the bleeding	Apply pressure over cotton wool taking care to avoid contact with the blood (see AIDS and hepatitis, page 24–5).
Severe cuts	To stop the bleeding	Keep applying pressure over a clean towel until qualified help arrives. Put on disposable gloves as soon as possible.
Electric shock	To remove from source of electricity	Do not touch the person until they are disconnected from the electricity supply. If breathing has stopped, artificial respiration will need to be given by a qualified person. Ring for an ambulance (see Calling the emergency services, page 3).
Dizziness	To restore the flow of blood to the head	Position the person with their head down between the knees and loosen their clothing.
Fainting	To restore the flow of blood to the head	Lie the person down with their feet raised on a cushion.
Nose bleed	To constrict the flow of blood	Sit the client up with the head bent forward. Loosen the clothing around the neck. Pinch, firmly, the soft part of the nose, until the bleeding has stopped. Make sure breathing continues through the mouth during this period. If bleeding has not stopped after half an hour, medical attention must be sought.
Burns	To cool the skin and prevent it from breaking	Hold the affected area under cold, running water until the pain is relieved. Serious burns should be covered loosely with a dry sterile dressing and medical attention sought.
Epilepsy	To prevent self-injury and relieve embarrassment after an attack	Do not interfere forcibly with a person during an attack. Gently prevent them from injuring themselves. prevent them from injuring themselves. Ensure the person's airways are clear and wipe away any froth which forms at the mouth. After the attack, cover with a blanket, comfort and give reassurance until recovery is complete.
Objects in the eye	To remove the object without damaging the eye	Expose the invaded area and try stroking the object towards the inside corner of the eye with a dampened twist of cotton wool. If this is not successful, help the person to use an eye bath containing clean warm water.
Falls	To determine if there is spine damage. To treat minor injuries if the fall is not serious	If the person complains of pains in the back or neck, then do not move them: cover with a warm blanket and get medical aid immediately. For less serious falls, treat the bruises, cuts, sprains or grazes as appropriate.
Bruises	To reduce pain and swelling	Apply cold compresses for 30 minutes using a towel wrapped round an ice-pack or very cold tap water. Keep the compress in place with a bandage. Replace it if it dries out.
Grazes	To clean wound and prevent infection	Soak a pad of cotton wool with antiseptic and gently clean the graze, working outwards from the centre. Replace the cotton wool regularly throughout the cleaning. Apply a sterile gauze dressing, preferably a non-adherent type, to protect the wound as it heals.
		If dirt or foreign matter has become embedded in the graze, the person should be referred to a doctor who may want to give a tetanus injection.
Sprains	To reduce swelling and pain	Apply cold compresses to the area (see treatment for bruises) and support the affected joint with a bandage firmly applied. Refer the person to a doctor.

Remember

It is important to protect against all diseases which are carried by the blood and tissue fluids. Many people feel most threatened by AIDS: this is mainly because of intense media coverage which has emphasised the high mortality rate. In fact, there is a much higher risk of cross-infection with hepatitis B, because the HBV virus is so resistant and can survive outside the body.

AIDS (Acquired Immune Deficiency Syndrome)

Aids is caused by a human immuno-deficiency virus (HIV). The virus attacks the body's natural immune system and makes it very vulnerable to other infections which eventually cause death. Some people are known to be HIV positive, which means that they are carrying the virus without the symptoms of AIDS. HIV carriers are able to pass on the virus to someone else through infected blood or tissue fluid, for example through cuts or broken skin. The virus does not live for long outside the body.

Hepatitis B

This disease of the liver is caused by a virus (HBV) which is transmitted by infected blood and tissue fluids.

The virus is very resistant and can survive outside the body. People can be very ill for a long time with a hepatitis B infection. It is a very weakening disease which can be fatal.

Strict hygiene practices are essential to prevent hepatitis B from spreading in the salon.

Emergency aid: Self-checks

1. Why should the First Aid kit contain an antiseptic?
2. Why is it advisable to wear disposable gloves when treating an open wound?
3. What help should be given to a client who is feeling dizzy?
4. What is the cause of fainting?
5. What is the correct treatment for a nose bleed?
6. What immediate action should be taken following a burn to the hand?
7. Whenever possible, why should furniture be removed from the area where a person is having an epileptic fit?
8. What should an eye bath contain to flush out the eye?
9. What are the signs that a person may have damaged their spine following a fall?
10. For what reason might an ice-pack be used when giving emergency aid?

Emergency aid: Activities

1. Find out where the First Aid kit is kept in your salon and who is in charge of first aid procedures.
   Ask if you can have a look at the First Aid kit. Check the contents to see if there is anything missing. If there is, inform the supervisor.
2. Working with a partner, role play emergency aid procedures for each of the following: a) nose bleed b) dizziness c) object in the eye d) fainting.

Working with colleagues

A successful business employs committed, hard-working staff who pull together as a team and are motivated towards the same goals.

A good employer spends a lot of time and thought recruiting new people to the business, making sure that all new employees fit in with the rest of the team.

Most people are behaving slightly unnaturally at interview and it is not until they have worked in the salon for a time that their true character and personality are revealed!

Most good working relationships develop easily. Others have to be worked at. Whatever the personal feelings of individuals towards one another, clients must never sense a bad atmosphere in the salon because of friction between staff.

You will spend a lot of time in the company of people you work with. You won't always like everyone, but that does not really matter. You must accept that people are different and that, at work, mutual respect is more important than being the best of friends.

If you can be described as the following, you will not have too much trouble earning the respect of your colleagues (and you will probably be very popular as well!):

- conscientious: working to the best of your ability and being thorough in everything you do
- dedicated: showing commitment to the job and being prepared to put in extra time when required
- self-motivated: keeping yourself busy and not always needing to be told what to do.
- determined: wanting to succeed and taking every opportunity to improve your professional skills and knowledge of the job.
- responsible: not needing to be constantly supervised or watched over, having the confidence of your colleagues to get on with the work.
- well presented: appearing smart and professional, always projecting a good image for the salon.
- sensitive: accepting that there is room for different views and opinions, never making tactless remarks which could offend.
- reliable: arriving in good time for work and not taking time off unnecessarily.
- co-operative: being helpful and supportive, making a positive contribution to the team effort.

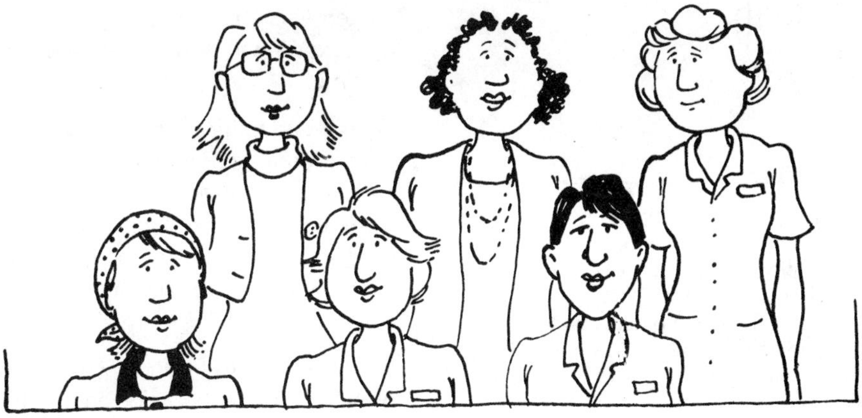

> *Remember*
> Skimping or leaving jobs lets down the rest of the team and lowers professional standards. A bad impression reflects on everybody.

> *Remember*
> You may be needed to help with outside demonstrations and other promotional activities which help to make the business a success.

> *Remember*
> Sometimes you will be required to take further training so that the salon can offer new treatments or services. Be grateful for the chance to learn new techniques - the more you can do, the more valuable you become as an employee.

> *Remember*
> Working closely with others can sometimes have its frustrations and tensions. You should always try to be sensitive to the feelings of others and act accordingly.

> *Remember*
> Reliability also means doing what you say you are going to do – not just talking about it !

> *Remember*
> It can be hard sometimes, but you must learn to leave your personal problems at home and always be cheerful with your clients and colleagues. Friends will want to share your problems, but not during working hours.

> Remember
> Some people work very well on their own but are not particularly helpful or supportive with their colleagues. A good team pools its resources and benefits from everybody's strengths.

- flexible: taking things in your stride, adapting to different situations and circumstances without complaining or showing resistance.
- warm and friendly: making everyone feel that you are really enjoy your work and that you have a genuine interest in others.

Everyone who works in a salon contributes to its success. Cleaners, receptionists, therapists, technicians and management all have roles which are different, yet essential to the operation. Take pride in your own work and value that of others. Once you have proved yourself as a member of the team you will have earned the respect of colleagues and the loyalty of your clients.

Professional code of ethics

As a beauty therapist, you will have much to gain by joining one of the professional membership associations which represents you and your industry. Technical and product up-dating, news bulletins, professional and social meetings with other professional beauty therapists will all be available to you, and also the benefits of preferential rates for professional insurance cover.

These associations are committed to advancing the beauty therapy profession and providing maximum protection for the public. They will work hard on your behalf. In return, you must be prepared always to conduct yourself according to the professional code of ethics and to maintain high standards of professional practice in all aspects of your work.

While each organisation produces its own code of practice, there are standard ethical rules which are common to all of them:

- never treating or claiming to be able to treat a medical condition
- showing respect for other professions by referring clients appropriately, for example to general practitioners, chiropodists, physiotherapists
- maintaining high standards of hygiene and safety in all aspects of work
- applying certain treatments only with the written permission of the client's general practitioner
- supporting, helping and showing loyalty to other professional beauty therapists, never actively 'poaching' another member's clients or criticising their work
- upholding the 'honour' of the profession at all times, for example when working on members of the opposite sex.

> Remember
> Be proud of your profession! Project an image which instils trust and confidence in both clients and work colleagues. Always treat other people as you would wish to be treated yourself.

Working with colleagues: Activity

1 Face the music time! Sometimes it can be very difficult to make judgements about ourselves. Being an effective team member really has more to do with how others see us, whether in employment or during training.

Working in pairs or small groups, list the essential qualities which have been identified and work out an appropriate rating scale, for example 1–5, with 1 being disastrous and 5 being excellent! Use this scale to grade each member against each quality. Talk quite openly about the scores you give. Justify the grades you award and be positive with the advice you give to colleagues on how they might improve on their team working skills.

It is important to listen to what is said about you! Accept any criticism in the spirit which it is given and treat it as a valuable aid to learning.

> Remember
> Being sensitive is an essential quality for members of a team. Choose your words carefully when criticising others and try to give helpful advice.

Chapter 2

Reception

After working through this chapter you will be able to:

- understand the importance of 'reception' to the success of a business
- describe the work of a receptionist
- describe the personal skills and qualities required to be successful at reception work
- carry out the correct procedures for looking after clients, recording appointments and dealing with enquiries, processing payments and handling and displaying retail stock.

The reception desk

The reception desk is the control centre for salon operations. Everybody's working day is planned according to the appointment book and then adapted as visitors come and go. Regular clients are welcomed back for treatments. Casual enquirers become new clients. The building up of a successful business starts at the reception, where good first impressions have lasting effects.

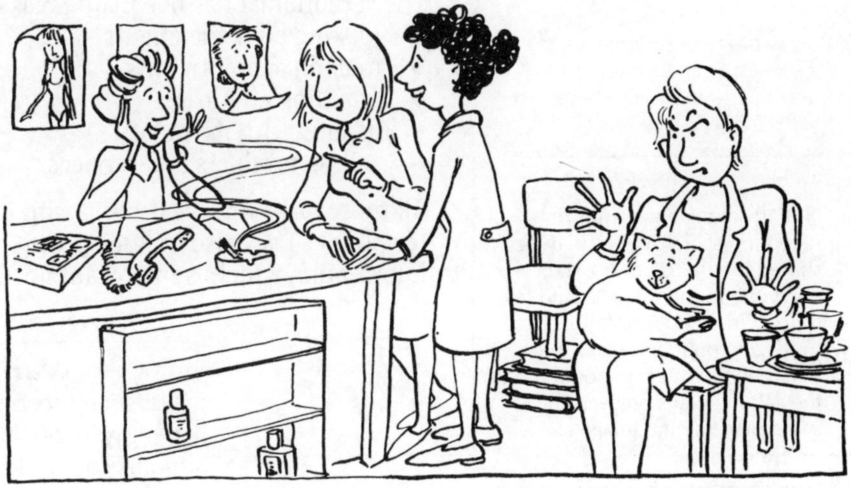

You should have spotted eight mistakes!

First impressions

Think of the last time you sat in a reception area waiting for an appointment. It could have been at the doctor's surgery, the dentist's or maybe the hairdresser's. Can you remember what you did while you were waiting:

- looked through the magazines? Were they current and in good condition?
- studied other people who were waiting? Did they look comfortable and relaxed?
- watched the receptionist? Was she busy, friendly and attentive?

- read notices on the wall? Were they eye-catching, interesting and well presented?
- kept your eye on the clock? Was the clock right and were people being seen to on time?
- examined the decor and furnishings? Were they clean, attractive and well maintained?
- listened in to telephone conversations! Were callers dealt with politely and helpfully?

If the answers to these questions were 'yes' then you probably felt comfortable with your surroundings and confident that you would receive a good, professional service.

> Remember
> Waiting time is not wasting time! Clients look and listen while waiting in reception. Good impressions bring the clients back. Good impressions lead to good business!

The reception desk: Activity

1 How does your salon area stand up to the test? Have a good look round. Consider the points covered in this chapter and, where appropriate, make a note of things to do. Do what you can as soon as you can and then see what your supervisor thinks of more ambitious ideas that you may have!

The receptionist

First impressions are lasting impressions. It is important that the receptionist presents a professional image of the salon and that each client feels 'special'.

The receptionist has five main areas of responsibility:

- looking after the clients
- making appointments
- handling enquiries
- dealing with payments
- selling products and services.

All these tasks involve dealing with clients either directly or over the telephone. They also include giving, receiving and recording information which is important for the business to run efficiently.

> Remember
> Not all salons have a full-time receptionist. The duties may be shared by the rest of the staff. Everyone in the salon should be trained in reception skills so that they can confidently take over when needed. It is important that the salon always presents the same professional image at reception.

> **Wanted**
> Full-time receptionist for busy beauty salon. NVQ level 2 qualification desirable. Good interpersonal and communication skills essential. Write or telephone personally for further details: 'Onyx', 15 Daisy Lane, Scunthrop. Tel: 09347.

Interpersonal skills

A person with the necessary personal skills and qualities can be trained in salon procedures and the administrative duties of reception work. A good administrator who does not relate well to people will not make a good receptionist. The interpersonal skills required include:

> Remember
> These skills are important for developing good relationships with both clients and colleagues.

- treating others with respect: making sure that everybody is treated the same and that personal feelings are not allowed to affect work
- being sensitive to other people's feelings: avoiding saying or doing anything which might offend somebody else, particularly if it involves their race or religion
- showing concern for others: always being caring and considerate, giving the right help at the right time.

Communication skills

Communication skills are used to convey and use information. They include:

- speaking clearly and confidently: making sure that information is accurate and well explained
- listening and hearing: ensuring that the facts are right
- reading and writing: recording information accurately so that it is understood easily
- using effective body language: appearing approachable, friendly and helpful even when not speaking
- personal presentation: projecting a professional image and pride in the job.

> Remember
> Receptionists are not allowed to have 'off' days! Whatever they may be feeling, their body language must convey the message 'Hello, nice to see you; how may I help you?'

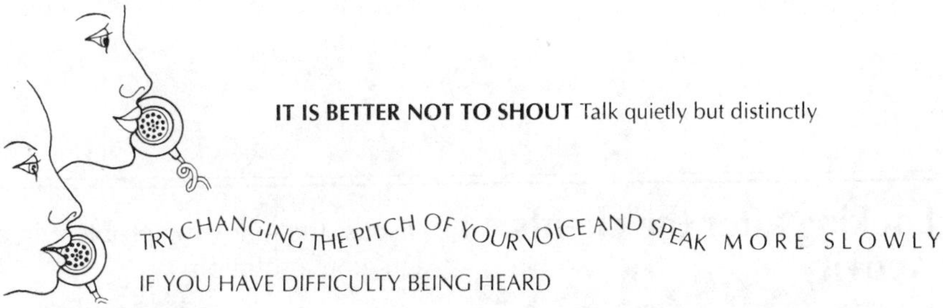
IT IS BETTER NOT TO SHOUT Talk quietly but distinctly
TRY CHANGING THE PITCH OF YOUR VOICE AND SPEAK MORE SLOWLY
IF YOU HAVE DIFFICULTY BEING HEARD

Tips for using the telephone

The receptionist: Self-check

1 Describe how a receptionist might use four different communication skills in her job.

The receptionist: Activities

1 See how the professionals do it: visit a local salon to obtain details of their treatments and a price list. Pay attention to the interpersonal and communication skills of the person who deals with you. Remember – you could be a prospective client. If you can, visit a few salons and compare the reception you get at each one.

2 Working with a partner or in small groups, take each of the interpersonal skills referred to in this chapter: discuss how a receptionist might need to use these skills in a range of situations. Remember that clients are not the only people a receptionist has to deal with.

Looking after the clients

The receptionist has to:

- welcome the clients and help them with their coats and belongings
- estimate the waiting period and inform the clients if this is to be longer or shorter than originally expected
- ensure the comfort and care of the clients while they wait, offering magazines and hospitality as appropriate
- after treatments help the clients with retail purchases and arrange a convenient time for their next appointment
- help the clients with their coats and belongings, confirm how nice it was to see them and accompany them to the door
- make sure the reception area is clean, tidy and pleasant for the clients
- keep the clients' records up-to-date and well organised.

> *Remember*
> Record cards should be kept in strict alphabetical order, using the clients' surnames. Where two or more clients share the same surname, the cards should be filed according to the initial letter of their first name.

Looking after the clients: Self-checks

1 In what order should the following clients' record cards appear in the filing system?
Sue Johnstone, Linda Johnson, Pat Jones, Sue Joiner, Eve Johnson, Mary Jones, Alice Jolson, Audrey Jolliff

2 State three ways in which a client should be made to feel 'special' at reception.

Looking after the clients: Activity

1 Discuss the following problem in a small group and see if you can agree on a solution:

Scenario A client arrives ten minutes late for her manicure appointment and explains, very apologetically, that she was held up by an unexpected visitor. The appointment book shows that another client is expected in twenty minutes.

Should you:

a) apologise and explain that there is not enough time left for a manicure and ask her to make another appointment
b) tell her not to worry, assure her that she can have the manicure and, when the next client arrives, explain that there will be a slight delay
c) explain to the client that she can have a manicure but that it will have to be 'cut down' so that it is completed within twenty minutes?

If your answer is (a), do you think that the client should be charged for the treatment she has not had? (After all, you were not able to offer the appointment to someone else.)

If your answer is (b), would it make any difference if the client expected for the later appointment is a regular or new client, visiting the salon for the first time?

If your answer is (c), should the client have the price of the manicure reduced because she has not had the full treatment?

Are there any other possible solutions to the problem?

Recording appointments

> Remember
> Sometimes clients have to cancel or change their appointment. When details are recorded in pencil, they can be rubbed out neatly and the space used for another client.

The receptionist has to:

- ensure that the reception desk is supplied with appointment cards, pens, pencils, ruler and a rubber
- prepare pages in the appointment book a few weeks in advance, to show the availability of each operator on a particular day
- as appointments are arranged, transfer details to the appointment book in pencil, stating the name of the client, their telephone number and the treatment or service required
- make out an appointment card for the client, recording details in pen and stating the date, day, time and operator's name

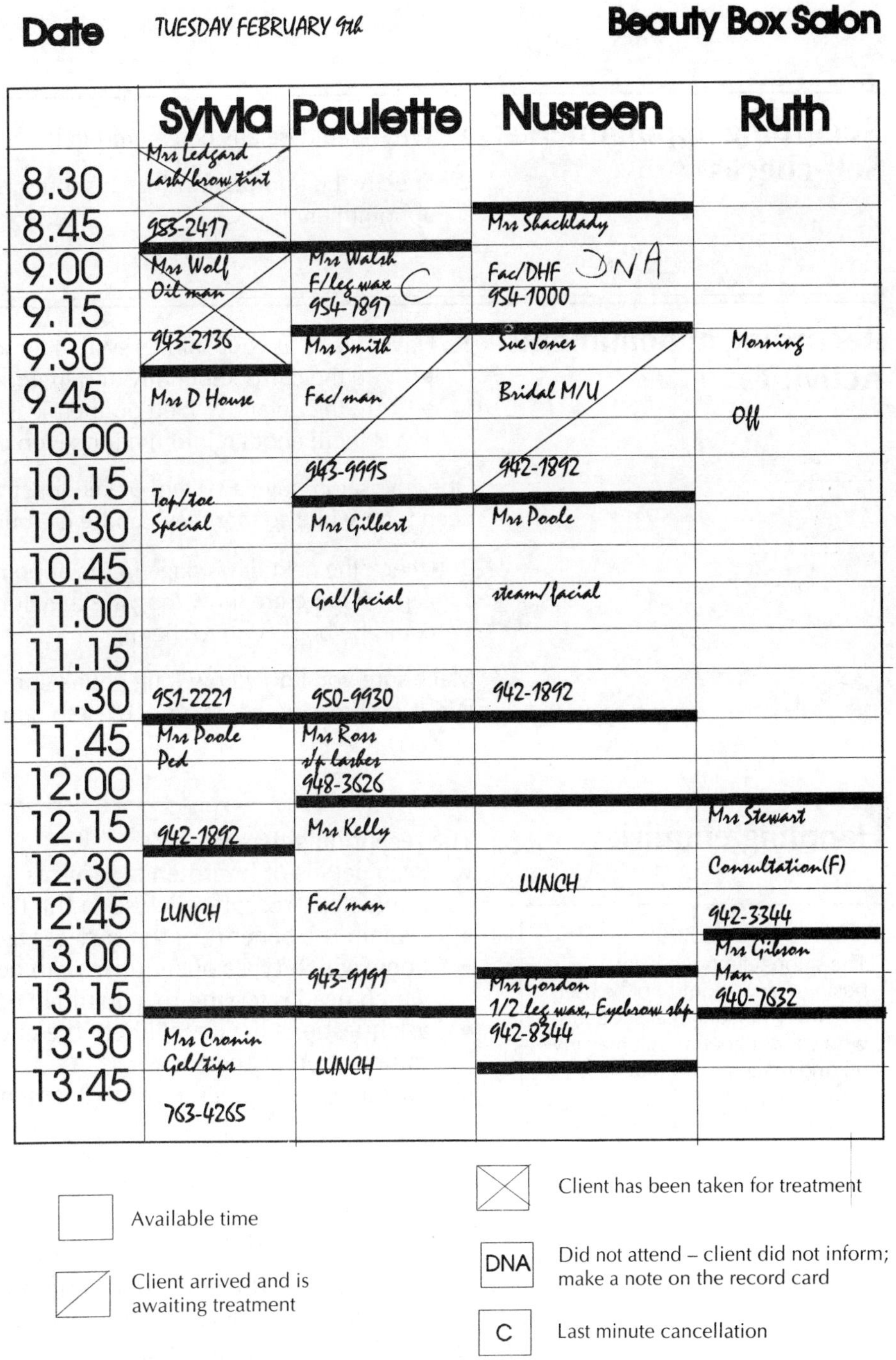
Date
TUESDAY FEBRUARY 9th
Beauty Box Salon
Sylvia
Paulette
Nusreen
Ruth
8.30
8.45
9.00
9.15
9.30
9.45
10.00
10.15
10.30
10.45
11.00
11.15
11.30
11.45
12.00
12.15
12.30
12.45
13.00
13.15
13.30
13.45
Mrs Ledgard
Lash/brow tint
953-2417
Mrs Wolf
Oil man
943-2136
Mrs D House
Top/toe
Special
951-2221
Mrs Poole
Ped
942-1892
LUNCH
Mrs Cronin
Gel/tips
763-4265
Mrs Walsh
F/leg wax
954-7897
C
Mrs Smith
Fac/man
943-9995
Mrs Gilbert
Gal/facial
950-9930
Mrs Ross
s/p lashes
948-3626
Mrs Kelly
Fac/man
943-9191
LUNCH
Mrs Shacklady
Fac/DHF
954-1000
DNA
Sue Jones
Bridal M/U
942-1892
Mrs Poole
steam/facial
942-1892
LUNCH
Mrs Gordon
1/2 leg wax, Eyebrow shp
942-8344
Morning
Off
Mrs Stewart
Consultation(F)
942-3344
Mrs Gibson
Man
940-7632
Client has been taken for treatment
Available time
DNA
Did not attend – client did not inform; make a note on the record card
Client arrived and is awaiting treatment
C
Last minute cancellation

A completed page of an appointment book

- check the accuracy of both sets of records before handing over the appointment card to the client
- record the client's arrival at the salon by drawing a diagonal line in pencil across their details in the appointment book
- when the client has gone through for treatment, draw a diagonal line across the first one to record that they are being attended to.

> Remember
> It is important that the appointment pages are kept neat and tidy. The correct codes and abbreviations must be used and the start and finish times of treatments made clear.

Clients who arrive unexpectedly may be treated provided that there is an operator available. The receptionist should always check first and then record the client's details in the appointment book.

In some salons the receptionist prepares a list for each operator which shows their schedule for the day. This is kept by the operator and provides a useful quick reference, particularly if an unexpected client arrives.

Recording appointments: Self-checks

1 Why should details be entered in the appointment book in pencil?

2 Specify the information which should be available at a glance in the appointment book.

Recording appointments: Activities

1 Have a look at your salon's system for keeping client records:
- Are the cards kept tidily and in good order?
- Are the details written on them easily understood?
- Is there enough information given on them?

Does the salon have a system of keeping track of clients who have not been for a while so that they can be encouraged back to the salon?

2 Check the next day's page in the appointment book: are there any gaps? If there are, how long are they for and what sort of treatments could be booked in to them?

Make sure you know how long your salon allows for various treatments. Write the times down on a price list to remind yourself.

Handling enquiries

> Remember
> The salon telephone is for business and should not be used for chatty personal calls. Clients who cannot get through may give up and make an appointment somewhere else.

The receptionist has to:
- keep details of treatments, services, products and price lists available at reception, close to the telephone
- explain the benefits of the services available to clients
- know which types of enquiries can be dealt with personally and which need referring to a qualified operator
- ask questions which will help the client to provide the right information in the answer
- take down messages accurately and pass them on, promptly, to the right person. Valuable time may be wasted responding to messages if details are missing or unclear.

Telephone enquiries

For many clients, the telephone is their first contact with the business. A good receptionist never forgets that all calls are from people, each one of whom is a prospective client.

Telephone answering techniques

You should always:

- answer promptly – on the second or third ring. This gives both sides time to prepare themselves without the caller becoming impatient
- be friendly – give the name of the salon and say who you are. Note the client's name so that you can use it in the conversation
- smile when you pick up the receiver. Your voice is you to a caller. Smiles definitely do travel down the telephone!
- be enthusiastic – ask how you may help the caller. Enthusiasm is infectious and shows you enjoy being helpful
- listen attentively – it is very off-putting for a caller if they can sense you are being distracted by someone or something else.
- leave a good impression. Remember that you are the salon to the caller. Repeat back to them any important points discussed and thank them for calling. Don't forget to use their name!

> *Remember*
> It is a good idea for the salon to have a telephone answering machine. This records messages outside business hours and is particularly useful for clients to use in the event of a last minute cancellation.

Handling enquiries: Activity

1 With a partner, role play a situation at reception which involves giving advice and arranging an appointment for a client over the telephone. If you are playing the part of the client, don't make life too easy for the receptionist! Give them the opportunity to use all their skills of tact and diplomacy – create a few problems!

Plan the background to your call so that you have got some answers ready. It may be useful to have a third person acting as observer who can feed back to you afterwards.

Dealing with payments

The receptionist has to:

- provide an itemised bill for the client
- handle cash payments
- give change from the till
- issue receipts
- supervise payments by cheque
- process credit and debit card payments.

Many salons have to charge VAT (Value Added Tax) to the client because their sales of products and services exceed a certain level. The tax is paid back later to the government. Some salons include VAT in their prices. Others total the bill and then add on VAT.

Using the till

Most salons have an electronic cash till which records payments, issues receipts and keeps money safe. The till may also provide a lot of other information which is useful to the business.

The till receipt shown below is fairly typical. Some tills have codes for each type of service and retail product, each operator's name and the method of payment used. The more details which can be provided through the till, the easier and less time consuming it is to collect information for the business records.

> *Remember*
> Never put money straight into the till drawer. Mistakes can be made which are difficult to deal with once the evidence of payment has gone. This is particularly important when handling notes.

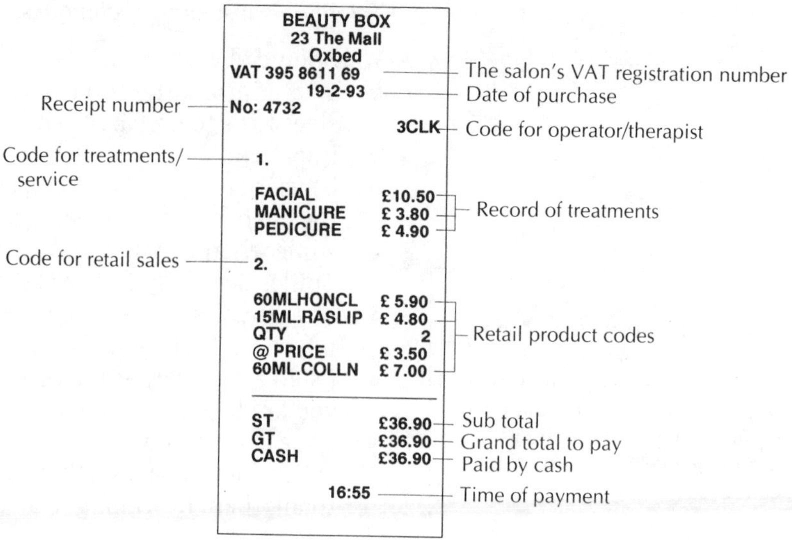

An itemised till receipt tells the client exactly what was paid for each item

> Remember
>
> The drawer of the till should never be left open after a transaction. The security of the money is the responsibility of the receptionist.

You will be trained how to use the till in your salon, but here is the basic procedure for dealing with cash payments:

1. Total the bill and inform the client of the cost.
2. Accept the payment gratefully and check that it is made up of legal currency, i.e. notes and coins produced in England, Scotland, Northern Ireland (not Eire), and Jersey. To check a bank note, hold it up to the light: a genuine note will show the water-marked picture of the queen's face.
3. Place the money on the till shelf.
4. Count out the change into your own hand.
5. Count out the change into the client's hand.
6. Ask the client to confirm that the change is correct.
7. Put the payment into the till.
8. Thank the client and give them their till receipt.

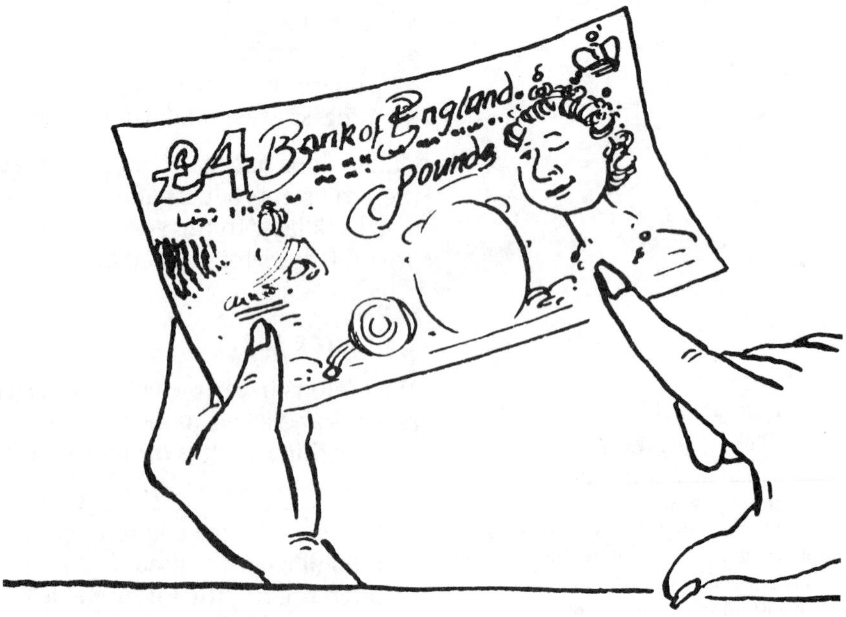

Unfortunately, forged bank notes are not this obvious!

> Remember
>
> The account number and signature on the cheque must correspond with those on the cheque card. If they do not, you should tactfully seek assistance from your supervisor.

Supervising payments by cheque

Many clients prefer to pay by cheque: make sure that the cheque is filled in correctly and that payment is guaranteed by a valid cheque card which covers the amount of the bill. It is the receptionist's job to ensure that the cheque is made out properly and that the information used is correct. The cheque card number must be written on the back of the cheque together with the receptionist's signature or initials before returning the card with a receipt to the client.

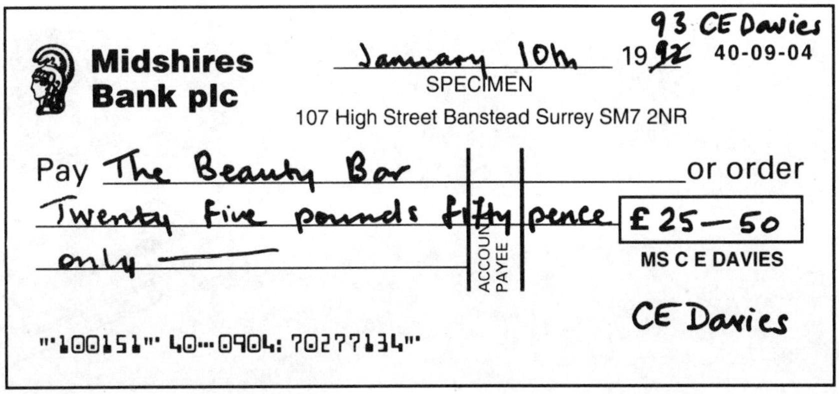

An initialled cheque showing correction

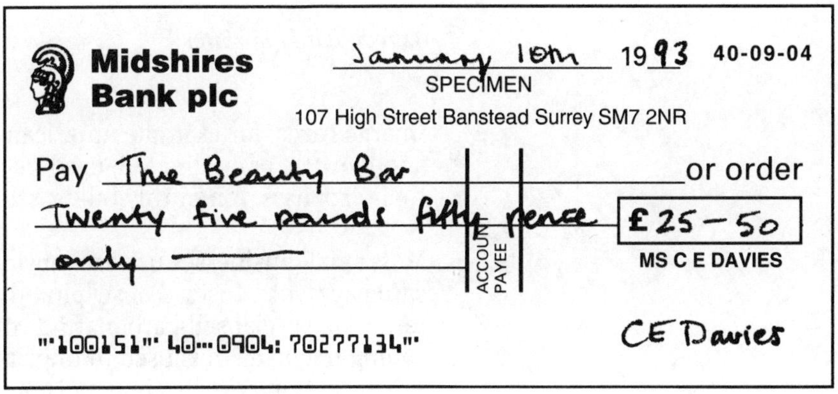

A correctly completed cheque

Processing credit and debit card payments

EFTPOS

EFTPOS (Electronic Funds Transfer at Point Of Sale) is an electronic payment system which cuts out the need for either cash or a cheque. The system is fast to use and there is very little paperwork. Customers use cards which are supplied by banks and building societies. In order to offer clients this facility the salon needs a special terminal through which the card is 'swiped'. The receptionist keys in the amount and the information is relayed automatically over communication lines to a central computer. Authorisation for payment comes from the computer which holds details of customers' accounts. When authorisation is given, payment is guaranteed.

A duplicate receipt is issued which the client has to sign. The receptionist compares this signature with the one on the credit or debit card. Both the client and the salon keep a copy of the receipt.

> Remember
>
> If you accept a stolen credit card in good faith, the issuing organisation will usually pay you the money.

Credit cards

Credit cards include 'Access' and 'Visa'. Money is transferred automatically from the client's credit account and is added to a bill which is sent monthly to the client. A proportion of the bill has to be paid back each month.

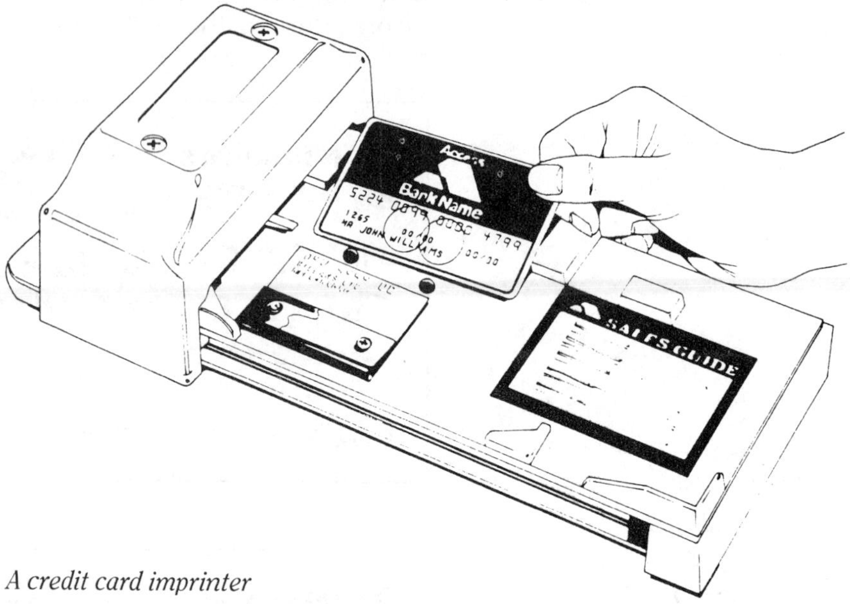

A credit card imprinter

Charge cards, for example American Express and Diners Club, are another type of credit card, used mainly by business people for paying their expenses. A monthly bill is issued which has to be paid off in full.

Most small businesses use an imprinter method of recording credit card payments. Instead of swiping the card through a computerised terminal, special self-carbonating vouchers are filled in and a manual sliding mechanism is used to imprint the card details on the vouchers. The receptionist writes in details of the sales and the voucher is signed by the client. Payment is authorised when the credit company receives a copy of the voucher. The top copy of the voucher is kept by the client as a receipt. The remaining copy is kept by the salon for accounting purposes.

Debit cards

Debit cards include 'Connect' and 'Switch'. Payment is made by automatic transfer of money from the client's bank account.

Cashing up

This is usually done by a senior member of staff at the end of each working day. Alternatively, cashing up may be the receptionist's responsibility, in which case there is usually a second person present.

BEAUTY BOX SALON

Cashing Up Sheet

Date: *Thursday May 1st*

Opening Float: *£25.00*

	IN	OUT	
CASH			
£50		*Milk*	*74p*
£20	*80.00*	*Window clean*	*£6.00*
£10	*50.00*		
£ 5	*25.00*		
Coins	*18.76*		*£6.74*
	£173.76		
CHEQUES			
Smith	*28.00*		
Jones	*36.00*		
Wray	*29.50*		
	93.50		
VOUCHERS			
	53.00		
SUB-TOTAL			
	320.26		
Payments	*6.74*		
	327.00		
Minus opening float	*25.00*		
GRAND TOTAL			
A	302.00	B Closing float	£25.00

A = The day's takings. This should correspond with the till 'Z' reading

B = After cashing up, an amount is set aside to be the opening float for the following working day

A cashing up sheet

Cashing up not only confirms the day's takings, it also shows whether the receptionist has handled and recorded payments correctly. A simple sum is done which produces a total which should balance with the till's 'Z' reading.

BEAUTY BOX
23 The Mall
Oxbed
VAT 395 8611 69
19-2-93
No 1732
GRAND TOTALS

TOTAL SALES	£302.00
CASH SALES	£173.76
CHEQUE SALES	£ 93.50
CREDIT SALES	£ 53.00
DISCOUNT	£ 00.00
RETURNS	£ 00.00
FLOAT	£ 25.00
PAID OUT	£ 6.74
DRAW BALANCE	£321.74
	2CLK
SALES TRTS	£ 65.00
SALES RETAIL	£ 82.00
	3CLK
SALES TRTS	£135.00
SALES RETAIL	£ 20.00
TOTAL TRTS	£200.00
TOTAL RETAIL	£102.00

CLIENTS = 11
VOIDS = 0

TIME 20.15

The 'Z' reading provides information for the whole of a trading period – usually one day

Money which is paid after the 'Z' reading has been taken must be included in the next day's figures when cashing up

This reading shows the transactions which have taken place and the total amount taken during a trading period

Following cashing up, some money is 'bagged up' for paying into the bank. An amount is usually kept back for the next day's float.

Remember

The float is an amount of money which is put in the till each morning to provide change for clients, and petty cash if that is not supplied separately. Petty cash is used to pay for small day-to-day purchases such as milk, pens, magazines, etc. It is important to keep records of petty cash payments so that they can be accounted for when cashing up.

Dealing with payments: Self-checks

1 Give three main functions of an electronic cash till.

2 Why should cash not be put straight into the till following payment?

3 What security measures should be taken when processing payment by (a) cheque (b) credit card ?

4 Why must receipts for petty cash payments be retained?

Dealing with payments: Activities

1 Make sure you know any special procedures in your salon for dealing with or recording payments. Have a go at filling in and processing a credit card voucher. Ask your supervisor to check that you have done it properly.

Make sure you tear up the voucher afterwards – do not put it through the till.

2 Have a good look at a till receipt and see if you can explain what the various codes mean relative to the amounts recorded.

Maintaining stock and the retail area

The receptionist has to:

- keep the retail area clean and tidy: the counter, shelves and stock should be dusted every day and, where possible, have regular changes of display. Stock which is grubby and dusty will lose its value
- inform clients of current promotions: the receptionist should draw the attention of clients to special offers and make sure that promotional material is displayed where it will catch the eye of the client
- carry out stock checks: stock checks should be carried out weekly, to monitor how well different products are selling and to make sure that popular lines are re-ordered before being sold out
- price the retail products: identical products must not be priced differently. Price tickets should be checked as part of the regular stock check. Old price tickets should be removed before putting on new ones so that a lower price is not disguised
- store stock correctly so that it does not deteriorate or become damaged. Keep fast moving lines at the front of the shelves and slower moving ones nearer the back. Do not block aisles or passageways with containers of stock; keep it in a locked cupboard or secure store room
- display stock attractively: displays should be set up with the minimum disruption to business. If all retail stock is to be displayed, extra space is needed for the fastest selling lines. Shelving should be clean, safe and undamaged and strong enough to take the weight of the products on display. Packaging should be displayed with the product. Take care with flimsy packaging and stack heavier goods lower down than more fragile items

> *Remember*
> Storing stock in straight lines makes counting easier.

> *Remember*
> Use 'dummy' stock under bright lighting: this way, the colour, texture and fragrance of products will not become spoiled.

> *Remember*
> Be careful when unpacking stock. Look out for sharp staple fastenings on boxes and avoid using a knife. Protect your overall when carrying large items and mind those nails! Paper and cardboard packages should be flattened before disposal.

> Remember
>
> The salon loses money on old stock which is sold off cheaply or thrown away. Products which are approaching their expiry date should be identified at the stock check and steps taken to sell them before it is too late. This may mean offering a special promotion, or reducing the price slightly as an incentive to buy.

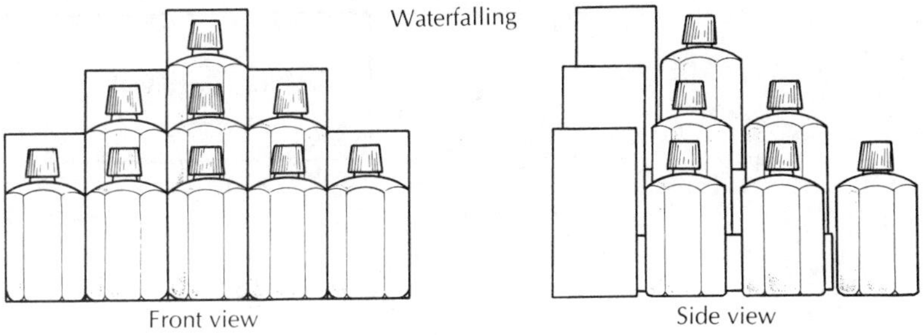

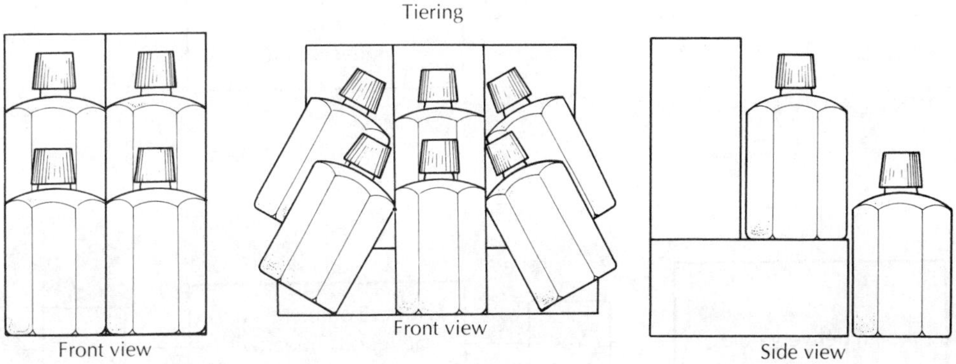

> Remember
>
> Take care when dismantling a display. Put back equipment where it will not become damaged and keep tools and accessories safe in a box.

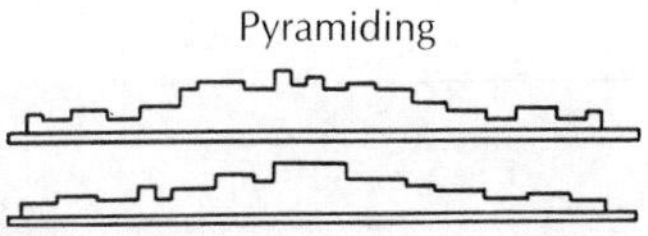

3 methods of stock display

- keep accurate stock records
  The quality of a product cannot be guaranteed once its expiry date has passed. Stock which has been stored beyond its 'shelf-life' has either to be sold off cheaply or disposed of.

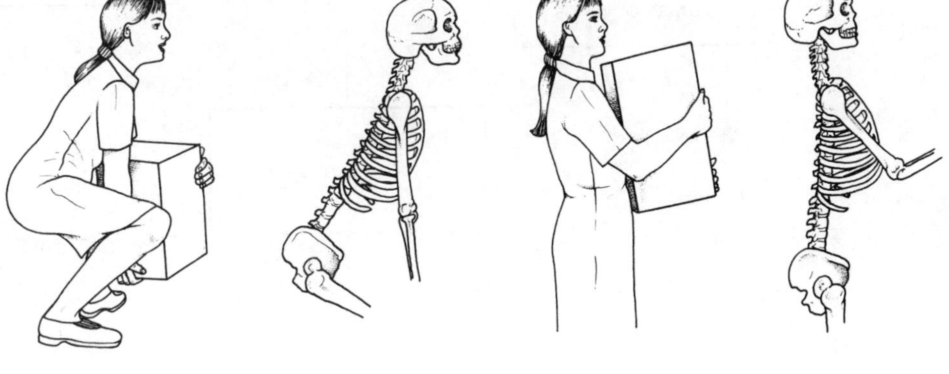

Correct lifting and carrying technique: avoid straining your back when moving heavy stock

- store stock in a cool dark place
- do not pile boxes too high
- when an order arrives, bring older stock to the front of the shelves and store new stock behind. This method of stock control is called FIFO, i.e. First In, First Out.

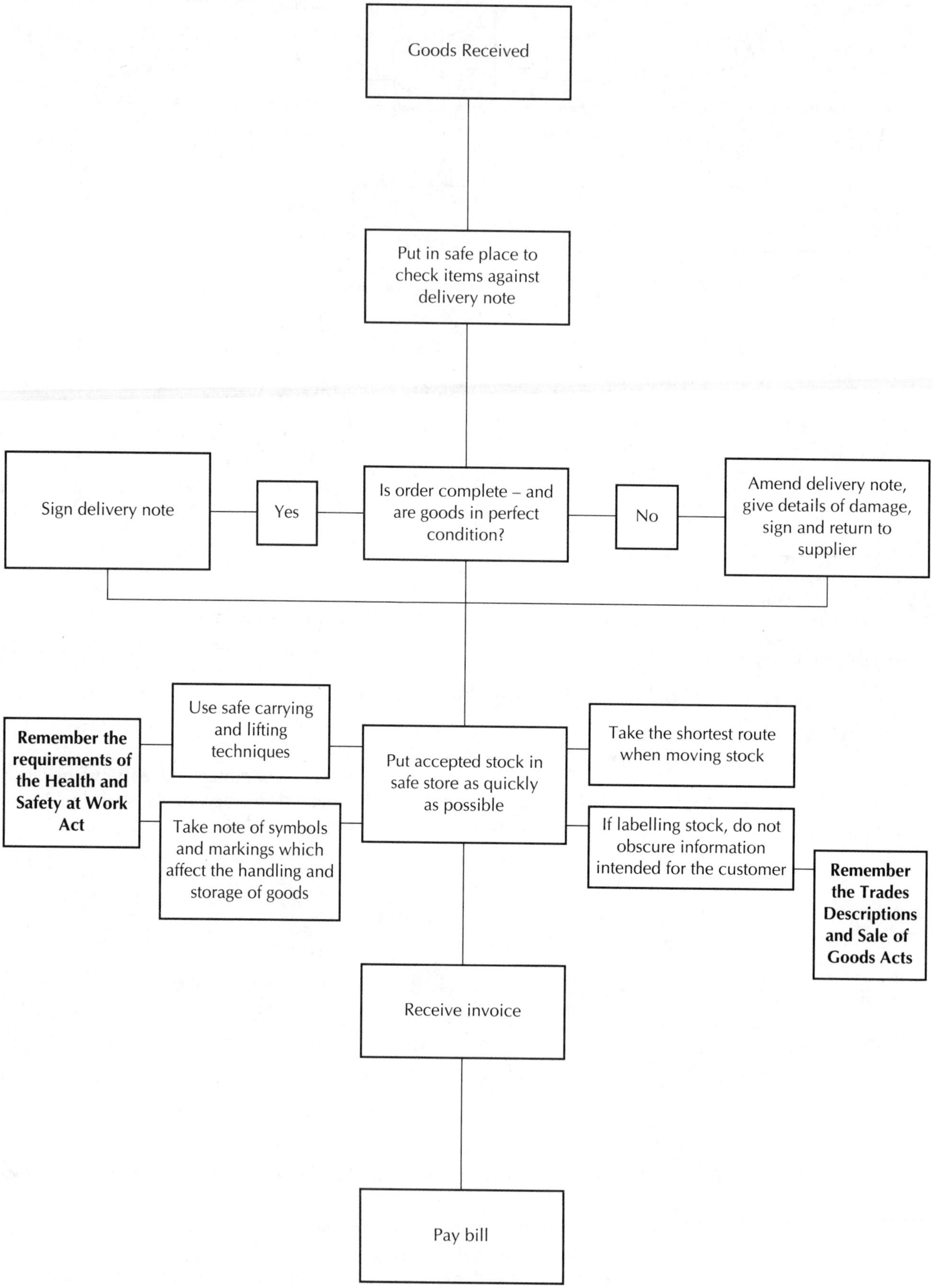

Distribution of stock

	STOCK LIST		STOCK LIST
1	Dermalesse Cleansing Oil 75ml	**21**	
2	Dermalesse Cleansing Milk 150ml	**22**	
3	Dermalesse Cleansing Cream 150ml	**23**	
4	Dermalesse Exfoliant 100ml	**24**	
5	Dermalesse Cleansing Milk 100ml	**25**	
6	Dermalesse Cleansing Cream 300ml	**26**	
7	Dermalesse Skin Freshener 150ml	**27**	
8	Dermalesse Skin Tonic 150ml	**28**	
9	Dermalesse Skin Freshener 300ml	**29**	
10	Dermalesse Skin Tonic 300ml	**30**	
11		**31**	
12		**32**	
13		**33**	
14		**34**	
15		**35**	
16		**36**	
17		**37**	
18		**38**	
19		**39**	
20		**40**	

The stock sheet lists the number of items in stock per product line. The details of a stock check are recorded on a stock sheet before being transferred to the stock book

STOCK BOOK

NO	PRODUCT CODE	PRODUCT	BASE STOCK	DATE: 29/2/93							DATE: 7/3/93						
				Counter stock	Stockroom stock	Total stock (*i*)	Order	Received	Total stock (*ii*)	Sold	Counter stock	Stockroom stock	Total stock (*i*)	Order	Received	Total stock (*ii*)	Sold
1	00191	Dermalesse Cl. Oil 75ml	10	6	2	8	2	/	8	2	4	2	6	/	2	8	/
2	00192	Dermalesse Cl.Mlk 150ml	10	4	2	6	4	/	6	/	4	2	6	/	4	10	2
3	00193	Dermalesse Cl. Oil 75ml	10	4	2	6	4	/	6	4	2	/	2	4	4	6	1
4	00194	Dermalesse Exfol 100ml	6	4	/	4	2	/	4	1	3	/	3	1	2	5	2
5	00195	Dermalesse Cl.Milk 300ml	5	2	2	4	1	/	4	2	2	/	2	2	1	3	2
6	00196	Dermalesse Cl. Crm 300ml	5	2	/	2	3	/	2	/	2	/	2	/	3	5	1
7	00197	Dermalesse Sk Frsh 150ml	8	4	2	6	2	/	6	4	2	/	2	4	2	4	1
8	00198	Dermalesse Sk Tonic 150ml	8	5	/	5	3	/	5	1	4	/	4	1	3	7	2
9	00199	Dermalesse Sk Frsh 300ml	5	2	1	3	/	2	5	1	3	1	4	1	/	4	2
10	00200	Dermalesse Sk Tonic 300ml	5	3	1	4	1	/	4	3	1	/	1	3	1	2	/
11	00201	Dermalesse Cr Mask 75ml	4	2	1	3	1	/	4	3	1	/	1	3	1	4	2
12	00202	Dermalesse Ampoules	6	3	/	3	3	/	3	2	1	/	1	2	3	4	1
13	00203	Maqui Base Ivory	6	2	3	5	1	1	6	2	3	1	4	2	1	5	/
14	00204	Maqui Base Cream	6	4	/	4	2	/	4	2	2	/	2	2	2	4	1
15	00205	Maqui Base Beige	6	2	/	3	2	1	4	/	3	1	4	/	/	4	2

Different colours may be used to record the figures in each column. This is useful if you need to find figures quickly. For example:
Stock = blue
Received stock = green
Orders = black
Sold stock = red.

The stock book identifies re-order levels, and the receipt and sales of stock

Maintaining stock and the retail area: Self-check

1 Give three reasons for carrying out regular stock checks.

2 What steps can be taken to avoid keeping stock beyond its shelf-life?

3 What is the main purpose of (a) a stock sheet (b) a stock book?

Maintaining stock and the retail area: Activities

1 Ask your supervisor if you can carry out a stock check using one of the salon's stock sheets. It would be helpful if a partner could do one as well so that you can compare your results. (Remember to check the contents of boxes. Regrettably, pilferers can be very cunning and may leave an empty box on the shelf to cover their tracks.)

2 Discuss the following with a partner and compare your answers with other members of the group:
   a) What could be the possible reasons for discrepancies at a stock check?
   b) How do you think seasonal variations might affect the allocation of space given to stock?
   c) When are the best times for changing displays and attending to stock?
   d) Why should the salon aim for a fast turnover of stock?
   e) What sort of things should be considered when fitting out a stock room?

Computers

Businesses are becoming increasingly aware of the benefits of computerised record keeping. All sorts of information, such as clients' details, stock records and sales figures, can be stored on a disk. The information can be retrieved easily by a trained person. Some manufacturers produce software (programs) specially for use in a salon.

If you use a computer, you should copy recorded information on to a second disk to provide backup in case of loss or damage to the main disk.

Computers: Activity

1 Not all beauty salons have a computer. If yours does or if you know of a salon that does, ask if you can have a word with the supervisor about the benefits of a computer to their particular business.

Find out what sort of computer is used and what the staff who use it think about it. Get details of the software which is used.

See if there are any plans to replace the computer. If there are, find out why and ask which replacement computer has been chosen. Get details of the staff training involved in computerising a salon.

Chapter 3

Selling products and services

After working through this chapter you will be able to:

- appreciate the importance of selling
- know how to make a sale
- understand basic consumer law
- deal with problems and complaints
- conduct a consultation
- fill in a client's record card
- relate the planning of a treatment programme to the sales of goods and services
- sell perfumes.

Selling in the salon

You should read all the information about the products you sell: you will need a good knowledge of the products and services offered by the salon so that you can confidently advise and make recommendations to the clients. Make sure you can explain the specific benefits of the treatments which are available. Ask a senior member of staff to explain anything you do not understand.

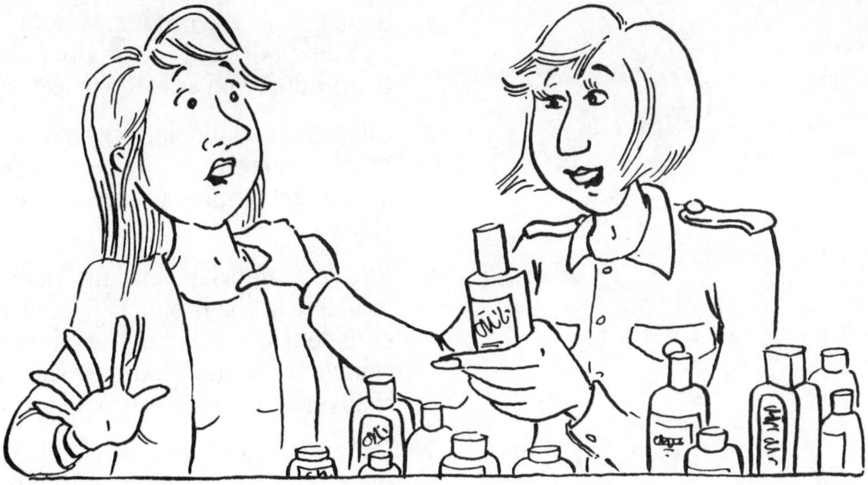

Some people worry about 'selling'. They feel that they might be pushing clients into spending money against their will: this is nonsense! Selling should be seen as an extension of the other professional services offered by the salon.

Clients trust the recommendations they receive in the salon. They expect, quite rightly, that the products on sale there will be of good quality and that they will get the best advice. Most clients admit quite freely to having wasted money in the past on purchases made elsewhere without the proper professional advice.

> Remember
> It is usual for staff to be paid a special rate of commission for retail sales and treatments on top of their basic wage. The profits from retail sales are usually higher than for treatments.

Making the sale

Selling is a very important aspect of salon operations. Profits made on the sales of products and services make the business successful. They also contribute greatly to the wages of the employees.

Here is some advice for successful selling. The techniques should be used by everybody who deals with clients in the salon. They apply to the selling of both products and services.

1. Find out exactly what the client needs. This means asking questions and listening carefully to the answers.

   Use closed questions to get short, straightforward answers (usually yes or no). These help to confirm or eliminate information and ideas. They are useful when planning advice for example, 'Do you have a regular nail care routine?' 'Have you ever tried wearing a ridge filler basecoat under your nail enamel?'

   Use open questions to invite fuller and more detailed answers. Open questions help to develop the conversation and provide more personal information, for example, 'How do you normally look after your hands?' 'Can you describe the problem to me?'

> Remember
> Maintain eye contact with the client when discussing the product. This shows confidence and the client will trust your advice.

> Remember
> A good system of stock control helps to ensure that there are always products available to sell. If an item comes out of stock, make a note of it in the order book and let the client who wishes to make the purchase know when the next delivery is due.

2. Give the client advice. Always relate the benefits of the product specifically to the client, for example, 'By using this enriched cuticle cream regularly, you will prevent these splits occurring (indicate them) and your nails will not be as brittle. You will soon notice a great improvement in the appearance of your hands.'
3. Always smile and talk confidently and positively about the product which you have chosen. Where possible, tell the client about your personal experiences with the product.
4. Explain how the product should be used. If possible, let the client feel, smell or hold the product. Remember If the client touches the product and asks the price, then the item is practically sold!
5. Close the sale. Look for signals that tell you the client has decided to take your advice and buy the product: head nodding in agreement, smiles and friendly eye contact are positive buying signals.
6. Where appropriate, explain the benefits of the different sizes available in the product. These will usually be linked to price. Be confident when giving the client the price. Hesitation or reluctance to mention the price will give the client the impression that you consider the product too expensive.
7. Gain agreement with the client. This is achieved either immediately or after a short period of 'thinking' time Do not be afraid of silences at this stage. Just keep quiet and wait patiently for the client to make a decision. Do not talk yourself out of a sale!
8. Use link selling to encourage your client to buy complementary products from the same range, e.g. cleansers and toners, eye creams and eye gels, nail enamels and base coats.
9. Once you have sold the product, wrap it up and process payment. As you hand over the purchase, check once more that the client understands how to use the product.
10. Enter details of the purchase on the client's record card.

Selling in the salon: Self-checks

1 State three ways of demonstrating confidence in a product when selling it to a client.

2 How can you tell when a client is ready to buy a product?

Selling in the salon: Activities

1 Role play a selling situation with a partner. One of you should be the client and the other one the receptionist. If possible, use the salon reception or make a small display of retail products to help set the scene. (Remember the steps to successful selling and practice using open and closed questions. An outside observer may be able to tell you at which point you seemed to have made or lost the sale.)

2 Know your suppliers! When a business deals with only a small number of suppliers, there is usually a special professional relationship with the salon. You should get to know the technical representatives who visit your salon. Find out which firms supply which products and details of the service they provide. Get an idea of delivery schedules so that you can give your clients a realistic idea of how long they may have to wait to purchase a product which is out of stock.

Handling refunds

A good salon ensures that clients have realistic expectations from their treatments and that they understand how to get the best results from products purchased for home care.

Nevertheless, you may, one day, be in the position of having to deal with a client demanding a refund to compensate for disappointment with the products or treatments received. As consumers of your products and services, clients do have legal rights under the Sale of Goods Act 1979. This legislation identifies the contract of sale which takes place between the retailer (in this case your salon) and the consumer (client) when a product is purchased. The law makes the retailer responsible for ensuring that the goods sold are free from defects. If they are found to be defective, the retailer must, strictly speaking, refund the money. (In practice, the retailer may offer to replace the goods.) Afterwards, it is the responsibility of the retailer, having now become the aggrieved party, to take up the complaint with the supplier.

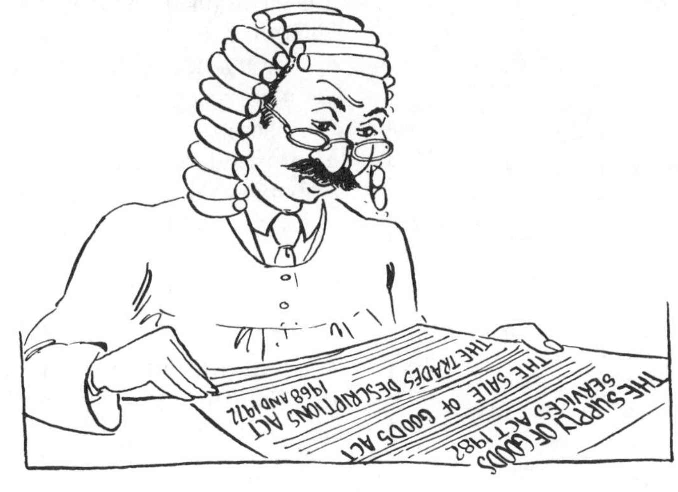

The Supply of Goods and Services Act 1982

This Act was passed to extend the protection given to consumers under The Sale of Goods Act to the provision of services, goods on hire and goods given in exchange for vouchers. A client disappointed with a beauty treatment could take action against the salon if it was proved that reasonable care had not been taken under the terms of the Supply of Goods and Services Act.

The Trades Descriptions Act 1968 and 1972

This act makes it a crime to describe goods falsely, and to sell or offer for sale goods which have been so described. It covers many things such as advertisements, display cards, oral descriptions and applies to quality, quantity, fitness for purpose and price. The part of the Act dated 1972 deals with the labelling of the country of origin: a product must be clearly labelled so that the consumer can see where it was made.

> Remember
> You must make sure that returned goods are acceptable for a refund or exchange. You are not obliged to compensate for careless breakage or misuse of a product by the client. Sometimes when a product is returned as faulty, you may suspect that you are not being given entirely truthful information. This can be a difficult situation to handle and you should seek the assistance of your supervisor.

A client requesting a refund should be questioned tactfully and goods which have been returned examined closely to determine the cause of the problem. As always, the client should be dealt with calmly, politely and sympathetically.

> Remember
> The salon will probably have a policy on client complaints and refunds. Make sure you know the established procedures.

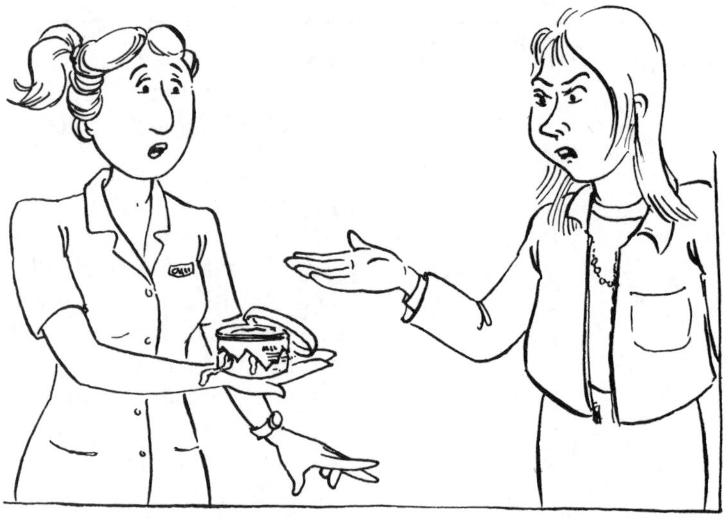

A client requesting a refund should be questioned tactfully to determine the cause of the problem

> Remember
> If a product which has been returned is faulty, the client is not required by law to produce a receipt. It is obviously reassuring to have evidence that the product was bought from the salon, but failure to produce a receipt does not jeopardise the client's rights as a consumer.

It is usual for the manager to supervise refunds. He or she will want to find out if the cause of the complaint is due to:

- negligence on the part of the salon: the client may have been given incorrect or incomplete advice. Alternatively, there may have been discrepancies with stock handling or stock control procedures
- misunderstanding by the client: sometimes, no matter how much you explain to a client, misunderstandings can occur. A product appears not to be working when, in fact, the client is not using it properly.
- defective products sold to the salon by a supplier: in this case, the terms of The Sale of Goods Act apply.

> Remember
> Exchanges will have an effect on stock levels, and refunds need to be taken into account when cashing up. Records should be kept of any refunds or exchanges so that stock differences can be reconciled and, where appropriate, accurate information can be passed on to the supplier of defective goods. Refunds must be recorded against the day's takings for the salon account.

Whatever the outcomes of the discussion, it is important that the client feels that they have been dealt with fairly and professionally. A satisfied client will probably come back and, hopefully, recommend you to others. A client who feels humiliated and badly treated is lost forever.

Handling refunds: Self-checks

1 What is link selling?

2 Name two pieces of legislation which protect the consumer.

3 Under what circumstances should a client receive a refund?

Handling refunds: Activities

1 Find out how your salon provides refund information through the till, and how your manager would deal with a supplier of defective goods.

2 If a product is returned for a refund, you will have to examine it carefully and ask questions before deciding whether there are genuine grounds for a refund. Working with a partner, take each of the following products, and assuming that they were all sold in perfect condition, discuss how you would recognise a suspicious situation:

- lipstick
- eye shadow palette
- eye pencil
- block mascara
- jar of skin care cream
- nail enamel.

Dealing with complaints

Remember
Do not pretend a mistake has not been made when you know very well that it has. Mistakes on the part of the salon must be acknowledged and rectified as soon as possible.

Despite everyone's attempts to provide an efficient, personal service for the clients, mistakes can occur. Depending on the circumstances and the mood of the client on the day, some mistakes can go by more or less unnoticed while others may result in the client becoming upset and complaining quite openly in the salon or at reception.

Whatever the cause, it is important to deal with complaints quietly, tactfully and, if possible, away from the rest of the clients. Here are some tips to help you deal with complaints:

- keep cool and be pleasant and polite with the client
- ask the client to come with you to a more private area of the salon.
- offer the client a seat: a comfortable client is more likely to calm down.
- give the client the opportunity to explain to you exactly what the complaint is about
- listen carefully and do not interrupt
- analyse the complaint and ask the client to clarify points which are not clear to you
- do not contradict or argue with the client
- always show concern and understanding for the client being upset, irrespective of who or what is to blame
- negotiate an acceptable solution to the problem. You may need to involve your supervisor by this stage
- do not be tempted to show anger, even if the client is being unreasonable
- explain your answer calmly and confidently, maintaining eye contact
- always apologise for the client being upset or inconvenienced

Remember
Contrary to popular belief, the client is not always right! However, if the situation is handled tactfully, a client will be prepared to accept that they are wrong without feeling embarrassed or offended.

- record details of the complaint and the action taken. Details of serious complaints must be recorded together with the action taken. These will be referred to if a client who has suffered damage seeks compensation from the salon.

Dealing with complaints: Self-check

1 Why should details of a client's complaint be recorded?

Dealing with complaints: Activity

1 Dealing with complaints is always a good basis for role play! Again, working with a partner and, if possible, an observer, create a realistic situation which might occur at reception when a client is unhappy with a service or product received. Have a 'supervisor' on hand in case your client gets out of control!

Selling perfumes

> Remember
> No two 'noses' are identical. The chemical reaction which occurs between the skin and a perfume means that the same fragrance may not always smell the same on different people.

Choosing perfume is a very personal matter and should not be rushed. Experienced buyers of perfume learn, by experience, the advantages of letting perfume samples settle on the skin before making a final decision.

The true fragrance of a perfume may take up to an hour to develop, so a client should not be expected to judge a perfume by its first impression.

How we smell

Smells are picked up by special nerve cells in the lining of the nose which connect directly to the brain. Perfumes are volatile, (they evaporate) and mix with the air that is breathed in through the nose.

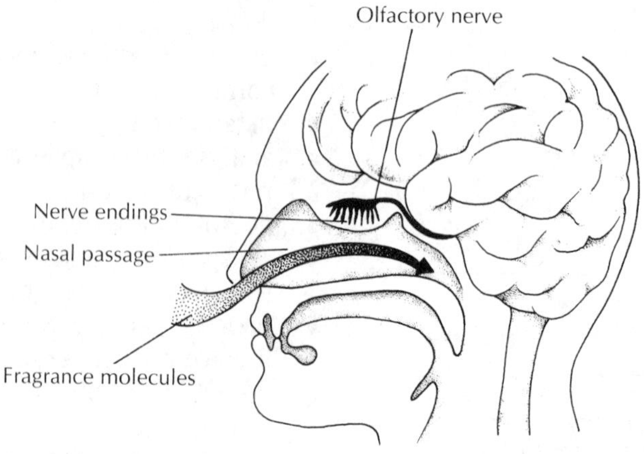

Different smells have different associations through their direct link with the brain

There is a special language used in the perfumery industry to describe fragrances:

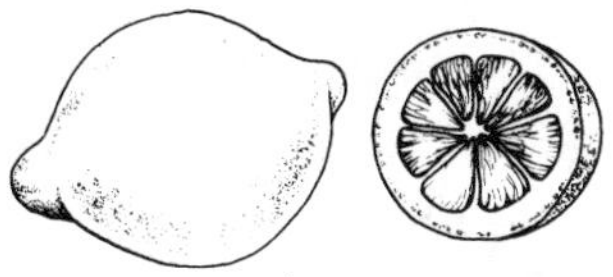

Lemon

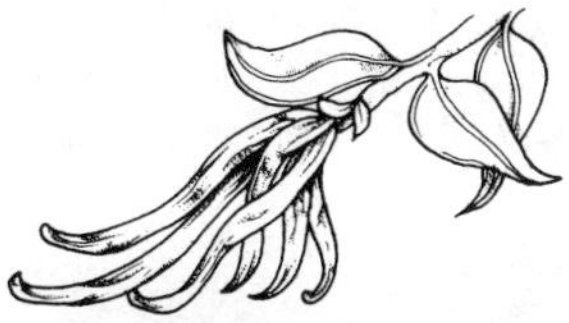

Vanilla

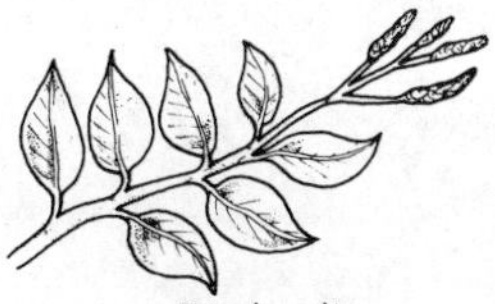

Patchouli

Type	Sources	Description
Floral	single blossoms, e.g. rose, lavender, lily of the valley	light, refreshing, sweet
Citrus	e.g. lemon, orange, lime, bergamot	sharp fresh, stimulating
Green	pine, cedar blended with mosses, ferns, grasses, flower stems	fresh, woody, crisp clean, dry, aromatic
Modern	usually contain synthetic oils which imitate floral, woody and herbal fragrances which are less easy to identify	bright, cheery, cool clean, fresh
Spicy	cinnamon, cloves, vanilla ginger, exotic flowers	heavy, pungent, sometimes described as 'leathery' in male fragrances
Sweet	very fragrant combinations, e.g. jasmine, gardenia	very sweet. Can be overpowering if applied heavily
Oriental	Eastern woods and grasses, sandalwood, patchouli	full-bodied, aromatic, heavy, sultry, exotic

The qualities of perfumes are often described to match the 'mood' of the fragrance, for example mysterious, classical, warm, intense, seductive, discreet. This language is used to full effect when marketing a fragrance.

Types of perfumed products

The strength of a perfume refers to the concentration of its base in alcohol or alcohol and water. The natural fragrances are extracted from their sources as oil. The more oil contained in a product, the more lingering the fragrance and the more expensive the product.

There are two types of raw materials used to make perfumes:

- natural: these are mainly essential oils obtained from the various parts of plants and flowers
- synthetic: *aldehydes* which can be blended quite effectively to imitate natural fragrances.

At one time, the finest perfumes contained ingredients obtained from animal sources, such as ambergris from the sperm whale and musk from musk deer.

These wild animals have now become endangered species and the risk of their extinction has prompted strong lobbying by environmental pressure groups. Synthetic alternatives are now widely available.

Perfume

The strongest concentration of a fragrance, perfume is long lasting and contains only a small amount of alcohol. A perfume is the truest version of a fragrance. It should be applied to the pulse points where the warmth of the skin helps to develop its character.

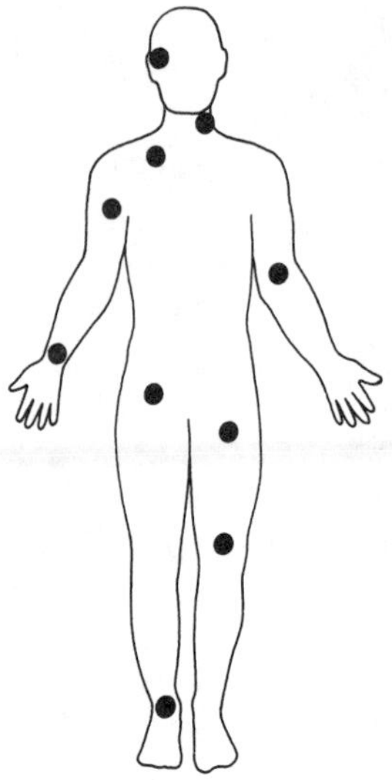

Location of pulse points

Eau de parfum

A lighter version of perfume, *eau de parfum* is suitable for use all over the body.

Eau de toilette/eau de cologne

The most dilute forms of a perfume, this is probably the most popular strength of fragrance. It is cheaper than perfume and is usually available as a spray or splash-on which is refreshing to use.

Fragrance notes

A fragrance keeps developing for some time after it has been applied. The true character of the perfume appears only when the alcohol content has evaporated and the other ingredients have settled on the skin.

A fragrance develops in stages called notes:

- top note: the impression made when the bottle is opened and the perfume is first applied
- middle note: the initial top note lingers and gives way to the middle note which carries the true character and richness of the perfume. This is the best stage of fragrance development. In a good perfume, the middle note lasts for 4-6 hours
- base note: composed of the longest lasting elements of the perfume, known as fixatives. On their own, the fixatives smell quite unpleasant, but they give permanence and depth to the other components of the perfume.

When only the base note remains, it is time to reapply the perfume.

> *Remember*
>
> The top should always be fastened tightly on a bottle of perfume which has been opened. Once the seal has been broken on a bottle, slow evaporation takes place which creates a less balanced perfume.
>
> Once a bottle of perfume has been opened it should be used up. Storing the perfume in a cool, dark place helps to prevent oxidation and spoilage.

'Why does this perfume smell different on me?' is not an uncommon question. It can be quite an expensive mistake choosing a new fragrance before testing it properly. The main problem is skin chemistry: if the pH of the skin is not normal, a reaction occurs which affects the development of the fragrance. Perfume lasts longer on an oily skin but tends to turn sweeter. A sharper, more citrus fragrance is usually more suitable.

Other factors which may affect the skin's reaction to a perfume are:

- smoking: apart from the smell of smoke and tobacco clinging to clothing and skin, nicotine can alter skin chemistry and reduce the staying power of perfume
- medication: in particular, the contraceptive pill can affect the skin's reaction to perfume
- menstruation: the perception of smells can change at this time
- Climate/environment: warmth makes perfumes evaporate more quickly. This speeds up the rate at which the base notes appear. Many perfumes are sweeter and heavier in tropical conditions
- Air pollution: perfume usually needs re-applying more often in a city-centre environment than in the country.

Testing a perfume

It is best not to confuse the perfume testing by sampling more than two products at once. The nose can become over-stimulated into a kind of numbness which makes it difficult to distinguish between the samples.

> *Remember*
> The sense of smell eventually diminishes by going backwards and forwards between the different fragrances.

When helping a client to choose between perfumes, always:

- test the lightest fragrance first
- use a spray: spraying helps the perfume to develop faster and helps the client to choose more quickly
- spray on the wrist, holding the bottle far enough away to avoid dampening the skin
- advise the client to give the alcohol time to evaporate before smelling the fragrance
- instruct the client not to smell the fragrance too closely and to avoid rubbing it into the skin: doing so may eliminate the top notes and interfere with the perfume's development
- perform the second test as soon as the client has made a decision on the first fragrance
- allow time for the client to make a final choice: offer advice only if it is requested.

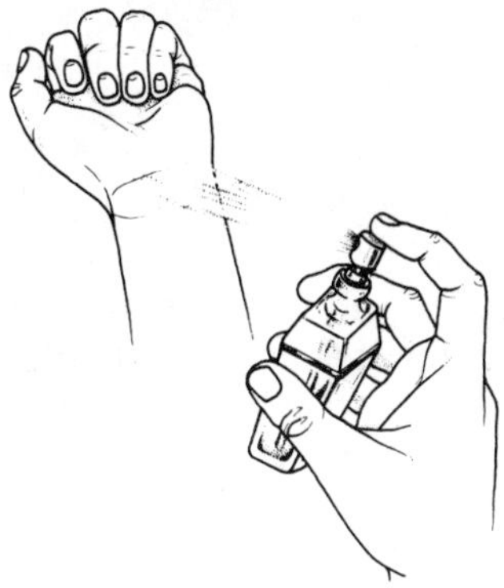

Once the client has made a decision, use the fragrance on her, but not too close to the face where it could 'suffocate'.

Spray the perfume outside the triangle which goes from the nose to the shoulders. Be careful not to spray perfume on jewellery, particularly pearls, or on fragile fabrics such as silk or crepe.

> Remember
>
> Applying perfume is a very important part of dressing. Perfume reflects personality, mood and occasion.
>
> Women often choose different perfumes for different occasions, for example a light fresh fragrance for day and a heavier, aromatic fragrance for evening.

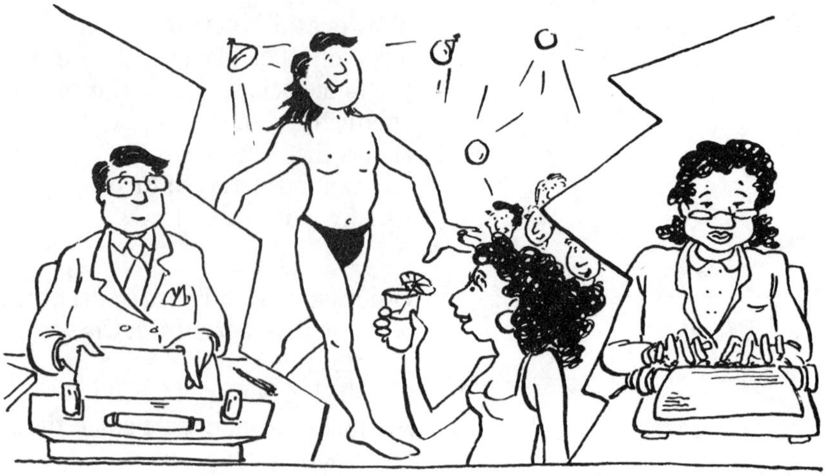

Fragrance-building

A layering effect can be achieved by using different forms of the same fragrance to produce a build-up effect. Fragrance-building actually works out more economically than using only the more concentrated versions of a fragrance. Selling related products from a range is called link selling. When selling a perfume, these could include:

- bath oil
- scented soap
- talcum powder
- deodorant
- shampoo
- body lotion.

Male fragrances are usually 'green', 'citrus' or 'spicy'. They contain ingredients which compensate for the 'sweetening' effects of a male skin which generally tends to be greasier than a female's. There are opportunities for fragrance building for men by selling a combination of some of the following products:

- after-shave
- foam shave
- shaving soap
- pre-electric shave (for preventing razor burns)
- deodorants
- body shampoo
- talc
- shower gel
- body lotion.

Perfume should not be applied over damaged or infected skin. Areas of abnormally 'active' cell growth, for example moles and warts, should also be avoided. Some people are particularly sensitive to ingredients contained in a perfume: they can actually feel bilious and quite unwell when they inhale the fragrance. Alternatively, they may experience a typical contact allergic dermatitis skin reaction. Whatever the adverse effects of the perfume, the client must stop using the product and, in the case of a skin reaction, apply a soothing antihistamine cream. If the condition does not improve, the client should seek advice from a doctor.

Photosensitisation

Perfume ingredients, for example bergamot oil, can make the skin very sensitive to ultra-violet light. The result can be 'sunburn' after only a very short exposure time: sometimes, brown patches appear on the neck where melanin has been produced following photosensitisation of the skin by applying perfume directly to the neck.

Perfume should not be worn when sunbathing or when using a sunbed.

Selling perfume: Self-checks

1 Why should a perfume not be judged by its first impression?

2 Why is it better for a perfume to be tested before being purchased?

3 Give two examples of natural ingredients which may be found in each of the following types of fragrance: a) green b) spicy c) floral d) oriental.

4 Distinguish between a 'perfume' and an 'eau de toilette'.

5 What are the 'notes' of a perfume?

6 What are the correct storage conditions for perfume?

7 Give two reasons why a perfume may smell differently on you than on someone else.

8 Why should a spray be used when testing a perfume?

9 What is 'fragrance-building'?

10 Why should perfume not be worn when lying on a sunbed?

Selling perfume: Activity

1 With a partner or a small group of colleagues, visit a perfume department and each test the same two perfumes on the wrists. Wait half an hour and then compare how the fragrances smell on each of you.

Try using the language of perfumes to write down a description of the fragrances. Compare your answers afterwards.

Assessing clients

The most successful salons earn their reputation by providing excellent personal service. A service can only be truly personal when the needs of the individual clients are understood, and treatments and advice are matched to those needs.

Clients have different reasons for attending a salon for beauty treatment:

- to complete their 'make-over' for a special event
- to keep their hands, skin or body in good condition
- to improve and control the appearance of certain conditions and disorders
- to make them look and feel younger
- to 'spoil' themselves as a special treat

- to relax and enjoy peace and quiet away from the children or the job!
- to boost their confidence and increase their feeling of personal well being.

There are probably many more reasons. Clients are individuals with their own particular needs and expectations. Once you have managed to find out why the client has come to the salon, you can plan your treatments accordingly. Whatever their reason for attending the salon, it is important for a consultation to take place with every client before treatment begins.

> Remember
> It helps to know if it is the client's first visit to the salon so that extra time can be allowed in the appointment book for a consultation. Alternatively, the client may book in for a consultation first and then come at a later date for treatment.

> Remember
> Clients are unlikely to understand many of the treatments fully until they have had them explained by a professional beauty therapist. They may think they want a particular treatment, but there may be alternative ones they do not know about which will be more beneficial for them.

> Remember
> The more you explain to the client, the more evidence you provide of your technical knowledge. The client will then have more confidence in your advice and trust in your professional judgement.

Giving a consultation

Information is obtained at the consultation by asking questions and by examining the area to be treated. Keep eye contact with your client, listen carefully and develop the answers they give you. This way, clients know you are sincerely interested in what they have to say.

The main aims of the consultation are to:

- put the client at ease
- gain the confidence of the client
- establish a good rapport
- find out what the client wants
- determine what the client needs
- ensure the client is suitable for treatment
- discuss the treatment options available
- answer the client's questions
- agree a treatment plan with the client
- sell the client appropriate treatments and products.

If you recommend a treatment or course of treatments, you must make sure that the client understands why they are necessary, what costs are involved and any particular conditions which are necessary for achieving success with the treatments, for example frequency of appointments, or specific home care.

> Remember
> The consultation is between you and the client. Any information you are given is confidential and must not be discussed with anyone else.

Filling in a record card

During the consultation, you will have to fill in a record card, but try to avoid writing and asking questions at the same time. You must take care to fill in the record card neatly. At some future date, the information you write down may be needed by someone else. It is no good if only you can read your writing!

One side of the card is used for recording the client's personal details and information related to treatment planning. The other side is for recording the dates of the client's visits to the salon with details of the treatments received and retail products purchased.

This side of the record card has the client's personal details. Some of these influence the treatments given and others provide useful practical information.

(i) The initial of the client's surname is printed in the top right hand corner of the card to enable it to be retrieved quickly from the index storage system.

(ii) The information given here is important for effective communication with the client. It is more polite to ask a client their date of birth rather than their age. Knowing this will help you to assess the condition of the skin and advise the most suitable treatments and home-care.

(iii) Details of the client's doctor may be needed in an emergency. Health and medication details are important to know when assessing the skin.

(iv) These details are necessary for making an accurate diagnosis and planning appropriate beauty care.

	BEAUTY BOX SALON		(i)
(ii)	Mr/Mrs/Ms Surname Forenames	Address Date of Birth	Tel. no Home Work
(iii)	Doctor's name Doctor's address	General state of Health Current medication	Recent illness/operation Allergies
(iv)	Basic skin type Skin tone Skin colour Muscle tone Problems Contra-indications	Skin history/treatment General comments	Recommended home care Date of consultation Given by Signed

A sample record card

(i) Shows the frequency and regularity of the visits/treatments.

(ii) Shows which treatments the client has received, including skin tests.

(iii) Details of the client's reaction to treatments may be recorded; the information may be important to recall for the next visit.

(iv) Client home care may be monitored by referring to details of the purchases made. This information is used for recommending further purchases.

(v) It is necessary to know which therapist has treated the client. This information may be needed when making a follow-up appointment or when referring to a previous treatment.

Date	Treatment record	Comments	Initials	Retail purchases
(i)	(ii)	(iii)	(iv)	(v)

This side of the record card records details on the client's visits to the salon

> Remember
>
> A new client needs advising exactly what to do. Give clear instructions so that there is no misunderstanding which could cause embarrassment later.

Examining the client

Clients are more satisfied when they feel they have been examined thoroughly. Information provided by the examination helps to provide an accurate diagnosis and more effective treatment plan.

The nature of the examination will depend on the body area concerned. Here are some general guidelines:

- instruct the client about which clothing needs to be removed. A gown should be offered if the client needs to undress down to underwear.

- ensure the client is warm and comfortable. Areas of the body not being examined should be supported and covered appropriately
- conduct the examination in private, peacefully and avoiding interruptions
- wash and dry your own hands before beginning the examination.
- cleanse thoroughly and dry the area to be examined
- examine the skin and nails in good light, preferably through a magnifying lens
- question the client to determine the specific cause of conditions you come across during the examination
- be pleasant and tactful when asking questions
- write down details of the examination as you go along
- find out details of previous treatments that the client may have had and how successful they were.

Remember
Use closed questions to help confirm or eliminate ideas. Use open questions to get fuller and more detailed answers.

You must be able to identify conditions which will not be made worse by treatment, those which can be treated and will be improved and those which must definitely not receive treatment (i.e. are contra - indicated).

Remember
Diseases and infections are contra-indicated to beauty treatments because of the risk of them spreading and also being made worse by treatment.

If you come across diseases and infections in the salon, you must tactfully explain why treatment cannot be given. You may need to refer the client to a doctor. Always emphasise how much you look forward to meeting the client again once the condition has cleared.

When you have completed the examination, there may be other points you wish to discuss with the client before recommending a treatment plan. For example, it is helpful to know how much time the client has available for attending the salon. You may have to amend your treatment plan and consider different options.

Remember
When you advise the client, you are helping them to make a buying decision, in other words you are selling them the best combination of treatments and products to match their needs.

By this stage of the consultation you will have assessed your client's needs. Now you must give advice on the treatments and products which are going to be of greatest benefit.

Remember the basic rules of selling:

- describe the treatments and explain how they work
- relate the benefits specifically to the client
- talk confidently and positively about the treatments
- discover and deal with concerns and expectations
- state the price confidently
- recognise and respond to buying signals
- do not rush the client into making a decision.

Remember
Do not forget to write in details of treatments and product sales on the client's record card.

A client who wants to say 'Yes', but acts indecisively may just need final reassurance from you. If you have recognised positive buying signals, let the client know you agree with their decision and explain why, for example: 'I think that gel nails are ideal for you. They look very natural and they will help to strengthen your own nails so that they can grow to a reasonable length.'

Remember
The more you explain to the client, the more evidence you provide of your technical knowledge. The client will then have more confidence in your advice and trust in your professional judgement.

Once you have gained agreement with the client, the sale is closed and the consultation has officially finished.

Assessing clients: Self-checks

1 Why do the client's wants not always match their needs?

2 What are the main purposes of a client consultation?

3 What information is recorded during the consultation?

4 Give an example of (a) a closed question and (b) an open question which might be used during an examination of the client's hands and nails.

5 Which particular aspects of the consultation are most likely to give a client confidence in your advice?

Assessing clients: Activity

1 Working with a partner, role play a consultation with a new client. Imagine that the client has received a gift voucher, entitling her to treatments and products from the salon up to a value of £25.00. She has never been to a beauty salon before and has no idea what to expect. She does not really know what she wants although she has fairly firm ideas of what she does not like about herself.

Enlist the help of a third person to give you feedback on how successful you are.

You will need to sound confident, so brush up on your knowledge of treatments and products before you act through this role play.

Chapter 4

Examining the face and neck

After working through this chapter you will be able to:

- carry out an examination of the face and neck
- understand the structure and functions of the skin
- recognise and respond to a full range of skin diseases and disorders
- identify basic skin types
- explain the effects of internal and external influences upon the skin
- give general home care advice
- appreciate ethnic variations in skin types
- understand the significance of bones and muscles on facial contours.

Assessing the client

The client's skin and facial features must be assessed accurately so that the best treatments and products can be recommended. A consultation provides the opportunity to examine the skin closely and to ask questions which help build a clearer picture of the client's needs.

Preparing the client

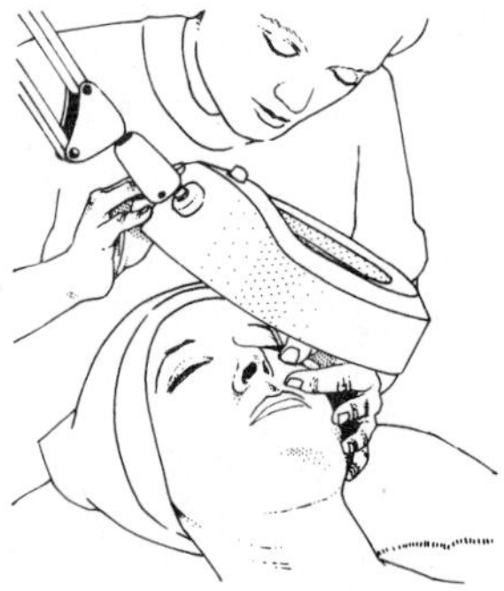

Skin inspection

> **Remember**
> Always examine the face in good light. Using an illuminated magnifier allows you to give the skin a detailed, close-up inspection.

The client's hair is secured off the face, and clothing protected with a cape, gown, towel or tissues. Earrings and necklaces are removed and kept safely for the client, make-up is cleansed off and the skin deep-cleansed, toned and dried.

Examining black skin

Some aspects of skin assessment are difficult on black skin because of the amount of pigment present. A more accurate assessment can be made if the examination is carried out under a Wood's light. This is an inspection lamp which produces deep ultra-violet rays. It makes different types of skin fluoresce (glow) characteristically in different colours and intensities.

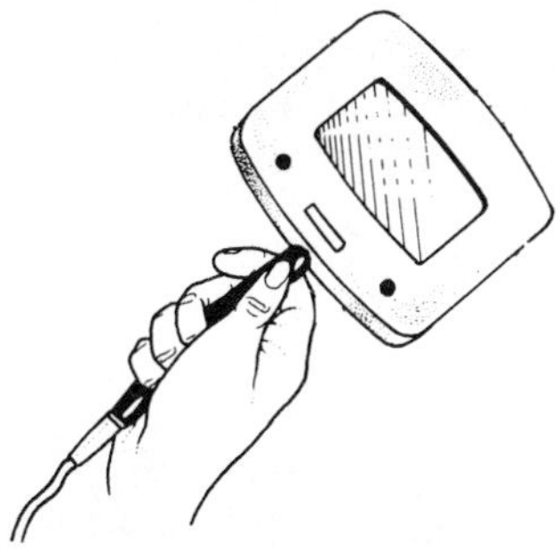

The Wood's light is most effective when used in a darkened room

The following table shows these differences.

Skin type	**Colour of fluorescence**
Balanced skin	purplish-blue
Dry skin	weak violet
Greasy skin	coral pink
Hydrated skin	strong violet
Thick stratum corneum	strong white
Thin stratum corneum	purple
Build up of dead skin cells	silvery white
Increased pigmentation	brown

The facial examination

By carrying out a facial examination, you will be able to:

- assess the client's skin type. This is important for choosing the correct skin-care preparations and giving the best home care advice
- recognise minor blemishes and abnormalities. Sometimes, the appearance of these may be improved with cosmetic treatments. They certainly will not be made worse by them
- identify contra-indications. If these are present, beauty therapy treatment must not be applied to the affected area. This is because there is a risk of spreading infection or of making the condition worse. The client may need referring for medical advice
- identify specific problems. Depending on the client's age, health and previous skin care, there may be conditions present which need particular attention. It may be necessary to adapt the basic salon procedures and to recommend special home care treatments
- note the client's colouring and facial features. These are particularly important when designing the make-up for a client. Cosmetics are chosen and applied to enhance the client's good points and minimise the bad ones. Sometimes, illusions need to be created to achieve balance. A good knowledge of facial structure is required to do this effectively
- test the elasticity of the skin. To do this, pinch the skin gently in each of the main facial areas. Skin with good elasticity is firm and will spring back into shape. Skin which has lost its elasticity is over-stretched and crepey and does not recover immediately from the pinch test. Without its elasticity, it forms wrinkles and sags. Clients need advising on the correct way of treating their skin to prevent it from becoming over-stretched. Great care is also taken when choosing and applying professional beauty treatments
- assess muscle tone. The muscles of facial expression produce characteristic lines on the face which become deeper and permanent with the ageing process. Some of the muscles cause the features to 'sag' when they lose their tone and the contours become less well defined. Beauty treatments help to minimise the effects of reduced muscle tone. The client may be taught facial exercises and advised how to prevent lines and wrinkles from getting worse. Other factors can cause the lines to appear prematurely.

The examination should start with a general assessment of the skin and then concentrate on specific areas of the face and neck until the whole area has been covered. The following diagram divides the face and neck into areas which have particular characteristics because of their structure. It is important to include all these areas in the facial examination.

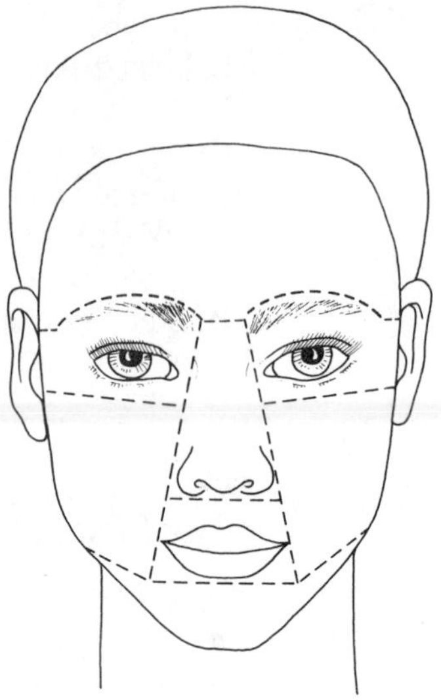

The facial map

A detailed description of the characteristics of these areas is given in the section on facial structure (pages 101–4).

Your assessment of the client is based on what you see and what you know. Remember that closed questions produce 'yes' or 'no' type answers. They help to confirm or eliminate ideas. Open questions require fuller answers which give more detailed information. Establish the client's skin history with general questions first, to find out their approach to skin care and to establish the basic skin type.

Examples of closed questions

- Do you have a skin care routine?
- Do you protect your skin in the sun?
- Do you ever use soap on your face?
- Do you wear a moisturiser under make-up?
- Is your general health good?
- Have you noticed any changes in your skin recently?
- Does your skin ever react to make-up products?

Examples of open questions

- How do you normally look after your skin at home?
- What are the main problems you have with your skin?
- Which skin care products do you use?
- How much make-up do you usually wear?
- How do you remove your make-up?
- What sort of environment do you work in?

Once a general assessment has been made, careful questioning at each stage of the examination helps to identify the specific causes of conditions which may be present.

> Remember
>
> The more practice you get, the more confident you will become at carrying out an examination and making correct judgements about the skin. Experience will develop your ability to recognise signs and follow them up with the most appropriate questions.

Assessing the client: Self-checks

1a) Give three reasons for examining the skin before recommending facial treatments.

b) Why is a Wood's light useful when examining black skin?

2a) State two possible consequences of giving beauty therapy treatment when there is a contra-indication.

b) What advice should be given to a client who is contra-indicated to a treatment?

3a) What are the general effects of ageing on the skin?

b) How would you expect the skin of a young client to respond to the 'pinch' test?

Facial structure

Facial contours are determined by the relative sizes, shapes and positions of the facial bones together with the muscles and fatty tissue which lie over them.

The skull provides the basic framework of the head. Consisting of 22 bones in all, eight of them make up the cranium, which extends over the front, top, back and sides of the head, seven contribute to facial structure and help shape the openings containing the eyes, nose and mouth and a further seven are situated more deeply in the facial cavities. They do not contribute to facial contour.

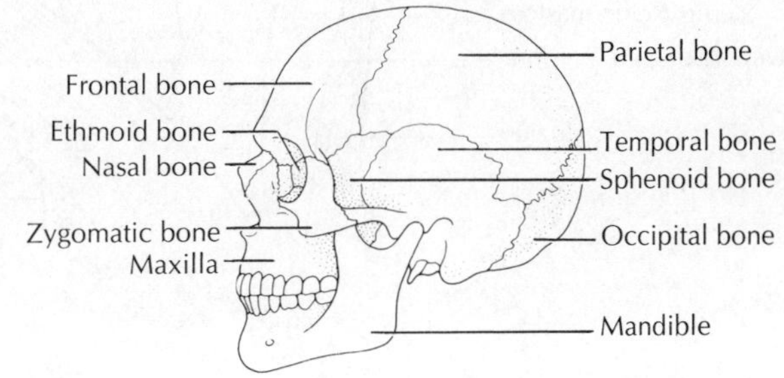

The bones of the skull

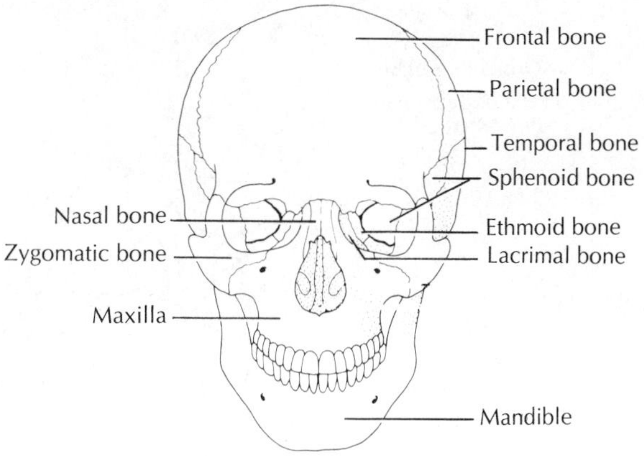

The facial bones

A knowledge of the deeper facial bones is not required.

> Remember
> There are ethnic variations in bone structure. For example, oriental people have less prominent zygomatic bones which give them flatter facial features than other races.

The mandible is the only moveable bone in the skull. It moves at hinge joints and is used for chewing and talking. The other bones meet at fixed joints called sutures.

The bone structure usually becomes more prominent with age when fat is lost from the face and the skin becomes less well supported.

Muscles of the face and neck

The muscles of facial expression insert into the skin. They are made up of fibres. The fibres of most muscles lie in parallel formation but special muscles called sphincters have fibres which surround openings. When these muscles contract, the openings close up.

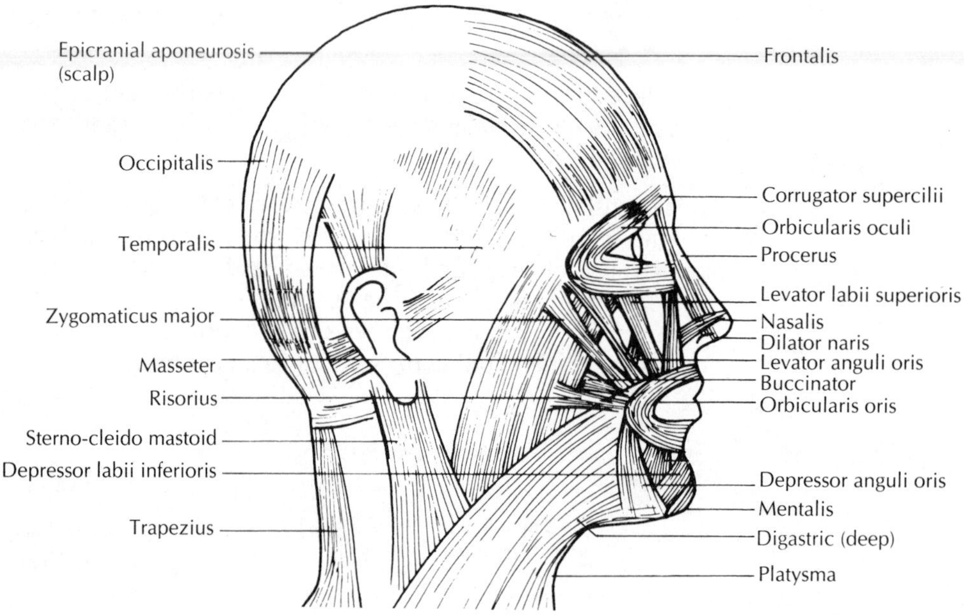

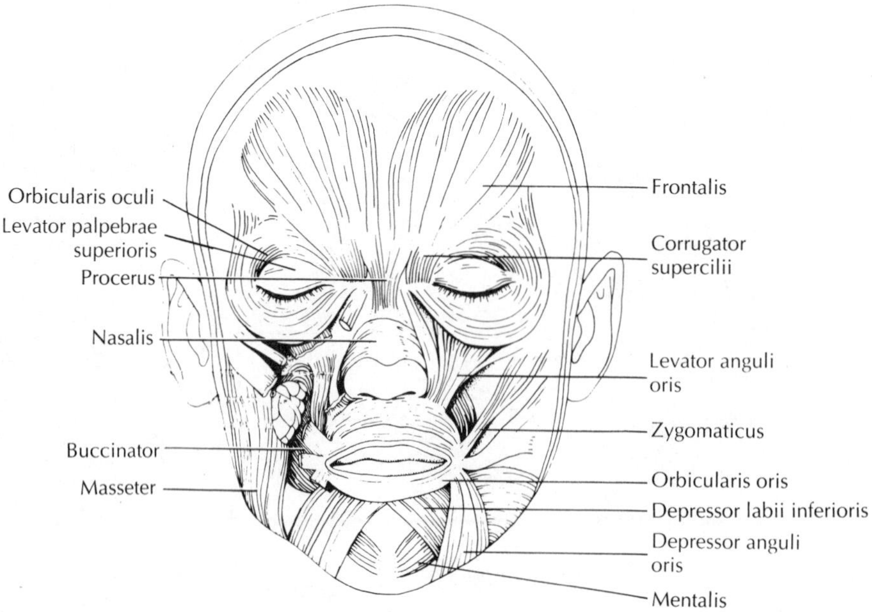

Muscles of the face and neck

Location and action of the muscles of the face and neck

Facial area	Name of muscle	Location	Action
Forehead	Frontalis (1)	Front portion of the occipito-frontalis muscle which covers the upper part of the cranium	Lifts the eyebrows causing the skin of the forehead to form horizontal creases
	Corrugator supercilli (1)	Interlaces with the frontalis muscle and is positioned below the inner corners of the eyebrows	Draws the eyebrows together producing vertical wrinkles between the brows, as in frowning
	Procerus (1)	Lies over the nasal bone and inserts into the skin of the brow and forehead between the eyebrows	Depresses the wider part of the eyebrows producing horizontal wrinkles over the bridge of the nose
Eyes	Orbicularis oculi	Sphincter muscles which surround the eye. Extend over the temporal region and downwards over the upper cheek	Close the eye. A strong contraction produces wrinkles which fan out from the outer corner of the eye (crow's feet) and beneath the eye
	Levator palpebrae (2)	Upper eyelid	Raises the upper eyelids
Nose	Dilator naris (2)	Sides of nostrils	Expand the nostrils
	Nasalis (1)	Over front of nose	Compresses nose, causing it to wrinkle
Mouth	Orbicularis oris (1)	Sphincter muscle which surrounds the mouth and forms most of the lips	Produces a small opening, as in whistling, and closes the mouth
	Levator labii superioris (2)	Run upwards from the upper lips	Lift the upper lip and assist in opening the mouth
	Depressor labii inferioris (2)	Run downwards from the lower lip	Draw down the lower lip and assist in opening the mouth
	Levator anguli oris (2)	Run upwards from the corners of the mouth	Lift the corners of the mouth
	Depressor anguli oris (triangularis) (2)	Run downwards from the corners of the mouth	Draw the corners of the mouth downwards
	Mentalis (1)	Lies over the chin and inserts into the lower border of orbicularis oris	Lifts the skin of the chin and turns the lower lip outwards
	Digastric (1)	A deep muscle located underneath the chin	Moves the bones involved in swallowing. The digastric is responsible for a 'double chin' condition
Cheeks	Buccinator (2)	Form the greater part of the cheek. The fibres cross the cheek and enter the lips, blending with orbicularis oris	Puff out the cheeks and help to increase the pressure in forced blowing. The muscles maintain tension in the cheek and are used to keep food between the teeth in chewing
	Risorius (2)	Placed horizontally in the cheeks, the muscles join with the corners of the mouth	Pull the corners of the mouth out sideways, as in smiling and grinning
	Zygomaticus (2)	Situated in the middle face, the muscles run downwards to the corners of the mouth	Pull the corners of the mouth upwards and sideways
Sides of the face	Temporalis (2)	Run down the sides of the face to the mandible	Aid mastication (chewing) by raising the mandible and closing the mouth
	Masseter (2)	Powerful muscles which run downwards and backwards to the angle of the mandible	Lift the mandible and exert pressure on the teeth when eating. The masseters are responsible for jowls which develop if the muscles lose their tone
Neck	Platysma (1)	A weak, superficial muscle which arises from the upper part of the chest and shoulders and covers the neck. The upper fibres pass over the mandible and blend with the muscles around the mouth.	Depresses the jaw and lower lip causing the skin of the neck to wrinkle (necklace lines)
	Trapezius (1)	A large, flat triangular muscle which covers the back and sides of the neck and the upper part of the back.	Assists with movements of the shoulders and upper arm. Tension causes the fibres in the upper back to harden or develop nodules
	Sterno-cleido mastoid (2)	Powerful muscles which run down each side of the neck towards the collar bone.	Flex the neck and rotate the head on one side. When used together, the muscles bow the head forward

Muscles with good tone remain in a state of tension even when they are relaxed. This helps to keep the contours firm and well defined. Muscles in poor tone become slack. When this happens, the contours drop and the appearance of the face changes.

Wrinkles and expression lines

When facial muscles contract, the skin to which they are attached falls into wrinkles and folds which form across the direction of the underlying muscle fibres. Where muscles interact with one another, the lines produced join together to form a curve. Skin which has good elasticity returns to normal once the muscle relaxes. Skin which has lost its elasticity develops permanent expression lines and wrinkles. This happens as a natural consequence of the ageing process, but can occur prematurely if the fibrous proteins in the skin become damaged.

Facial structure: Self-checks

1a) What is the biological name for the cheek bones?
b) Which is the only moveable bone in the face?

2a) Why does bone structure become more prominent with age?
b) How does a knowledge of the client's bone structure influence beauty therapy treatments?

3a) What are dropped contours and how are they formed?
b) Explain the relationship between muscles, skin and wrinkles.

Facial structure: Activities

1. Using a diagram of the facial bones for reference, look in a large mirror and feel your way around your own face. Try to identify the main bones which give contour and locate the position of the moveable joint.
2. Don't let a face pass by you without trying to analyse its muscle tone! Whether reading, watching television or sitting on a bus, study as many faces as you can. Look for tell-tale expression lines, wrinkles and dropped contours. Try to identify the specific muscles involved.

The blood supply

Blood carries food, oxygen and water to the body's tissues and takes up the waste products of their activities for excretion by the kidneys, lungs and skin. Blood circulates around the body in vessels. The heart is the pump which drives the blood through the circulation.

Types of blood vessels

Arteries

Arteries carry blood from the heart to the tissues. Large arteries are elastic and pulsate with the heart beat. They drive the blood on through the system. Arteries sub-divide into arterioles.

Veins

Veins carry blood from the tissues to the heart. Thinner than arteries, they have valves to keep the blood flowing in the right direction. Veins sub-divide into venules.

Capillaries

The walls of these tiny vessels are thin and porous. They consist only of a single layer of cells. Capillaries join arterioles with venules. The gaps between the blood capillaries and the cells contain tissue fluid. The interchange of nutrients and waste products takes place through this tissue fluid.

> Remember
>
> The superficial capillaries dilate to regulate the temperature. This turns the skin pink. Capillaries which have been over-stimulated become damaged. They remain permanently dilated or broken and appear as a network of fine red lines underneath the skin.

Fluid leaks out of the capillary walls and bathes the tissues. The nutrients contained in the fluid penetrate the walls of the cells. Waste products leave through the walls of the cells and enter the tissue fluid before passing into the capillary network and then on to a large vein.

Although some of the tissue fluid containing waste products returns to the blood capillaries, much of it is collected up by a second set of vessels which form the lymphatic system.

Lymphatic vessels

Lymphatic vessels are present in the tissue spaces as blind-ended tubes which remove proteins and surplus fluid from the tissue spaces. In this way, swelling is prevented. The vessels contain lymph, a fluid made up of cells (mainly lymphocytes) and plasma (a watery fluid containing some proteins). Lymphocytes are special cells which fight off infection.

The lymphatic vessels create a network through the tissue spaces in very close proximity to the blood vessels. Lymphatic glands or nodes are found at intervals along the path of these vessels. The nodes 'filter' foreign bodies and quickly produce lymphocytes to deal with them. When there is a severe infection, this activity causes the glands to swell. Eventually, the large lymphatic vessels empty their contents back into the blood circulation.

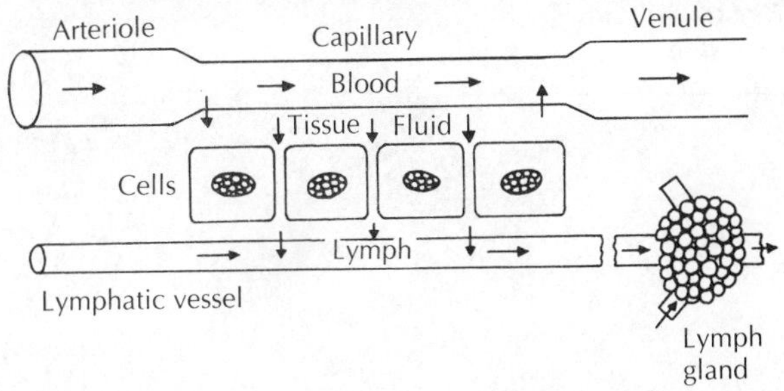

Tissue fluid exchange

The blood supply to the face and neck

The external carotid artery is the main vessel supplying blood to the upper part of the neck and face. It sub-divides into branches which supply different areas. These include the following arteries and veins.

The facial artery

The facial artery lies between the superficial and deeper muscles and supplies the upper and lower lips and facial muscles.

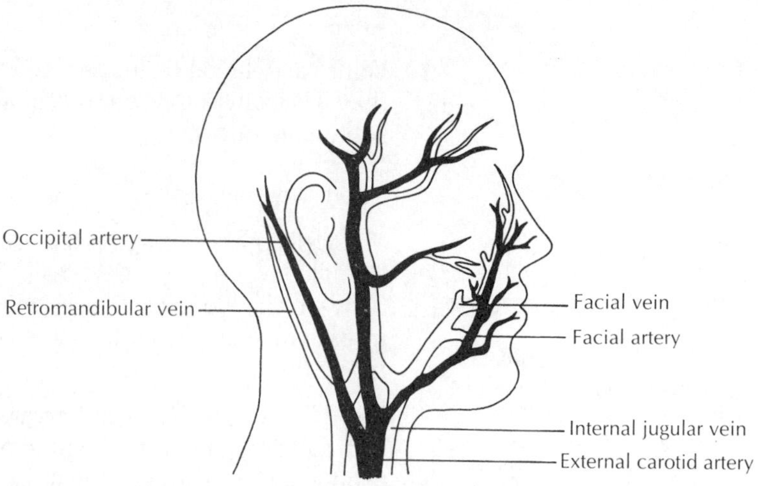

The main blood vessels supplying the head and neck

The occipital artery

The occipital artery supplies the upper part of the neck and back of the scalp.

The superficial temporal artery

The superficial temporal artery supplies the face by its transverse facial branch.

The internal jugular vein

This vein is the main vessel draining blood from the face and neck. Blood is supplied to it by smaller veins which drain different areas. These include:

- the facial vein, which drains the front of the scalp and the superficial structures of the face
- the retromandibular vein, which drains the face below the jaw and the back of the scalp.

> Remember
>
> Many beauty therapy treatments stimulate the supply of blood to the skin and speed up the rate of lymphatic drainage. This increases the nutrition of the skin's surface layers and prevents the build up of toxins and waste products in the skin.

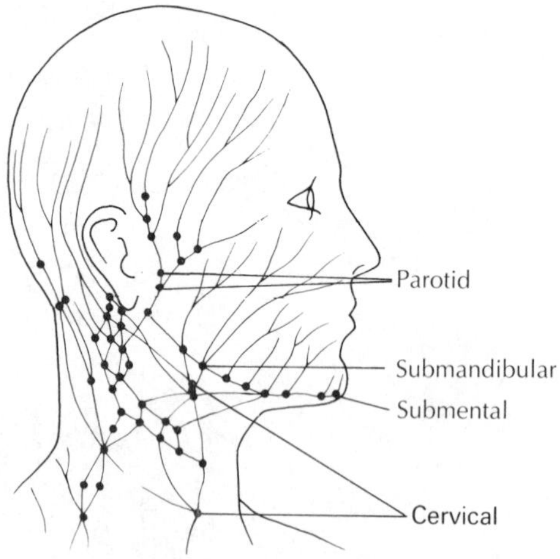

Lymphatic circulation: lymph drains from the chin to the submental nodes, from the middle part of the cheeks and face to the submandibular nodes and from the sides of the cheeks and forehead to the parotid nodes

Lymph from the left side of the head and neck eventually passes through the thoracic duct and empties in to the left subclavian vein

Lymph from the right side of the head and neck eventually passes through the right lymphatic duct and empties in to the right subclavian vein.

The blood supply: Self-checks

1a) What are the main functions of blood?
b) Distinguish between arteries and veins.

2a) Explain the relationship between blood, tissue fluid and skin cells.
b) Why do lymph glands swell?

3a) Name the main artery which supplies blood to the face and neck.
b) Name the main vein which drains blood from the face and neck.

4a) Name the two main ducts which drain lymph from the head and neck.
b) What are the benefits to the skin of beauty treatments which stimulate the flow of blood and lymph?

The blood supply: Activity

1 Find a willing friend, and using an eyebrow pencil to draw on their skin, locate the position of the main lymph nodes of the face and neck. Learn the names of the lymph nodes and ask your friend to test your knowledge using the skin markings.

The skin: some basic facts

Skin covers an area of between 1.2 and 2 square metres. and accounts for approximately 12% of our total body weight. It moulds to and moves with our body, creating a boundary that separates our insides from the outside world. Constantly in contact with its surroundings, the skin has to be tough enough to withstand both physical and chemical assault yet sensitive enough to respond to subtle changes in the internal and external environment.

The skin is working all the time, even when we are asleep, helping to protect and regulate body processes which keep us healthy. Healthy skin provides some protection from:

- mechanical injury, for example from bumps and knocks
- chemical damage.
- radiations
- invasion by micro-organisms
- sudden temperature changes
- excessive water loss
- penetration by foreign materials
- allergens.

Problems occur if the natural protective functions of the skin break down.

A closer look at the structure of the skin helps us to appreciate what is going on beneath the surface and why it is important to keep the skin in good condition.

The structure of the skin

The skin consists of two layers. The epidermis forms the outer protective covering of the body. The dermis provides the 'packing' material which supports all the other structures. A subcutaneous layer, made up of fatty tissue, cushions the internal organs against shocks and acts as an insulator and source of energy when required. This fatty layer separates the skin from underlying muscles.

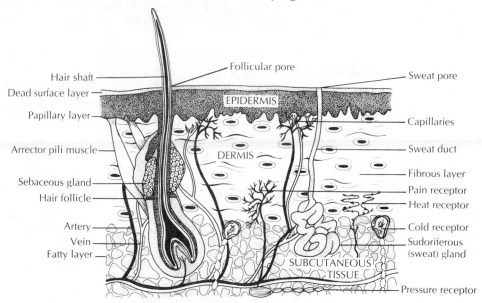

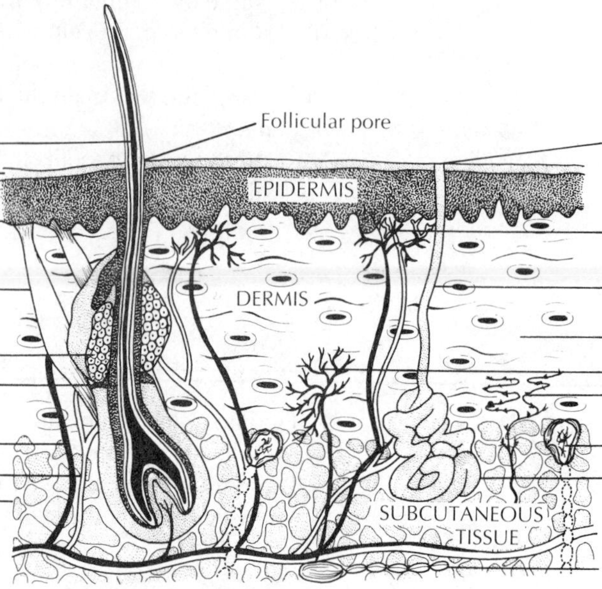

Cross-section through the skin

The structure of the skin

Position	Structure	Function
Epidermis: upper portion of skin	Consists of five layers. Cells in bottom layer are living. They reproduce by mitosis (each cell divides into two) and carry on moving upwards through the layers until they eventually die and harden at the surface	Protection
Dermis: Lies beneath the epidermis Papillary layer situated at the interface of the dermis with the epidermis Reticular layer situated beneath papillary layer	Papillary layer: undulating (wavy) tissue. The upward projections are called dermal papillae. They contain blood and lymph capillaries and nerve endings Reticular layer: dense and fibrous. Contains the main components of the skin. The protein fibres are produced mainly from fibroblast cells contained in a 'ground substance'	Papillary layer increases surface area of reproductive cells and provides living layers of epidermis with vessels which supply nourishment and remove cellular waste Reticular layer protects and repairs injured tissue. The fibres allow skin to bend and fold over underlying muscle activity: • Collagen: gives skin its strength and resilience • Elastin: allows the skin to stretch easily but quickly regain its shape • Reticulin: keeps all the other structures in place
Subcutaneous layer: lies beneath the dermis	Fatty layer of skin. Cells called *lipocytes* produce lipids which are the fat cells from which subcutaneous tissue is formed	Cushions muscles, bones and internal organs against shocks and blows Acts as an insulator and source of energy when required

The structure of the skin *continued*

Position	Structure	Function
Sudoriferous glands: situated in the dermis Eccrine glands are present all over the body, being most numerous on the palms of the hands and soles of the feet Apocrine glands are found mainly in the armpits, nipples, anal and genital areas	Eccrine glands: coiled glands which produce sweat, a watery fluid containing some salt and urea. Sweat passes upwards through a duct and eventually reaches the skin's surface through a sweat pore Apocrine glands: fewer in number and larger than eccrine glands. They open up into hair follicles and produce a thicker secretion than eccrine sweat	Eccrine glands help to regulate body temperature by producing sweat which evaporates off the skin's surface and cools it down when it is hot. Eccrine sweat removes some waste materials from the skin and also contributes to the protective acid mantle which coats the surface of the skin Apocrine glands are under nervous control and respond to emotional, psychological and sexual stimuli. They are considered a sexual characteristic
Hair follicles: situated in the dermis. Present all over the body except on the palms of the hands and soles of the feet	Formed from a depression of epidermal cells. Sac like structures which contain hairs. Outer layer of follicle is fibrous and has very good supply of blood and nerves. Inner layer formed from two layers of cells called the inner and outer root sheath The base of the hair follicle degenerates and rebuilds during the cycle of hair growth and replacement. It contains a dermal papilla which supplies blood to the base of the hair The follicle opens at the skin's surface at a follicular pore	Produce and contain the hairs during their life cycle Help provide nourishment for the hairs
Hairs: contained in follicles in the dermis. Present over most areas of the body but do not grow on the lips, palms of the hands or soles of the feet	The length of hair showing above the skin's surface is called the shaft The portion lying in the follicle is called the root The enlarged base of the root surrounding the papilla is called the bulb Hair is made up of the protein keratin. It consists of three layers. The outer layer is made up of scales which overlap upwards and interlock with scales on the follicle lining to keep the hairs in place	Protect against friction and damage from the external environment Hair is a sexual characteristic
Sebaceous glands: situated in the dermis adjacent to hair follicles. They are not present on the palms of the hands or soles of the feet Some glands open directly on to the skin's surface	These lobulated glands produce sebum, a fatty substance containing waxes, fatty acids, cholesterol and dead cells The sebum passes through a duct and up the hair follicle from where it passes on to the skin through a follicular pore	Sebum lubricates skin and hair and combines with sweat to form the protective acid mantle of the skin. Sebum also helps to waterproof the skin. It retains natural moisture in the skin and provides some insulation
Arrector pili: muscle which connects the side of the hair follicle with the base of the epidermis	Made up of muscle tissue which contracts in response to sensory stimulation. Contraction of the arrector pili makes the hair stand on end which pulls the surface of the skin up into 'goose bumps'	The action of raising the hairs provides some protection from attack and helps to trap heat next to the skin when the body is cold

The structure of the skin *continued*

Position	Structure	Function
Blood vessels: arteries and veins run through the dermis and subcutaneous layer Arteries sub-divide in to arterioles. They form a network of capillaries which supply the various componenents of the skin Veins sub-divide in to venules	Arteries carry oxygenated blood. Their walls are muscular and elastic. Blood is pumped around the body in arteries Veins carry de-oxygenated blood. Their walls have valves which stop blood from stagnating or flowing backwards Capillaries are very fine vessels made up of a single layer of cells. Some materials can pass in and out through the thin walls of the capillaries The surface blood vessels dilate in response to heat and contract in response to cold	Arteries carry oxygen and nutrients to the skin via the capillaries The veins remove waste products The surface capillaries help to regulate body temperature When the vessels dilate, heat is lost from the body through the skin. When the body is cold, the vessels contract and heat is retained Components of the blood produce clots which prevent further blood loss and infection through broken skin following injury
Nerves: contained in the dermis and subcutaneous tissue. Different types of nerves are distributed according to where they are needed most Special 'sympathetic' nerves supply blood vessels, sweat glands and the arrector pili muscle	Made up of white or grey nerve fibres which terminate in sensory nerve endings. The nerve endings or 'receptors' are specially shaped and positioned to respond to a range of different stimuli: heat, cold, pain, pressure, touch	Nerve stimulation causes a reaction which triggers an appropriate response from the body

The skin as a barrier

If harmful organisms or chemicals penetrate the dermis, they get transported round the body by the blood, causing a widespread problem. If adequate moisture levels are not maintained within the living layers of the skin, the cells shrivel and die. The epidermis is structured to provide a barrier which keeps out the bad and keeps in the good.

The epidermis

The outer skin, the epidermis, is made up of a type of body tissue called *stratified* (layered) *squamous* (made up of scales) *epithelium* (covering). An organised production line converts living cells at the base of the epidermis into dead, hardened, compacted layers of protein (keratin) on the outer surface.

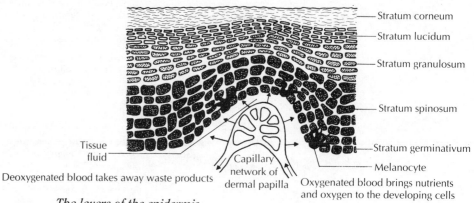

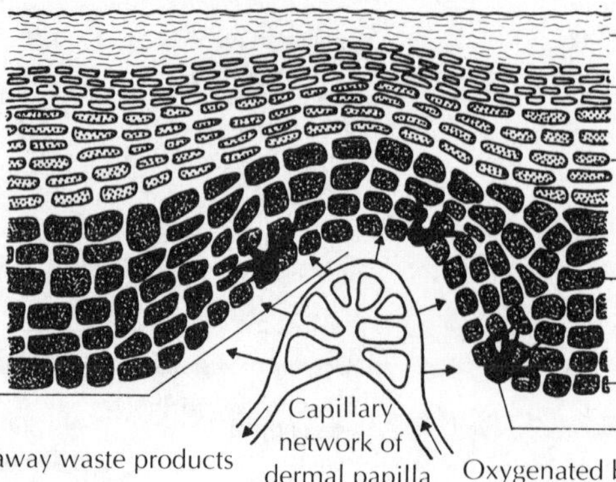

The layers of the epidermis

The rate at which new cells are generated by the epidermis depends on the body's available energy. Regeneration usually occurs during the 4 hours after midnight when body metabolism has slowed down. It takes about 200 days for a cell to mature in the epidermis. The life time of the mature cell is 7-20 days and the replacement time for the stratum corneum between 32 and 36 days.

The epidermis is never more than 1 mm thick. It is thickest on the palms of the hands and the soles of the feet where it needs to withstand the friction caused by gripping and walking. It is thinnest on the eyelids where it must be light and flexible. The cells of the epidermis are packed more loosely in the upper layers. This is to prepare them for shedding (desquamation) which occurs continuously and helps to remove debris and micro-organisms which might otherwise settle on the skin and cause infections.

The epidermis also provides a barrier to the harmful ultra-violet rays in the sun. If these rays reach the dermis, they destroy the protein framework of the skin. Sometimes they cause skin cancer. Sunlight is the commonest cause of skin cancer.

Melanin

Melanin is the dark pigment which produces a sun tan. It protects the deeper layers of the skin by absorbing the sun's ultra-violet rays.

The cells which form pigment are called melanocytes. They are spider-shaped with long irregular arms which reach out from the cell body. The arms of each melanocyte link it with approximately ten of the surrounding cells. Melanocytes inject pigment granules, *melanosomes*, into the neighbouring cells, spreading pigment across the skin. Melanocytes make up about 1% of all skin cells. Everyone has approximately the same number of melanocytes in their skin, regardless of its colour: differences in skin colour are due to the amount of melanin the cells produce. This, in turn, depends on how much ultra-violet radiation they must absorb. The more melanin there is in the body, the more efficient this absorption becomes and the better the protection given.

The stratum corneum thickens when exposed to strong sunlight, presenting a further barrier to the penetration of ultra-violet rays.

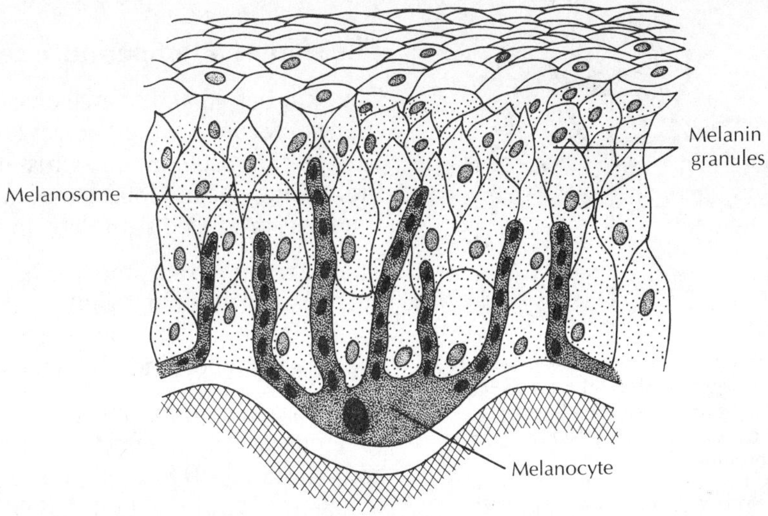

Melanocytes, melanosome and pigment production

Sebum

If the epidermis is to be effective as a barrier, it is important that its surface is kept intact - breaks in the skin provide entry to the deeper layers. *Sebum* is the natural lubricant of the skin which helps to keep it supple. It also keeps the surface cells compacted and obstructs the passage of substances through the skin. Made up of fatty substances and the remnants of dead cells, sebum provides a greasy coating which helps to insulate the skin and prevent natural moisture loss. Sebum also helps to block the mouths of hair follicles so that bacteria can not enter.

Sebum is generally regarded as being waterproof. This is not quite true. Some of the components of sebum are good emulsifiers which help the greasy film to mix with water, particularly after prolonged contact with hot water. Sebum delays the penetration of water and aqueous solutions through the stratum corneum. A more effective barrier to water is created by a thin, fatty layer which exists beneath the stratum corneum.

Now, perhaps, you can understand why the skin underneath the tips of the fingers and toes goes very soft and wrinkled after soaking in a hot bath. The keratin in the stratum corneum absorbs water and the skin swells above the barrier zone. The patterns created follow the lines of stress in the skin which also produce our fingerprints.

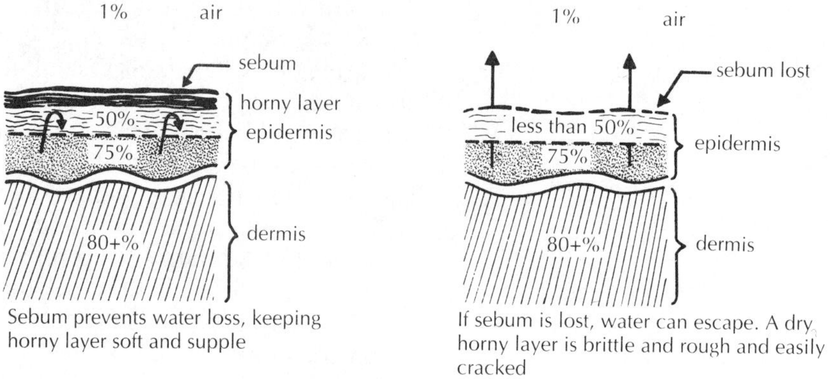

The distribution of water and the barriers in the skin

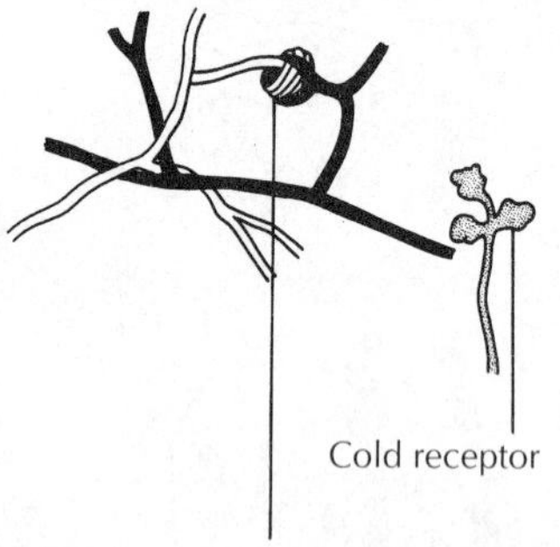

The reaction of blood vessels to cold

The skin as a temperature regulator

The skin has an abundance of specialised nerve endings called *thermoreceptors* which detect cold and heat. These receptors interact with the *hypothalamus*, a cluster of nerve cells at the centre of the brain. Changes in blood temperature are detected and the nerve impulses produced stimulate an appropriate response

There are more receptors in the skin to detect cold than there are to detect warmth. Cold receptors are most abundant in the hands, feet, eyelids, nose and lips. If these areas are not insulated in cold weather, the skin soon becomes dry, chapped and sore.

The internal systems are so finely balanced that even a slight variation in temperature can affect them. The body is maintained at approximately 36.8 °C (98.6 °F) so that our vital organs can work efficiently. We are all familiar with some of the changes that occur if our body temperature rises above or below normal.

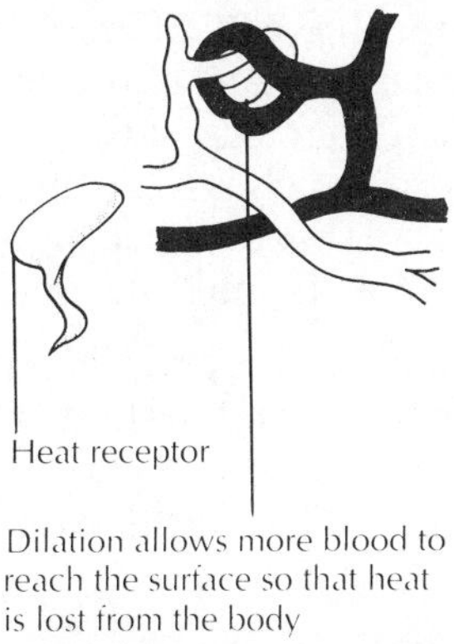
Heat receptor
Dilation allows more blood to reach the surface so that heat is lost from the body

The reaction of blood vessels to heat

In these situations, the body's activity is concentrated on working to restore a normal internal working environment by controlling the amount of heat lost from its surface. Heat is carried around the body by the blood. The superficial blood vessels expand to lose heat, turning the skin pink. They contract to reduce heat loss, making cold skin appear pale and, sometimes, even blue.

There are special connections between veins and arteries which intermittently substitute for capillaries when blood has to be re-routed. The middle section has a thick, muscular wall which, when it contracts, restricts blood flow to the extremities and reduces heat loss. When the skin is warm, this area dilates so that blood can reach the surface to shed heat.

When the body is hot, the sudoriferous glands respond to the hypothalamus by producing sweat. Sweat is composed almost entirely of water which evaporates from the skin's surface, drawing excess heat out of the body.

The life on skin

The skin provides a home for many different types of bacteria and yeasts which coexist quite happily. They actually help the skin to stay healthy by taking up space which might otherwise be invaded with

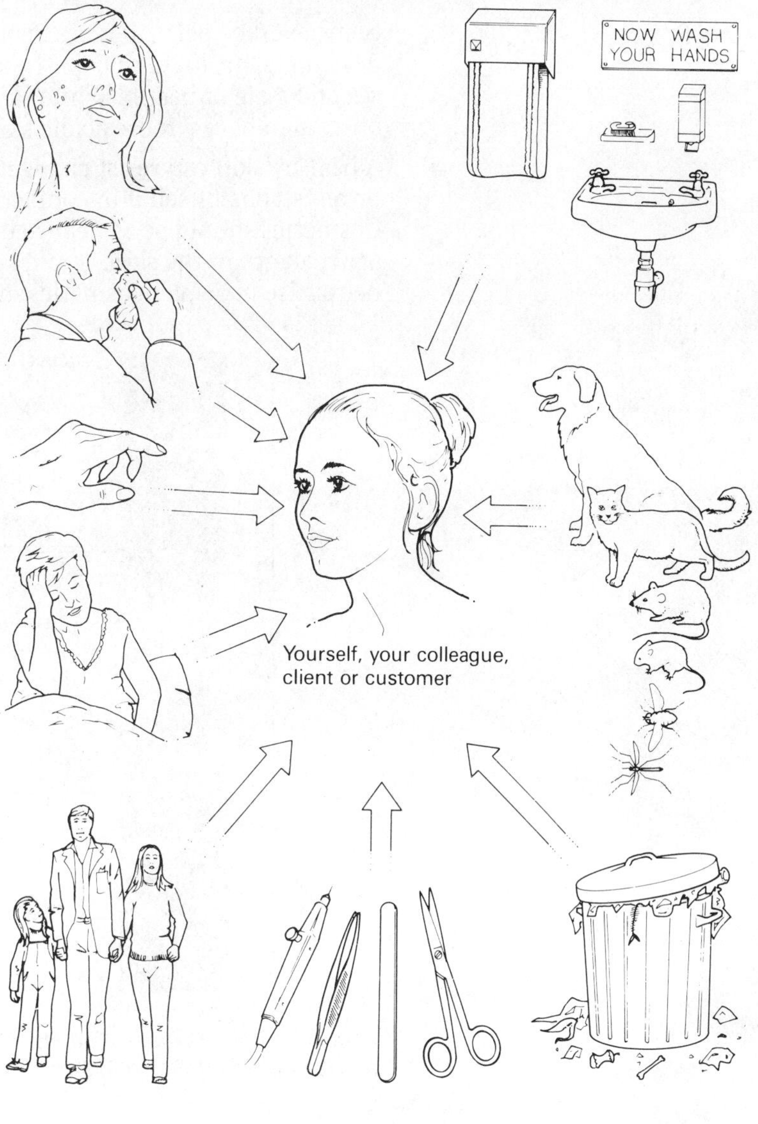
NOW WASH YOUR HANDS
Yourself, your colleague, client or customer

Bacteria are spread from person to person by touch and by picking up infected skin cells which have been shed

more harmful organisms. Different populations thrive in different conditions. For example the relatively greasy centre panel of the face supports different communities from the much drier skin of the forearm. Everyone has a unique flora of bacteria which is as distinct to a microbiologist as fingerprints are to a detective. Bacteria occupy most of the skin's surface. They are acquired at birth, multiply rapidly and remain for life.

It has been estimated that, within a day of birth, bacteria in the armpit number approximately 36 000 per square inch. By day nine, the bacterial population levels off at approximately 490 000 in the same area.

Protection from disease

Infections occur when the skin becomes broken and invaded, or when the acid mantle which coats the skin surface breaks down. Made up of sebum, sweat and keratin, this mantle creates a slightly acid coating to the skin which supports the least harmful bacteria but keeps them fairly inactive.

When the skin is slightly acid, the resident organisms consume anything nutritious on its surface. By removing all traces of 'food', these large populations make it difficult for new organisms to become established.

Some average pH values are: facial skin: 5.4-6.2; forehead, backs, limbs: 5; armpits, groin, toes: 6-7. The values vary according to a person's age, sex and state of health. White skins tend to be more acidic than black ones. Men have a more acidic skin surface than women.

A healthy skin can resist changes in its pH value. It can readily adjust or re-establish itself if in contact with acids or alkalis for short periods. Cosmetics should be as near neutral as possible so as not to upset the acid balance of the skin. It takes approximately one hour for the skin to neutralise incorrect cosmetics, two hours for detergents.

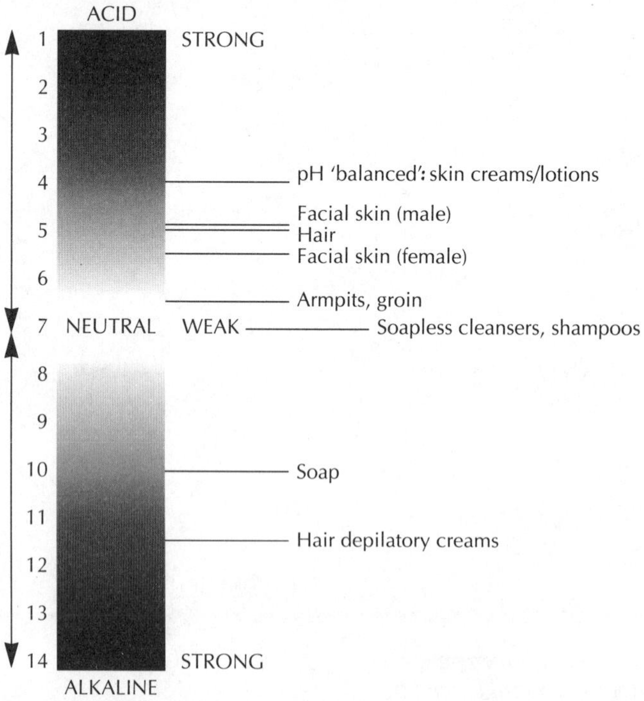

Some average pH values: The pH scale 1-14 measures acid/alkaline values: pH7 is neutral, pH1 strongly acidic and pH14 strongly alkaline

The high-fibre skin

The protein fibres in the dermis support the skin. They keep all the various components in place and prevent them from being damaged. They also make the skin tough and help it to change shape over underlying muscle activity. Collectively, the fibres are known as *connective tissue*.

Collagen fibres give the skin its resilience, firmness and strength. The fibres are arranged loosely in the skin and, although not elastic themselves, allow the skin to stretch without tearing. Healthy collagen is flexible, mostly unlinked, and is able to absorb water. Collagen also builds scar tissue to heal skin damaged by cuts and abrasions.

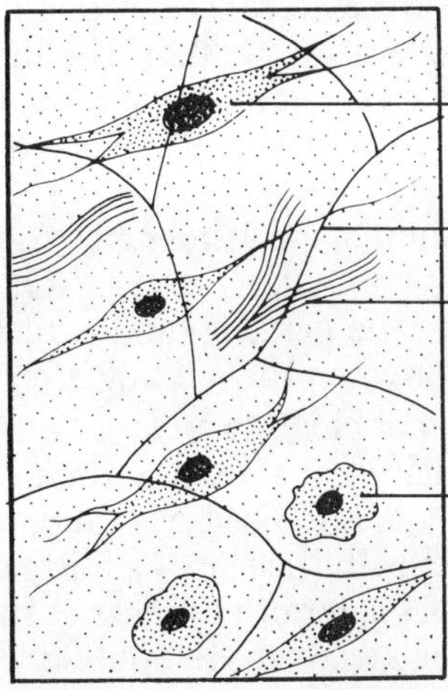

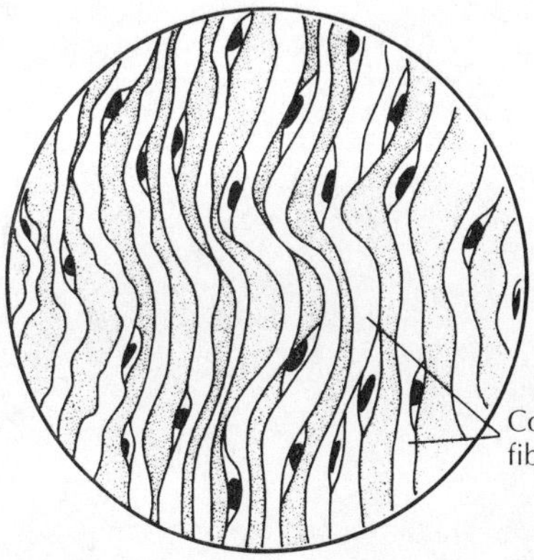

Protein fibres

Elastin fibres branch out to form a loose network throughout the supporting connective tissue. These fibres are elastic: they stretch easily and return to their former length when tension is removed. Elastin fibres are found everywhere but are most numerous on the face and scalp.

Reticulin fibres run through and between the other fibres and structures in the dermis, helping to support them and keep them in place.

The skin's fibres are contained in a firm jelly called the ground substance which is rich in nutrients and contains the fibroblast cells which produce collagen and elastin. Ageing gradually slows down the production of new cells and the fibres become rigid and inflexible.

Skin on the attack

If the living layers of the skin are penetrated or damaged, special cells in the dermis move into action to eliminate the invader and initiate cell repair. The mast cells release *histamine*, a signalling substance which triggers off a 'pain' reaction and dilates the blood capillaries in the area. The extent of the histamine reaction depends on the nature of the injury.

> Strong histamine reaction – pain, swelling, inflammation, pimples, pustules, blisters.
>
> Mild histamine reaction – itching and slight erythema (reddening) of the skin.

Histamine reactions

- Itching: caused by stimulation of just a few pain nerve endings. Itching is a symptom of many disorders and is the skin's way of drawing attention to a problem so that appropriate action can be taken. Scratching relieves the irritation of itching but care should be taken to avoid breaking the skin or infection may occur.
- Erythema: reddening of the skin caused by dilation of the blood capillaries in the dermis layer of the skin. The rate of blood flow is increased, which speeds up the removal of irritant or penetrant from the area and the transport of repair materials to clear up the damage.
- Pain: caused by stimulation of a considerable number of pain nerve endings; it is a feature of many skin diseases. A build up of fluid in the area puts pressure on the nerve endings which subsides once the infection is cleared or when the irritant is removed.
- Swelling: the stimulation of blood to an area causes seepage of serum through the capillary walls into the tissues. Serum is the watery component of blood. Localised swelling produces a bubble of the colourless fluid beneath the skin – a blister. More widespread swelling produces a large blister or puffiness of the skin.
- An increase of fluid in the area helps to dilute the irritant and 'cushion' the deeper layers of the skin from injury.
- Inflammation: the reaction of body tissues to infection or injury. The blood supply to the area is increased, bringing extra white blood cells which promote healing. The area becomes red, swollen, hot and tender. Any disorder that is an inflammation ends with -it is, for example *dermatitis*, inflammation of the skin.
- Pustule: a raised, inflamed spot on the skin which contains pus. Pus is a yellowish liquid that forms when the body fights bacteria. It consists of white blood cells, dead and living bacteria, fragments of dead tissue destroyed by bacteria and serum. Pus is sometimes greenish in colour depending on the type of bacteria present.

The skin: Multiple choice quiz

Choose the correct answer from the given alternatives.

1 The main function of the epidermis is:
a) insulation
b) absorption
c) regulation
d) protection.

2 The dermis is a:
a) fatty layer
b) fibrous layer
c) dead layer
d) barrier layer.

3 The arrector pili is a:
a) muscle
b) blood vessel
c) nerve ending
d) hair.

4 Sweat is produced by the:
a) sebaceous glands
b) epidermal cells
c) keratin
d) protein fibres.

5 Connective tissue is made up of:
a) fat cells
b) epidermal cells
c) keratin
d) protein fibres.

6 Fat cells are stored in the
a) subcutaneous layer
b) epidermis
c) dermis
d) papillary layer.

7 The sensations of touch, pain and changes in temperature are transmitted by:
a) capillaries
b) muscles
c) collagen
d) nerves.

8 The dermal papillae contain blood capillaries and:
a) sebaceous glands
b) hair follicles
c) nerve endings
d) fatty tissue.

9 The protein found in the epidermis is called:
a) melanin
b) keratin
c) reticulin
d) elastin.

10 Collagen fibres are:
a) waterproof
b) elastic
c) sensitive
d) strong.

The skin: Self-checks

1 Five of the following statements are true and five are false. Decide which is which and then write down an explanation for each of your answers.
a) The epidermis is dead.
b) Black skin has twice as many melanocytes as white skin.
c) The dermis contains more water than the epidermis.
d) A healthy skin is slightly acid.
e) Sweating is bad for you.

f) Healthy skin is free from bacteria.
g) The pores are spaces between loose skin cells.
h) Sebum helps to protect the skin from sunburn.
i) The skin is nourished by blood.
j) Ageing slows down the rate of skin cell replacement.

2 Explain each of the following responses of the skin to injury:
a) itching
b) erythema
c) pain
d) swelling
e) inflammation
f) pustule.

The skin: Activity

1 Make a large copy of the diagram of a section through the skin. Use different colours to identify the various parts and then try to label them without looking at the book. No cheating!

Skin blemishes and abnormalities

The following conditions affect the appearance of the skin but they are not infectious and cannot be caught from or passed on to anyone else. They do not contra-indicate beauty therapy treatments.

Disorders of pigmentation

Pigmentation disorders are caused by irregularities in melanin production and can usually be concealed quite effectively with cosmetic camouflage.

Melanoderma

Melanoderma is a general term for patchy pigmentation of the face. It usually describes an increase in melanin caused by applying a cosmetic or perfume which contains a light-sensitising ingredient. This means that the area of skin to which the product is applied becomes extra sensitive to ultra-violet. Bergamot oil, used in the perfumery industry, is one such ingredient. Some drugs have a similar effect.

An increase in pigmentation can also follow inflammation and is sometimes the cause of irregular brown patches on the skin following sunburn.

Freckles (ephelides)

Freckles are tiny, flat, irregular patches of pigment which occur commonly on the face, arms and legs of fair-skinned people, particularly those with blond or red hair. Instead of being deposited evenly throughout the skin, the melanin appears in small clumps.

Freckles become more noticeable on exposure to strong sunlight. They often increase in size and join up to form larger pigmented patches. The skin between freckles contains little or no melanin, so burns easily in the sun. The use of a good sunscreen should be recommended.

Lentigines

A lentigo is larger and more distinct than a freckle. It is sometimes slightly raised but not as much as a pigmented mole. Lentigines do not darken or increase in number on exposure to sunlight.

Chloasma

Chloasma is a smooth, irregularly shaped patch of brown pigmentation which occurs when there is increased production of the melanocyte stimulating hormone (MSH). This often occurs on the face during pregnancy and the condition is especially marked on the temples. A similar reaction occurs as a side effect of taking the contraceptive pill, in which case the neck and mouth may also be affected. The discoloration usually disappears once the balance of hormone levels is restored.

Vitiligo (leucoderma)

In vitiligo small patches of skin appear white due to the destruction of melanocytes in the basal cells of the epidermis. Sometimes, the patches converge to create larger ones. Vitiligo is most noticeable on dark-skinned people. The white patches burn easily in the sun, in contrast with the surrounding skin which tans normally. Areas affected by vitiligo should be protected with a total sun block or kept out of the sun altogether.

Albinism

People with albinism are called albinos. They have no melanin at all; consequently their skin and hair are white and their eyes are pink. Albinos have to take extreme care when out in the sun due to the increased risk of damage to their skin and eyes from the effects of ultra-violet rays.

Skin blockages

The pores are openings in the skin which allow sebum and sweat to flow freely onto its surface. Obstruction of the pores may occur through increased glandular activity, when sebum or sweat are produced at a faster rate than the skin can accommodate, or when a barrier is created over the pore. Skin blockages are unlikely to occur if a good skin care routine is followed.

Blocked pores

This term usually describes a build-up of sebum in the openings of hair follicles as a result of excessive sebum production. Over a period of time the pores become stretched. The blockages need releasing to prevent an accumulation of sebum further down the follicle. Special pore-cleansing treatments may be given as part of a salon facial.

Sebaceous cyst (steatoma or wen)

A cyst forms when sebum retained behind a very small, tight pore collects in the duct of the gland and then in the gland itself, which stretches and forms a swelling under the skin. The swelling may appear as a small nodule or may grow to be the size of a small egg. If a small cyst is squeezed, the released contents have a very characteristic rancid smell which is produced by resident bacteria. Large cysts must not be squeezed due to the risk of skin damage. They are not harmful, but may be surgically removed under local anaesthetic.

Comedones (blackheads)

Comedones occur when sebum becomes trapped in a hair follicle. Cells from the epidermal lining of the upper follicle mix with the sebum, forming a hardened plug at the surface. The characteristic black tip of the comedone is due to oxidation in air of the exposed sebum and, also, melanin contained in the deposited skin cells. The sebum beneath the blackhead is pale and has a soft, cheesy consistency.

Comedones occur commonly on greasy skin. Their effects on the walls of the follicle, the sebaceous duct and the gland itself depend on the amount of sebum being produced and the length of time the pore remains blocked. Comedones become inflamed when they are a symptom of acne (see page 84).

Comedones may be removed after the skin has been cleansed and softened. Care should be taken during their removal to prevent damaging and infecting the skin.

Milia (whiteheads)

Milia appear as small, solid, white pearly nodules and are formed when a fine cuticle of skin grows over the mouth of the hair follicle, obstructing the passage of sebum onto the surface of the skin. Milia often occur around the eyes and above the cheekbones of people with dry skin. They can be exposed and removed from the follicle with a sterilised needle, but great care is required to minimise skin damage and prevent infection.

Miliaria rubra (prickly heat)

Prickly heat is most likely to occur in very hot, humid weather and particularly affects fair-skinned people visiting the tropics. The increased amount of sweat produced by the body is not able to evaporate and, instead, the skin becomes soggy. Keratin plugs form in the tiny sweat pores, blocking the further flow of sweat up to the skin's surface. When sweating occurs, the blocked sweat duct ruptures in to the epidermis forming a vesicle, which is like a small blister, within the epidermal layers. Small hard lumps called papules appear on the skin's surface accompanied by intense itching. Treatment consists of cooling the body and keeping the skin dry.

Haemangioma

Haemangioma is a number of conditions caused by permanent dilation or damage of the superficial blood vessels. They contra-indicate stimulating beauty treatments but are not affected adversely by those which have a cooling ,soothing effect on the skin. Haemangioma can usually be successfully camouflaged with make-up.

Dilated capillaries

Dilated capillaries result from a gradual loss of elasticity in the walls of the vessels where they fail to contract back after stimulation. The superficial capillaries remain permanently dilated making the skin a pronounced pinky-red colour. The cheeks and nose are the areas most affected but people with extremely fine skin may have a more widespread condition.

This usually follows many years of exposure to weather conditions, harsh rubbing of the face when washing and general lack of protection. Internal stimulants such as alcohol, spicy foods and very hot drinks can also be a factor. People with dry sensitive skin are most likely to have dilated capillaries.

Split capillaries

Sometimes the walls of the vessels weaken so much that they rupture and blood leaks out in to the surrounding tissues. The individual capillaries can be seen quite distinctly and usually respond well to treatment with diathermy by a trained electrologist. This treatment cauterises the blood vessels, blocking off the flow of blood.

Spider naevus (stellate haemangioma)

'Spider' accurately describes the appearance of this condition, where fine capillary 'legs' radiate out from the 'body' which is a central dilated vessel. Spider naevi occur most often on the upper part of the face and cheeks, particularly in pregnancy when oestrogen levels are raised. They respond well to treatment with diathermy.

Port wine stain

A port wine stain is a bright purple, irregularly shaped flat birthmark which may be quite small or may cover extensive areas of the body. The colour is thought to be due to blood capillaries which have been damaged by pressure upon them during the foetal stage of development. A port wine stain grows with the body. It does not regress and may cause particular distress if located prominently on the face. Cosmetic camouflage usually has very successful results.

Tumours of the skin

A tumour is formed by an overgrowth of cells. Almost every type of cell in the epidermis and dermis is capable of benign or malignant overgrowth. Tumours are lumpy and, even when they cannot be seen, can be felt underneath the surface of the skin.

Benign (non-cancerous) tumours do not contra-indicate beauty therapy treatments but special care is needed to avoid over stimulation and disturbance of the skin cells in the area. Many benign tumours appear at birth or shortly afterwards and are referred to as birthmarks. The majority of these tumours remain harmless but some may undergo changes later in life and so are potentially dangerous.

Malignant (cancerous) tumours are definitely contra-indicated to beauty therapy treatments. If you suspect a client has a malignant growth they are unaware of, tactfully recommend a prompt visit to their doctor. Malignant tumours appear more commonly in old age but can develop as the result of changes in an existing tumour.

Moles

Moles vary in size and may be raised or flat, pigmented or a normal skin colour. Their surface can be smooth or rough, hairy or hairless. Moles are usually harmless. They have a very good blood supply and the individual vessels can often be seen quite prominently in the smooth, raised, skin coloured type.

Pigmented moles are not usually present at birth but develop over the years of childhood and, sometimes, even later. They are caused by an overgrowth of melanocytes in the basal layer of the epidermis at its junction with the dermis. As time goes by, the cells drop into the dermis and become permanently lodged there. The majority of pigmented moles are harmless but some may become malignant, particularly if they are over exposed to strong sunlight.

Malignant melanoma is a deeply pigmented mole which is life-threatening if it is not recognised and treated promptly. Over exposure to strong sunlight is a major cause and the incidence of the condition is increasing in young people with fair skins.

Some melanomas develop on areas of previously healthy skin not normally exposed to sun. This makes their early detection easier, and medical treatment by radiation, excision or chemotherapy is usually quite successful.

Changes to look for

> **Remember**
> The most dangerous moles are the smooth, slightly raised, very dark brown, bluish-black or greyish ones which measure less than 2 cm across. Hairy moles are usually safe but it is wise to cut the hairs rather than pluck them to avoid disturbing the skin cells.

Medical advice should be sought if any of the following changes occur in the appearance of a pigmented mole:

- an increase in size
- breaking up of the defined edge of the mole
- the formation of new, tiny moles around the borders of an existing one
- a deepening of pigmentation
- bleeding or crust formation
- inflammation around the mole
- pain, tenderness or itching are also signs that should not be ignored.

Rodent ulcer (basal cell epithelioma)

This malignant tumour starts off as a slow growing pearly nodule, often at the site of a previous skin injury. As the nodule enlarges, the centre ulcerates and refuses to heal. The centre becomes depressed and the rolled edges become translucent, revealing many, tiny blood vessels. Rodent ulcers do not disappear. If left untreated they may invade underlying bone.

The medical treatment of rodent ulcer is very successful. This form of cancer does not spread to other parts of the body. Although rodent ulcers are more common in people over the age of 50, they are occurring more frequently in younger age groups as a result of over exposure to sunlight.

Squamous cell epithelioma

This tumour is also malignant and arises from the prickle cell layer of the epidermis. It is hard and warty and eventually develops a heaped-up, cauliflower-like appearance. The tumour is very slow growing and medical treatment is usually very successful if the condition is diagnosed before it spreads.

Scars

> *Remember*
> Scars are necessary to keep the surface of the skin intact and to protect it from invasion.

Scars are formed from replacement tissue during the healing of a wound. Depending on the type and extent of skin damage, the scar may be raised and shiny (hypertrophic), rough and pitted (ice-pick) or fibrous and lumpy (keloid). Alternatively, a scar may show as loss of skin tissue. When the protein fibres in the dermis are damaged by a cut, burn, injury or disease, they knit together differently as the skin tries to repair itself. The deeper and more extensive the injury, the more fibres are affected and the thicker and lumpier is the resulting scar. Scars do not usually grow hair or have skin sensations.

> *Remember*
> As a general guideline, beauty treatment should not be given over scar tissue which is less than six months old.

Scars heal at different rates on different people. You should take care that beauty therapy treatments are not given over a scar which has not completely healed. The general signs of healing are:

- the scar is not painful
- the scar is sealed and dry
- there is no inflammation.

Skin blemishes and abnormalities: Self-checks

1 Describe the appearance and give one cause of each of the following:
a) chloasma
b) comedone
c) milium
d) dilated capillaries
e) port wine stain
f) malignant melanoma.

2 a) Explain how a scar is formed.
b) How can you tell when a scar has healed?

Skin disorders

> *Remember*
> It is wise for a client who is being treated medically for a skin disorder to get the written consent of his or her doctor before having beauty therapy. The consent letter should be kept safely with the client's record card.

> *Remember*
> Do not give stimulating beauty therapy treatments to skin which is troubled by psoriasis. If the condition is present in a very mild form, the client may have basic skin care and make-up treatments.
>
> Make sure that the plaques are not disturbed during treatment or bleeding may occur and the skin will be open to infection.

The following conditions are not infectious but they may contra-indicate beauty therapy. The decision to go ahead with treatment depends on the severity of the condition. Occasionally the symptoms flare up, making the skin particularly sensitive and unsuitable for treatment. Sometimes secondary infection may be present which would also contra-indicate treatment.

Psoriasis

In this condition there is an abnormally rapid rate of cell turnover in the epidermis. It may take only four days for new cells to reach the stratum corneum. When the cells reach the surface, they clump together producing round or oval dull, red plaques of different sizes, covered in silvery scales. The skin feels very rough and, if the scales are removed, tiny spots of bleeding occur.

Psoriasis is an inherited condition. It occurs on areas of skin which do not have much underlying flesh such as the limbs, elbows and knees. The scalp and face are sometimes affected. The symptoms flare up prominently in the teens and twenties and then later in life, in the fifties and sixties. They seem to be more severe as a result of shock, stress or illness but often fade away as quickly as they appear. The specific cause of psoriasis is not known.

Psoriasis sufferers have to be very patient and persevere with medical treatment. This usually consists of regular applications of coal-tar pastes which are messy to use, smell foul and stain clothes and bedding. Many patients respond well to PUVA (Psoralen-UVA) therapy which uses the photo-sensitising properties of various plant extracts to intensify the healing properties of UVA rays.

Acne vulgaris

This is the most common of all skin disorders and affects the face, shoulders, upper back and chest. The main symptoms are greasiness of the skin, blackheads, whiteheads, papules and pustules. There may also be inflammation.

Acne usually appears at puberty when the body starts producing more sex hormones. It takes some time for the correct balance of hormones to be achieved. When there is an excessive amount of male hormones (androgens) produced, the sebaceous glands become over-active and the skin appears very shiny. This condition of excess greasiness is called *seborrhoea*.

Bacteria which are present in the hair follicle break down the sebum and fatty acids are released which irritate the wall of the follicle. The epidermal lining thickens, narrowing the upper end and opening of the follicle so that sebum builds up further down. When the follicle pore becomes completely enclosed with hardened skin cells, a whitehead results. When the pore becomes blocked with hardened sebum, a blackhead (comedone) is formed.

> Remember
> Secondary infection occurs if bacteria invade through breaks in the skin. This may be caused by picking spots and squeezing blackheads.

Papules develop as the follicle and sebaceous gland swell with trapped sebum. Sometimes the contents of the follicle escape into the surrounding dermis, causing inflammation and pustules. In cases of severe acne, inflamed, painful cysts occur which often heal leaving permanent scarring and pitting of the skin.

Acne cannot be cured but it can be controlled. The medical treatment varies depending on the severity of the condition but usually includes de-greasing, medicated skin care and antibiotics. The condition may last for between eight and twelve years. It is usually most severe in females of about 17 and males of about 19. After these ages, the acne gradually improves and usually disappears completely by the age of twenty five.

Treatment of clients with mild acne

A client with mild acne may be given facial treatments in the salon but inflamed pustules contra-indicate beauty therapy. The beauty therapy treatment of acne should concentrate on gentle de-greasing of the skin and careful releasing of skin blockages. Very strong drying agents should be avoided as they irritate the skin, causing it to harden and thicken over the mouths of hair follicles. This makes the removal of skin blockages difficult and increases the formation of whiteheads and blackheads. Skin with mild acne should be warmed and softened before blockages are removed.

Rosacea

Rosacea usually affects people over the age of thirty, some of whom may have been troubled previously by acne vulgaris. The skin appears very flushed over the nose, cheeks and forehead. A characteristic butterfly shape is produced by the blood vessels which are dilated in these areas. The increase in skin temperature stimulates the production of sebum, making it appear greasy. Open pores, papules and pustules are often present in rosacea but blackheads are not a feature. In severe cases, the sebaceous glands may become so enlarged that the skin appears very coarse and lumpy.

> Remember
> Provided that the superficial blood vessels have not become permanently damaged, cooling and soothing beauty treatments will help to tone down the redness of skin with rosacea. Inflamed pustules contra-indicate beauty therapy treatment.

Rosacea often begins as occasional flushing in response to stimulants such as hot foods and drinks, spicy food, strong coffee, alcohol and exposure to cold, wind and sun. Chronic flushing may be brought on by stress, hormonal disturbance or permanently damaged blood vessels. There may be long periods of remission. Medical treatment consists of antibiotics and, sometimes, tranquillisers for anxiety to help reduce facial flushing.

You should not apply any stimulating facial treatments to a client troubled by rosacea. Handle the skin very carefully and keep it cool.

Skin disorders: Self-checks

1 a) Why should special care be taken when treating a client with a mild form of psoriasis?
b) Why are stimulating treatments not suitable for a client with psoriasis?

2 a) Explain why acne vulgaris appears most commonly in teenagers.
b) What general advice should be given to a client who has acne?

3 a) What are the main characteristics of rosacea?
b) What special care is required when treating a client with rosacea?

Infections of the skin

Skin infections are spread by direct contact, or indirectly, by touching a contaminated article.

> Remember
> All skin infections contra-indicate beauty therapy treatment. If the skin of your hands is infected, you are contra-indicated to giving treatment.

Skin infections caused by viruses

Warts are small, solid growths of skin tissue. The virus invades the stratum. germinatum of the epidermis and causes abnormal keratinisation. There are different types of wart. The ones which affect the hands and feet are described in Chapter 9 (Manicure and hand treatments) and Chapter 11 (Pedicure). The warts which affect the face and neck are:

- plane warts: very small, smooth and skin-coloured or light brown, these occur on the face in clusters and sometimes disappear spontaneously without treatment.
- seborrheic warts: these start to appear at middle age and begin as a brown thickening of the skin which grows to approximately 3-25 mm across, darkens and develops a rough, greasy surface.
- filiform warts: these appear on the face neck and eyelids as thin strips of skin up to 3 mm in length with a hard tip. Filiform warts may occur singly or in clusters.

> Remember
> Do not confuse filiform warts with skin tags which are tiny, loose, painless growths of skin which sometimes develop on the eyelids and sides of neck. They usually appear in middle age, are quite harmless and should be left alone. If skin tags are annoying because they catch on clothing or jewellery, they can be surgically removed under anaesthetic by a doctor or cauterised by a trained electrologist.

Most warts eventually disappear spontaneously without treatment, but special pastes and paints are available which must be used carefully. Persistent warts may be treated medically by freezing or burning and digging out with a curette.

Cold sore (herpes simplex)

> **Remember**
> The blisters contain the virus. A cold sore is most infectious when the blisters have formed and shortly afterwards, when they break and weep.

This condition usually recurs at the same site of the face, either the lips, cheeks or side of the nose. The virus lies dormant in sensory nerve cells and is activated only by stimuli such as a bad cold, menstruation, sunburn, infection or general debility. The onset is usually sudden: tingling, burning and itching may be felt for a few hours before blisters appear.

The skin usually becomes infected with bacteria, causing pain. Crusts form which take approximately 10-14 days to heal. Application of a spirit-based lotion helps to dry out the condition and prevent secondary infection of the skin.

Shingles (herpes zoster)

Shingles is a very painful condition which produces a rash and blisters along the path of a sensory nerve. Scales form after a week and the rash disappears after two or three weeks, leaving some scarring. Pain may persevere for quite a long time after the skin symptoms have disappeared.

Only people who have had chicken pox develop shingles. The chicken pox virus lies dormant in the nerve cells and becomes activated in middle age or later. Medical treatment usually consists of the prescription of an anti-viral drug and strong painkillers.

Skin infections caused by bacteria

Boil (furuncle)

This is a local pocket of infection which starts around the base of a hair follicle. The follicle and surrounding skin cells are killed by bacteria and form pus. The amount of pus keeps increasing until, eventually, it bursts through the skin and escapes. Sometimes, several follicles in an area are infected, producing a carbuncle. This causes an extensive pustular infection with several heads which burst.

Boils are most likely to occur on hairy areas prone to friction, for example the neck. They are often brought on by general debility and over-tiredness when the body's resistance is low. A heating poultice may help to draw out the infection. If the boil is persistent and very painful, it may be lanced by a doctor, who will probably also prescribe oral antibiotics.

Impetigo

A highly contagious skin infection, impetigo is particularly common in children but can be caught easily by adults. The nose and mouth are the areas of the face most frequently affected. Impetigo starts off as a red spot. This becomes a blister which quickly breaks down and discharges, causing yellow crusts to develop. The crusts spread and other spots then develop near the earlier infection. Oral antibiotics, prescribed by a doctor, help to speed up recovery. The sores may be treated by bathing with an antiseptic solution or applying an antibiotic ointment.

Conjunctivitis

This infection affects the very thin skin which covers the white of the eye and the inner surface of the eyelids. Conjunctivitis is the commonest cause of red and sticky eyes. Although the main cause is bacterial, the condition can be provoked by a virus or irritants such as a foreign body, tobacco smoke or eye cosmetics. Sometimes it may be an indication of an allergy.

Bathing the eyes with warm water helps to soothe and relieve any stickiness. If the eyes feel very gritty and redness persists after three days, a doctor may prescribe antibiotic drops or ointment.

Stye

> Remember
> Infections of the skin around the eyes are usually caused by the spread of bacteria from the nose and mouth. Cross-infection should be avoided by washing the hands after touching the face and not sharing face cloths and towels with other people.

This is a small boil in the glands at the root of the eyelashes. It is a common, unsightly and uncomfortable condition but can usually be treated without medical help. A stye begins as painful swelling and redness of the eyelid. After a few days, pus forms and discharges from the swelling on to the margin of the eyelid. The regular application of hot compresses helps to bring the stye to a head and speed up the recovery process. If the stye has not burst after three days, a doctor may recommend the use of an antibiotic ointment.

Skin infections caused by fungi

Ringworm (tinea corporis)

Ringworm is a highly contagious condition. The fungus lives on the dead horny outer layer of skin and is found, more commonly, on warm, moist areas of the body. Red pimples appear and spread at the edges, producing red rings with a clearing of normal skin colour in the centre. Scales and pustules usually develop over the rings. Ringworm can spread to the face from other infected areas of the body, such as the feet and head. Domestic animals and cattle are also a source of the infection.

Ringworm continues to spread for several weeks or months. During this time it can be treated with an anti-fungal preparation bought from the chemist. A doctor may prescribe anti-fungal cream or ointment and antibiotic tablets.

Infestations of the skin

Infestations such as scabies and pediculosis are disorders involving invasion of the skin by tiny animal parasites which live off human blood. They are highly contagious. Secondary infection often occurs as a result of breaking the skin through scratching.

Scabies

Commonly known as 'the itch', scabies is caused by a female mite, *sarcoptes scabiei* (see page 14), which becomes fertilised on the skin surface and then burrows into the skin to lay its eggs. The eggs hatch after four days and the mature mite appears on the skin surface ten days later. Characteristic greyish ridges track the routes of the burrows in the skin. Itchy pimples appear as an allergic reaction to the mite, the eggs and larvae. These become more uncomfortable at night when the body is warm. Persistent scratching produces inflammation and coarsening of the skin.

Scabies appears most commonly between the fingers, the insides of the wrist, the palms of the hands and the soles of the feet. Treatment is medical and consists of applying a preparation to kill the parasites followed by an anti-bacterial cream.

> Remember
> Towels and bedding which have been in contact with pediculosis should be disinfected before being laundered in the normal way.

Pediculosis

Pediculosis is a skin irritation caused by a tiny insect parasite, the head louse, which invades the scalp and lays its eggs (nits) which become attached to the hairs. The nits are a characteristic silvery grey colour. There is intense itching at the site of the infestation and blisters and sores invariably appear as a result of scratching.

Preparations are available at the chemist for treating pediculosis. A doctor may prescribe antibiotics to treat a secondary bacterial infection.

Skin infections and infestations: Self-checks

1 State the cause of each of the following skin infections or infestations:
a) wart
b) stye
c) ringworm
d) impetigo
e) furuncle
f) cold sore
g) conjunctivitis
h) scabies.

Skin infections and infestations: Activities

1 Visit your study centre and find a dermatology book which contains photographs of the skin diseases and disorders described in this chapter. Make notes of any additional information you find which helps to increase your knowledge and understanding of these conditions.

2 Make out a chart which summarises the appearance, cause and treatment advice for each of the skin conditions described in this chapter. You can then use the chart for quick reference and as a learning aid.

Allergies

> Remember
> Substances which cause allergies are usually harmless to the majority of people and only affect those who are hypersensitive.

An allergic reaction occurs when the body tissues react abnormally to a substance with which they have been brought into contact. The contact may be external (by touch) or internal (by inhaling, eating or drinking). Asthma, hay fever, eczema and urticaria are all due to allergies. Allergies can develop 'over night'. A person may have been exposed to a substance or used a product for years without any previous problems.

Allergic reaction

There are millions of tiny cells scattered throughout the tissue linings of the body called *mast* cells. They produce and store chemicals including *histamine*. Histamine is responsible for producing the symptoms of tissue damage. The mast cells also carry special antibodies which react with certain substances and trigger off an allergic reaction.

When the offending substance (*antigen*) penetrates the body, a chemical reaction occurs between the antigen and the antibody, and histamine is released in to the surrounding tissues. The reaction which occurs depends on the tissues which are affected:

- eyes: watering of the eyes, irritation and swelling of the eyelids
- nose: irritation, sneezing, runny nose, nasal blockage
- lungs: wheezing, breathlessness, tightness of the chest
- intestine: stomach pains, diarrhoea
- skin: irritation, itching, inflammation, swelling, rash, blisters.

Allergies affecting the skin

Some substances, particularly if they have a similar chemical composition, are more likely than others to provoke an allergic reaction in people who are hypersensitive. All products containing the offending substance will cause an allergic response, even if the substance is present only in tiny amounts. An allergic reaction of the skin may be local or more widespread depending on whether the skin has been irritated or sensitised by the offending substance. *Primary irritation* results from the direct action of the irritant upon the skin and occurs when the substance contacted is exceptionally harsh or concentrated, or when there is repeated contact with an irritant substance which gradually breaks down the skin's natural protective mechanisms. Primary irritation causes inflammation and itchiness of the skin. The condition is called *contact dermatitis* and usually shows up quite quickly on the area of skin to which the substance has been applied.

Irritant substances will produce a dermatitis reaction in most people if adequate precautions are not taken to protect the skin. Examples of common irritants are:

- detergents
- disinfectants
- water
- solvents
- bleach.

Depending on the concentration of the substance, how promptly remedial action is taken and how sensitive the skin is, the symptoms may develop into *contact eczema*, also known as *contact allergic dermatitis*. When this happens, the live skin cells become damaged and release histamine. This causes fluid to collect in the tissues, the skin swells and blisters appear which eventually burst, weep and then scab over. The symptoms may take up to 48 hours to appear. Some common causes of contact eczema are:

- armpits: perfumes, antiperspirants, deodorants
- trunk: nickel fastenings and elastic on underwear
- head and neck: cosmetics, hair sprays, plants
- hands: washing powders, dyes, flowers, rings, bracelets, watch straps, gloves
- feet: dyes and chemicals in leather shoes and boots.

> Remember
> Contact eczema (contact allergic dermatitis) is the most common allergic reaction of the skin to cosmetics.

It is obviously very important to avoid using any product which contains a substance known to harm the skin. The cause of a dermatitis reaction may be determined quite easily because the reaction is fairly immediate. An allergic reaction, however, is delayed and it is usually more difficult to isolate the cause.

A doctor may prescribe antihistamine tablets and a cortisone cream for relieving the symptoms of an allergic skin reaction. When the specific cause of the allergy is not known, the patient is usually referred to a dermatologist, a doctor specialising in skin problems.

> Remember
> Allergies are not always restricted to the area of skin contact. The offending substance may penetrate the skin or circulate in the blood stream causing a more widespread reaction of the body.

Sensitisation

Sensitisation is the 'true' allergic reaction and involves a delayed response. On first contact with the offending substance, there is no obvious reaction but the skin becomes *sensitised*. It recognises the substance as alien and produces special antibodies which wait in readiness for the next time contact is made. Subsequently, the symptoms of eczema occur at the site of contact with the substance.

> Remember
> Always check if your client suffers from any allergies before making your selection of products. If the client complains of irritation or you see the skin reacting to a product you are using, remove it immediately and enter details on the client's record card.

Urticaria

Certain foods can produce allergic symptoms of the skin. Dairy produce and wheat-based products sometimes cause an eczema reaction. Strawberries, lobster and shellfish are often the cause of urticaria (nettle rash or hives). In this condition there is intense irritation of the skin. Swollen areas of pale skin occur surrounded by red weals. The weals may appear anywhere on the body and vary in size from a tiny pimple to a large patch, several centimetres across. They last for 8–24 hours and fade without trace. Urticaria can also be caused by an allergy to certain drugs (for example aspirin, penicillin), flowers or an insect sting.

Allergies: Self-checks

1 a) Describe the appearance of a typical allergic skin reaction.
b) List six common causes of contact allergic dermatitis.
c) State two main differences between eczema and urticaria.

Basic skin types

Skin is usually described as being balanced, dry, greasy or combination. In addition, it may be sensitive, dehydrated, mature, congested, blemished or infected.

> Remember
> A balance of oil and moisture secretions maintains the acid mantle of the face between pH 5.6-5.8 (female) and pH 5.1-5.3 (male). This means that, provided that the skin is not broken, it has a good resistance to bacterial and fungal infections.

Balanced skin

Balanced skin is exactly what it says it is: it has a good balance of oil and moisture secretions which keep the skin soft, supple and flexible. Desquamation and cell generation take place at the same rate, so that there is an even replacement of the surface layers. This helps to keep the skin smooth and clear. The pores are small, the texture fine and even and the colour healthy. The skin feels slightly warm to touch due to its good blood supply. A balanced skin rarely develops spots and blemishes and, when it does, it usually heals well.

Maintaining a balanced skin

The main aim of skin care is to create or preserve the characteristics of a balanced skin. A balanced skin is a healthy skin. The therapist can use a wide range of treatments and products to help 'balance' any skin type, but, ultimately, the clients must understand what they have to do to keep the skin healthy.

The following advice is intended for all clients, irrespective of their skin type:

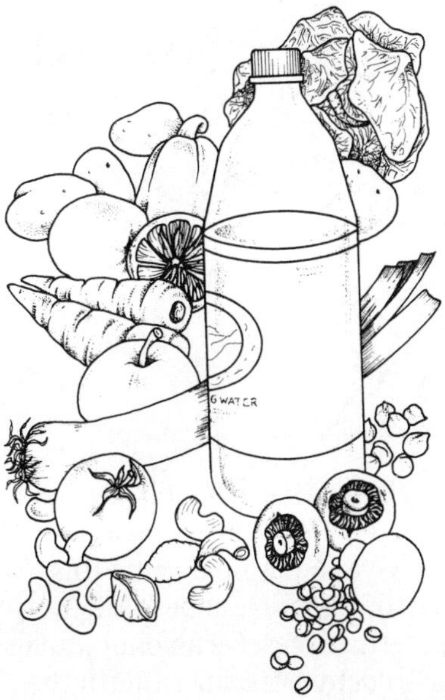

1 Eat a balanced diet which includes plenty of fresh vegetables, fruit and fibre. Foods containing vitamins A, B and C are particularly important for healthy skin. So are proteins and the essential fatty acids.
   - Good sources of vitamin A: milk, eggs, butter, margarine, fish-liver oils, (e.g. cod, halibut).
   - Good sources of vitamin B: cereals, pulses, meat, milk, wholemeal flour, leafy vegetables.
   - Good sources of vitamin C: fresh fruit, particularly blackcurrants, strawberries, oranges, lemons and grapefruit, fresh vegetables, particularly sprouts, cauliflower, cabbage, tomatoes and potatoes.
   - Good sources of protein: meat, fish, milk, eggs, beans, peas and lentils (pulses), edible seeds, nuts and oil-containing fruit.
   - Good sources of essential fatty acids: polyunsaturated vegetable and nut oils, soft margarines.

2 Drink plenty of water: this helps to maintain a healthy water balance in the body and speeds up the elimination of waste and toxins which can affect the skin.

3 Get enough sleep: remember that the rate of skin cell repair and replacement increases when we are asleep. Tiredness and exhaustion deprive the skin of the energy it needs to recover and regenerate.

4 Protect the skin: a balanced skin can easily become dry if it is not protected from the weather, extremes of temperature, central heating, sunlight, pollution and cosmetics. Wear a moisturiser to create a barrier between the skin and outside elements. Whenever possible, avoid exposing the skin to strong sunlight, otherwise use a suitable ultra-violet screening product.

5 Exercise regularly: apart from stimulating the flow of blood and supply of oxygen to the body tissues, regular exercise speeds up cell division and helps to build collagen. Keeping the body fit minimises stress and its effects upon the skin.

6 Keep the skin clean: do not allow dirt and grime to build up which could block the pores and irritate the skin.

7 Avoid harsh treatment: do not pull or stretch the skin. Be gentle when washing the face and using skin-care products. Remember that blood vessels are very near the surface of the skin and can become damaged quite easily. Avoid using perfumed products on facial skin or those with an alcohol or alkaline base which are very degreasing.

8 Do not smoke: besides being extremely hazardous to general health, smoking produces gases (mainly carbon monoxide and nitrogen oxide) which are carried round the body in the blood stream in preference to oxygen. As a consequence the cells do not receive enough nourishment. The skin suffers oxygen starvation. Other chemicals produced in the body by smoking interfere with the protein fibres in the skin and deplete the body of vitamin C which is essential for healthy skin.

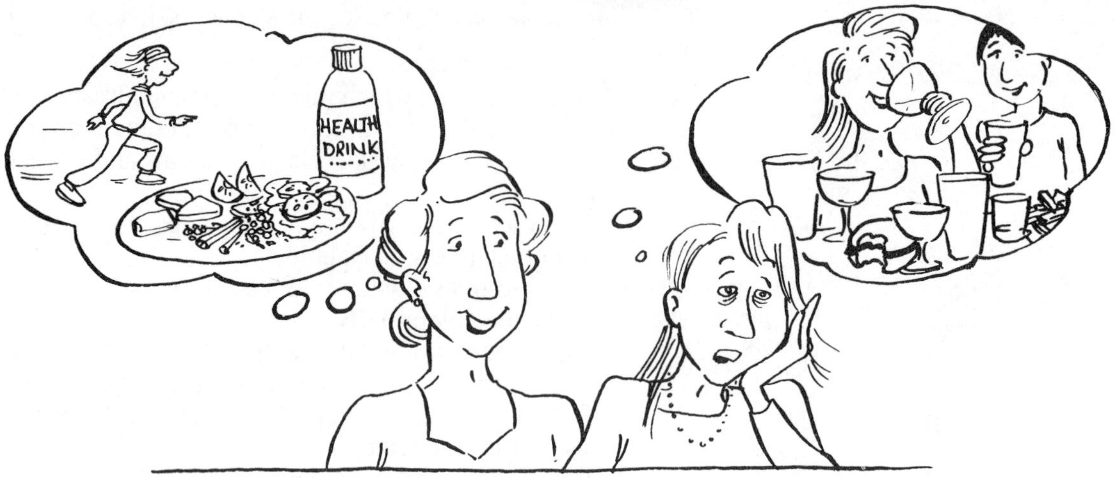

9 Control alcohol intake: alcohol raises the blood pressure and causes the blood capillaries to dilate. Over a period of time this can cause the walls of the capillaries to rupture and become permanently damaged. In the short term, excessive alcohol intake produces chemicals in the body which dehydrate the skin. In the longer term, puffiness of the tissues, coarsening of the skin texture, deepening of lines and wrinkles and chronic redness of the skin occur.

10 Monitor the skin: a balanced skin becomes drier with age as the body processes slow down. Keep a look out for early signs of changes in the skin so that cosmetic skin care can be adapted to compensate for them.

Dry skin

Dry skin has a matt, uneven texture. This is because there is not enough sebum to lubricate the surface cells and keep them compacted. In the absence of a greasy coating, natural moisture becomes lost from the upper layers. The surface cells curl up and flake. The skin lacks suppleness and often feels tight. Dry skin is usually thin and fine with no visible pores. It forms fine lines and wrinkles prematurely, particularly around the eyes. Dilated capillaries appear commonly on the cheeks and nose due to the lack of protection which is usually provided by sebum. Dilated capillaries appear red on fair skins.

Causes of dry skin

1 Hormone imbalance: a dry skin occurs naturally when the balance of male to female sex hormones circulating in the blood is lower than normal. Androgens are the male sex hormones, responsible for activating the sebaceous glands. Oestrogens are the female sex hormones. A level of oestrogen in the blood higher than normal inhibits the production of sebum.

Oestrogen has water-attracting properties which influence the amount of moisture held in the skin. If the amount of oestrogen circulating in the body is reduced, so is the amount of moisture which is available for the skin.

During the natural ageing process, there is a gradual reduction in the levels of sex hormones produced by the body. This affects the amount of sebum produced and the skin's ability to retain moisture.

2 Incorrect skin care: using harsh products strips the skin of its natural surface lubricant. If the body does not produce enough sebum to replace it quickly then the surface of the skin becomes dry, parched and irritated. Harsh products include lotions containing alcohol, alkalis, detergents and abrasives.

3 Central heating and air conditioning: these create a dry environment which takes water from wherever it can. Plants and skin are susceptible to moisture loss with similar effects! Skin which is not protected adequately against central heating and air conditioning loses its moisture to the atmosphere.

4 Extremes of temperature: when the weather is very hot or very cold the air is usually dry. Unless the skin is protected well it gives up its moisture in the same way as if it is exposed to central heating. The output of sebum is reduced on skin which is exposed to cold windy weather so there is less protection from moisture loss.

5 Over-exposure to sunlight: the sun's rays overheat and dehydrate the tissues. The effects occur not only in the surface layers but also deeper in the dermis. Sensible sunbathing consists of building up exposure times, keeping sensitive areas of skin covered and wearing a sunscreen product of an appropriate factor. If these precautions are not taken, the skin suffers considerable damage.

6 Prolonged illness: during periods of ill health, blood and lymph are diverted away from the surface tissues towards the diseased areas of the body. This reduces the amount of fluid circulating in the epidermis which leads to dehydration of the skin. Illnesses producing a high body temperature dehydrate the surface tissues. Some medicines, for example antibiotics, can cause the skin to become dry.

7 Crash dieting: water intake is reduced considerably during over-stringent dieting. This results in the body drawing on its reservoir of moisture in the skin to maintain its essential water balance. *Anorexia nervosa* is a serious diet related disease where little or no food is eaten. The production of sex hormones stops, causing changes in the body which include dehydration and thinning of the skin.

8 Smoking: smoking dilates the surface blood capillaries. This raises the temperature of the skin and can cause dryness in people who smoke heavily. The chemical toxins produced by smoking affect, adversely, the protein fibres of the skin and the way in which they hold moisture in the dermis. Prolonged smoking has degenerative effects on the walls of arteries and restricts the flow of blood to the skin.

9 Drinking too much alcohol: alcohol raises the blood pressure and, over a prolonged period, causes permanent damage to blood vessels. Chemical toxins build up in the body causing the protein fibres to harden and lose their water - binding properties. Dehydration is a short-term side effect of excessive alcohol intake. The body responds to high concentrations of chemicals in the blood by drawing water from the skin in to the circulation.

Greasy skin

Greasy skin produces more sebum than is needed to give the normal amount of lubrication and protection. Consequently, its surface appears shiny, thick, coarse, dull and often grimy. A build up of sebum in the ducts and hair follicles stretches the pores. Depending on how the skin is cared for, the pores may be open or blocked. Bacteria can penetrate open pores causing pustules. Blocked pores often result in comedones (blackheads). The thicker coating of sebum on the skin delays the rate at which desquamation takes place. Instead of being shed evenly, the cells remain 'stuck' down on the surface, accumulating more dust and grime. Meanwhile, new cells continue to be produced in the epidermis so that the overall thickness of the skin increases. This, together with the extra fatty content of the epidermis, gives the skin a sallow appearance.

Causes of greasy skin

1. Hormone imbalance: a greasy skin occurs naturally when the balance of androgens (see page 92) is higher than normal. A greasy skin commonly occurs at puberty before the balance of sex hormones has settled down.
2. Ethnic background: grease absorbs ultra-violet light. People who are natives of countries with hot sunny climates produce more sebum to help screen the skin against the damaging effects of ultra-violet.

> Remember
> Skin which produces an excess of sebum can still become dehydrated if it is not treated correctly.

Combination skin

Any combination of skin types may exist on the face where different areas show different physical characteristics. The most common combination consists of normal to dry skin over the cheeks and sides of the face, with a greasier T-zone down the centre panel. There are more sebaceous glands present on the centre panel of the face and they are situated nearer the skin surface.

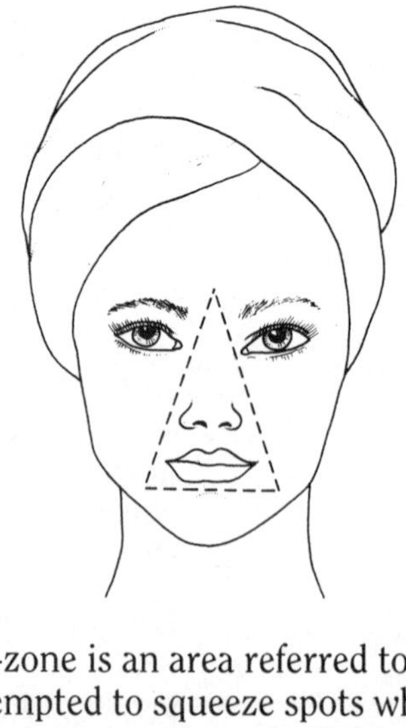

The danger triangle

Within the greasy T-zone is an area referred to as the 'danger triangle'. The client may be tempted to squeeze spots which occur there. This should be warned against very strongly. Behind this area are important blood vessels which connect with the brain. Fatalities have resulted from deep-seated bacterial infections behind the danger triangle caused by skin damage.

Sensitive

All healthy skins are sensitive, but this term is used in beauty therapy to describe a condition where the skin is hypersensitive, i.e. it over-reacts to even the mildest stimulus. The skin flushes very easily, causing redness which may appear in patches or as a clearly defined network of dilated capillaries. Skin which has been neglected over a number of years may have permanently dilated capillaries which are more pronounced when the blood supply is stimulated.

Dry skin types are the ones most likely to be sensitive. This is not surprising as they lack the protection normally given by sebum. Other types of skin can also be sensitive, however, particularly if the stimulus is an ingredient of a cosmetic or skin-care preparation.

Dehydrated

Dehydrated means lacking in moisture. The skin looks dull and parched and may feel tight and itchy. Dry skin is dehydrated but any skin type may suffer temporary dehydration if it is not properly protected and cared for.

Mature

This describes skin which has lost the firmness and suppleness of youth. It is lined and crepey, with some loss of underlying muscle tone. Skin normally ages very gradually and is described as mature once the changes brought about by ageing have become established.

White skins mature much sooner than black skins. Dry skin types mature sooner than others.

Congested

Congestion can often be felt as well as seen. The pores become blocked and waste accumulates beneath the upper layers of skin. The texture feels coarse and lumpy. Whiteheads and blackheads may be present.

The skin becomes congested when sebum and sweat are prevented from flowing freely onto the surface. This may result from inadequate cleansing of the skin, when stale make-up and other matter builds up in the mouths of the hair follicles and the sweat pores.

Another cause of congestion may be that in a humid atmosphere, sweat does not evaporate readily and this creates a build up in the ducts which carry sweat from the glands to the surface of the body. Very fatty skin care products can also clog up the pores.

If the skin's surface is not kept soft and supple, the upper layers of the epidermis harden over the openings in the skin, preventing the flow of sebum and sweat.

Blemished

Any irregularity in the colour or texture of the skin is called a blemish. A blemish may be permanent (for example a pigmented birthmark) or temporary (for example a pustule).

Blemishes must be identified correctly before recommending treatment. Most of them are harmless, many improve with beauty therapy, but there are others which must not be treated in the salon.

Infected

The appearance of infected skin depends on the nature of the infection. Bacteria, fungi and viruses affect the skin in different ways and each infection has its own distinctive characteristics. Inflammation, swelling, irritation or pain, discoloration or pus are all general signs of infection.

Strict hygiene precautions need to be taken when dealing with infected skin.

Skin characteristics: ethnic variations

The most obvious physical distinction which can be made between people of different racial origins is that of skin colour. The variety of colours is enormous, ranging from palest cream to darkest blue-black. Although we inherit our skin colour from our parents, its basic shade and tone results from years of evolution and adaptation to climatic conditions. In people native to hot sunny climates, the colour of the skin, together with variations in its thickness and structure, provide extra protection against damage from ultra-violet and the heating effects of sun on the body. A thicker epidermis with a generous sebaceous coating helps to screen out UV rays. As dark skins absorb more heat than pale skins, the larger and more numerous sweat glands of a person with black skin help to keep them cooler and more comfortable in intense heat.

> Remember
>
> People with fair skins run the greatest risk of severe sunburn, premature ageing and skin cancer. It is very important to know the best ways to protect the skin in hot sun if there is not enough melanin present to give natural protection. Sunlight is not the only threat to fair skins, which need additional protection in any extreme weather conditions.

The characteristic 'muddy' tone of a Latin complexion, while not always deeply coloured, usually has sufficient melanin present in its epidermis to enable the skin to tan quickly without burning in hot sun.

The natives of countries with a relatively mild climate do not need the same amount of protection as those living in regions with extreme climatic conditions. As a result, fairer skins are usually thinner with less active sebaceous glands. Unfortunately this means that there is very little natural protection for people with fair skins who move to or take holidays in hot sunny countries.

Ethnic variations in skin types: General characteristics

Skin type	Origin	Colour	Other features
White: Caucasian	British Scandinavian E/W Europe N America S Australia Canada New Zealand	Basic colour pale buff. Relatively small amount of melanin present. Some skins appear pinkish while others have a yellowish (sallow tone)	Hair usually red, blonde, 'mousey' or brunette Eyes usually grey, green or blue Prone to freckles (especially redheads) Skin comparatively thin, translucent and fragile Fewer and less active sebaceous glands Very limited natural defence to sunlight Greatest risk of severe sunburn, premature ageing and skin cancer (redheads with freckles most at risk)

Ethnic variations in skin types: General characteristics *continued*

Skin type	Origin	Colour	Other features
Oriental/ Light Asian	China Japan Middle East	More melanin present. Skin basically creamy coloured with tendency to yellow and olive tones	Skin very rarely shows blemishes and defies normal symptoms of ageing Oriental skin particularly remains trouble free with sparse facial and body hair Sebaceous glands less active Scars are more likely to occur and hyper-pigment causing uneveness, troughs, pits and hollows on the skin surface
Mediterranean/ Latin	Italy Spain Greece Portugal Yugoslavia S America Central America	Sallow skin with some reddish pigment. Far more melanin present which obscures the colour of blood vessels	Skin tends to have generous coating of sebum and additional fatty tissue Although oily, rarely suffers from spots, blackheads or acne Quite tough, and ages later than fairer skins Tans easily and deeply without burning Tendency to excessive hair
Dark Asian	Pakistan India Sri Lanka Malaysia	Very dark skin colours, deeply pigmented with melanin which do not reveal the blood capillaries	Smooth and supple with minimal wrinkling Ageing symptoms do not usually start until well after 40. Protein fibres degenerate much more slowly Sweat glands larger and more numerous. The sweat gives a sheen which is often mistaken for oiliness
Afro-Caribbean/ African: *Black*	West Indies Africa		Sebum fattier, sebaceous glands larger, more numerous and closer to skin surface, open pores Thick, tough skin which desquamates easily and forms keloid scars when damaged

Skin colour

The colour of skin depends on the degree of absorption and reflection of light from its surface. When light hits the skin, the epidermis absorbs some of it and reflects the rest. The reflected light is converted into a colour sensation. The colour produced is a combination of three main factors:

- melanin: the natural pigment produced by special cells in the epidermis. The intensity of light absorption is relative to the amount and type of melanin present in the skin: eumelanin -dark brown/black, pheomelanin-yellowish red
- fat: fatty material in the skin frequently has the fat-soluble vitamin carotene dissolved in it. Carotene is taken into the body in the diet and is contained in green vegetables and carrots. It has a yellowish colour and people who follow a vegetarian diet often have sallow skin because of this.
- blood: the influence of the blood on skin colour depends on the thickness of the epidermis and whether the vessels are dilated or contracted. The superficial capillaries add pink to the overall skin colour.

In black skins, fat and blood have virtually no influence on skin colour due to the density of melanin pigment. The paler the skin, the more significant the contribution of blood and fat.

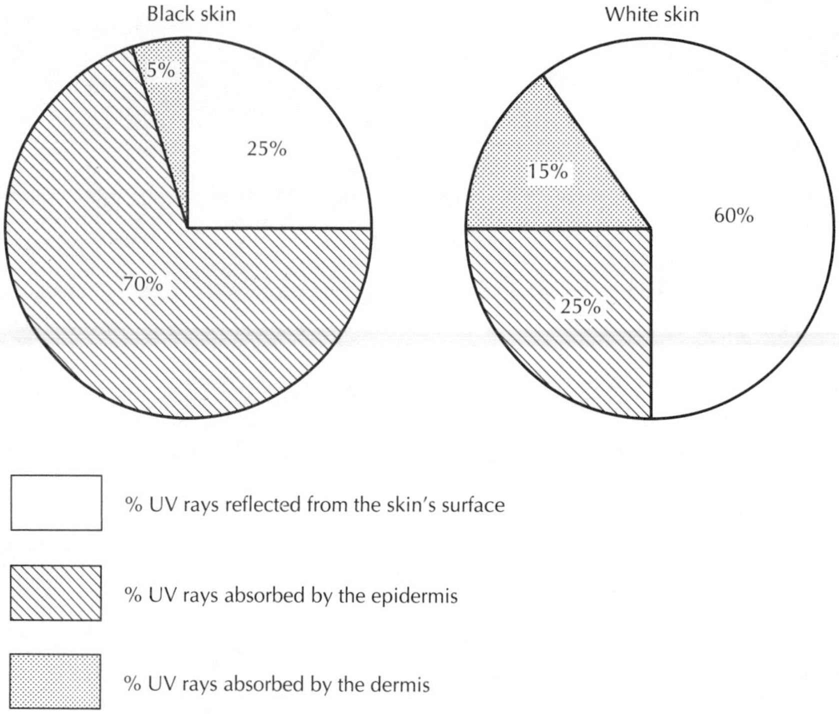

Percentage of UV light reflection and absorption by black and white skin

How melanin is produced

The normal natural skin colour relies on a constant process of melanin production. Melanocytes, present in the germinating layer of the epidermis, inject coloured granules, melanosomes, into adjacent keratinocytes. These cells then carry melanin upwards through the layers of the epidermis to produce a dense layer of pigment. The shade of the skin is determined by the size, maturity and distribution of the pigment granules:

- size: melanosomes are larger in dark skin than in fair skin.
- maturity: the melanosomes go through various stages of development before reaching maturity. Only fully matured cells transfer melanin with them into the keratinocytes. In dark skin, all the melanosomes produced reach maturity. In fair skin, not all the melanosomes reach this state. The melanocytes in dark skins are always in an active state, unlike those in fair skin which need stimulating into activity.
- distribution: the epidermis of dark skins is more densely packed with melanin than fair skins.

Sometimes the transfer of melanin into the keratinocytes is blocked. When this happens, no colour is produced.

Developing a suntan

The production of extra melanin in the skin involves chemical processes which take between 36 and 48 hours following initial exposure to sunlight. In fair people, it takes considerably longer to produce enough melanin to protect the skin.

This is not always appreciated by holiday-makers anxious to make a start on developing their tans as soon as they reach their sunny destination. All too often, the sore pinkness of sunburn during the first few days of a holiday is mistaken for the initial stages of sun tan development. This is not the case.

> Remember
> Burning and tanning are two separate processes. Burning is neither essential nor desirable before tanning. Sunburn causes extensive damage to living cells.

People with active melanocytes in their skin develop a tan much more readily than those whose melanocytes are inactive. Increased intensities of ultra-violet develop the colour of the melanin and speed up the rate at which the pigment bearing cells travel up to the surface of the skin. People with inactive melanocytes burn in the sun if their skin is not well protected.

Ultra-violet rays

The sun gives out heat, light and other rays which travel towards the earth. Most of the harmful rays are absorbed by the atmosphere. The ones that reach Earth are made up of visible light (white light or daylight), infra-red (produces heat) and ultra-violet. It is the ultra-violet which produces a suntan. Ultra-violet is made up of rays of different wave lengths:

- UVA: these rays have a long wave length and work on melanin granules already contained in the upper epidermis. They produce a rapid tan in people who tan easily. UVA rays speed up the ageing processes of the skin. They damage the protein fibres which make the skin firm and supple. Sometimes they cause allergies. UVA rays are thought to enhance the effects of UVB.
- UVB: these rays have a medium wave length and are strong enough to penetrate cells, making them produce more melanin. They also cause thickening of the epidermis. The tan produced by UVB rays takes longer to appear than with UVA: the melanin producing cells have to be stimulated into activity before working their way up through the layers of epidermis. However, the resulting tan lasts much longer. UVB rays cause sunburn and are known to be a major cause of skin cancer in people with fair skins. The gradual thinning of the ozone layer is causing more UVB rays to reach the earth.

> Remember
> The ozone layer is a layer of ozone gas which exists high up in the atmosphere, about twenty miles away from the earth's surface. The ozone layer prevents much of the ultra-violet produced by the sun from reaching Earth. Other gases, such as those produced by aerosols, rise up and replace or break down some of the ozone. This makes the layer a less effective barrier to the sun's rays.

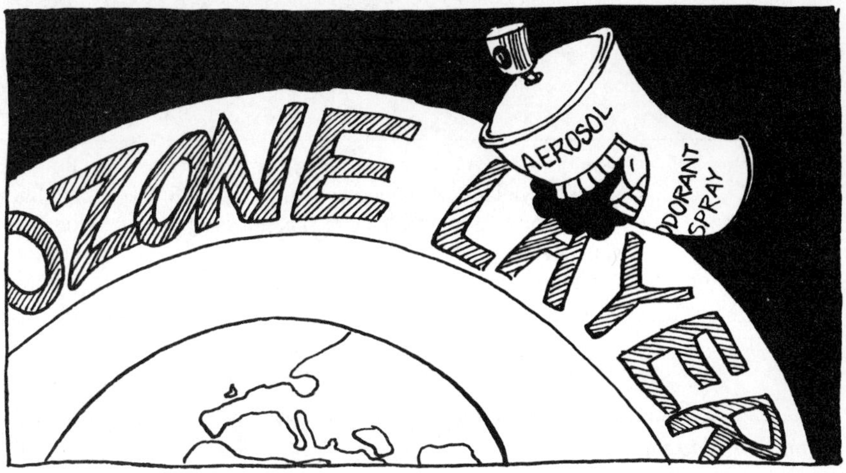

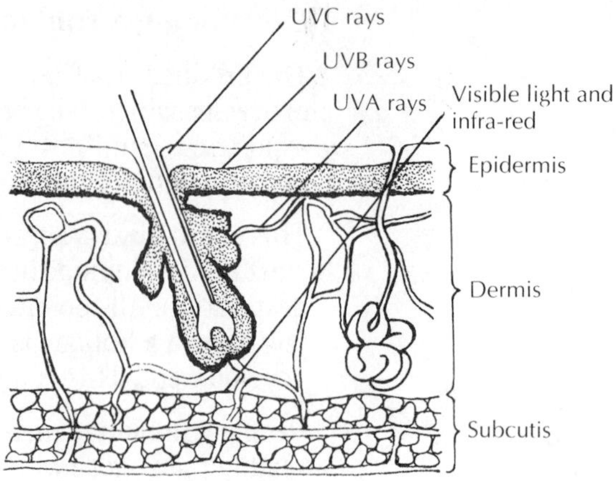

Penetration levels of UV rays through skin

- UVC: these rays have the shortest wave length and 'cut off' before they reach the earth. They do not reach the skin. UVC rays are very destructive. They are often used in sterilisation procedures because they destroy living cells. When the ozone layer is intact, it acts as a barrier to UVC rays.

Type	Features	Advice
Easy tanner	Skin quite fair but sallow; goes red at first then tans very easily. The melanocytes are active: exposure to strong sunlight speeds up the rate at which they produce melanin	Remember that there is a risk of burning on initial exposure to strong sunlight. Don't rush into prolonged sunbathing sessions without proper protection. Build up exposure times and wear a suitable sunscreen. Reapply it regularly. Remember that areas of the body which are usually covered will need extra protection from the sun. Always apply after-sun skin care to compensate for moisture loss.
Fast tanner	There is already a lot of melanin developed in the skin, so it can tan very quickly; the fast tanner very rarely suffers sunburn	There is always a slight risk of burning at first if sensible precautions are not taken. Avoid over-exposure. Protect the skin with a suitable sunscreen and reapply it regularly. Always apply after-sun skin care
No hoper!	Very pale skin which does not contain enough active melanocytes to produce a tan. The skin burns very easily. Sometimes small clusters of melanin appear as freckles and the skin burns in between them	Accept that you are not going to get a tan and be sensible about protecting the skin in the sun. Wear loose light clothing a good sunscreen (preferably a total sun-block) and a big hat. Stay n the shade as much as possible. Congratulate yourself on how well you are nursing your collagen through prolonged youth by keeping it away from harmful ultra-violet!
Slow tanner	Skin quite fair. Very little developed melanin in the skin. Melanocytes need activating by UVB to stimulate melanin production. Skin goes red very easily but tans eventually. Initial impatience invariably leads to burning which prolongs the overall time required to develop a healthy looking tan. Freckles may increase in size and join up to produce larger, brown patches	Build up exposure times gradually. Avoid sunbathing when the sun is at its hottest (usually between midday and 2 p.m.). Use a suitable sunscreen and reapply it regularly, particularly before and after going in the sea. Use after-sun products to soothe the skin and keep it moisturised

Which tanning type are you?

Sunbathing can damage your health!

Sunlight is the major cause of skin cancer, and it is not only older people who are at risk: in Australia, children as young as 13 have died of skin cancer because they did not wear a sunscreen. These were people who were used to living in a sunny climate and took it for granted. Only black skins have built in protection against the ravaging effects of strong sunshine: if you were not born with black skin, wear a sunscreen suitable for your skin type. This will reduce the amount of UVB rays which penetrate the skin and will enable you to stay out in the sun for longer without getting burned.

Characteristics of skin by facial area

Forehead

The skin of the forehead contains very little fat and fits closely to the broad, flattish frontal bone underneath. There are numerous sebaceous glands present and the area is contained in the greasy T-zone of a typical combination skin. Pimples, pustules and blackheads characteristic of greasy skin often affect the forehead. These become aggravated if the hair is also greasy and worn with a fringe.

Horizontal creases develop across the forehead as the muscles and skin lose their tone. Deep vertical creases between the eyebrows are also a sign of ageing but can occur as the result of prolonged eyestrain and stress.

Eyes

The area surrounding the eyes consists of two moveable skin folds, the upper and lower eyelids. The skin of the eyelids is very thin and does not usually contain fat. There are very few sebaceous glands so the skin easily becomes dehydrated and develops lines, wrinkles and crepiness before any other part of the face. The skin underneath the eyes becomes even thinner with ageing and the blood supply network shows through as a reddish blue colour. Glands can also be seen as tiny, skin-coloured lumps.

The contour of the eye area changes where the lower eyelid meets the upper cheek. Ageing causes a rift to develop between the two as support is lost from the dermis. Eventually, a broad, thin skinned, semi-circular depression cleaves itself into the tissues below the eye, causing a deeply shadowed groove.

Dark circles beneath the eye are a common complaint and can worsen on excessive exposure to sunlight, particularly if plain glasses are worn which focus light on the lower lid and upper cheek. The eyelids and eye sockets are danger zones in the sun as reflected rays bounce onto them from the frames of sunglasses. Tiredness and ill health can also cause dark shadows beneath the eyes. The condition can also be inherited and is common in races with a very sallow complexion.

Tiredness, hay fever, sinus problems and catarrh congest the tissues around the eyes and make them swell up. Very greasy and heavy creams clog up the pores and lead to fluid retention and puffiness. This is particularly a problem when the cream is left on overnight and seeps into the eyes. Heavy creams also drag the skin, encouraging it to slacken.

Rubbing and pulling the skin around the eyes also causes wear and tear, and constant rubbing can result in split capillaries and over-stretching of the skin. Milia (whiteheads) often occur near the eyes.

Crow's feet lines develop over the orbicularis oculi muscle and fan out over the temples and the upper part of the cheek. They are a characteristic of ageing and are much more noticeable on skin which has thickened as a result of weathering. Crow's feet can be caused prematurely by any prolonged habit of screwing up the eyes, in bright sunlight or when smoking. Laughing and smiling are the most acceptable causes of crow's feet!

Nose

The nose is the most prominent of the facial features and varies in width and shape between individuals and different races. Only the upper part of the nose is constructed from bone; the main part of it is made up of cartilage which is soft and flexible.

The skin of the nose is abundantly supplied with sebaceous glands which are larger than normal and situated near the surface. The nose is contained in the T-zone of a typical combination skin and generally has a tendency to greasiness with the associated problems of open pores, blocked pores and comedones (blackheads). Spots and pustules often occur here. The creases at either side of the nostrils accumulate grease and sweat and make-up often builds up in them if they are not cleansed thoroughly. The prominence of the nose exposes it to the effects of sunlight and harsh winds. If adequate protection is not worn, the capillaries in the skin dilate and often rupture, leaving a permanently red nose. Split capillaries can also result from pressure put on the nose when rubbing too harshly, perhaps when washing the face, or during a heavy cold with continued blowing.

Indentations at either side of the upper part of the nose are characteristic of people who wear glasses. Constant friction between the skin and the heavier types of frame can rupture the underlying blood vessels.

Cheeks

The skin of the cheeks is smooth, firm and plump in youth but gradually, as moisture, fat and support are lost from the deeper layers, the cheeks lose their full contour and the underlying bone structure becomes more prominent. It is usually only people who are overweight that do not develop a more gaunt appearance as they get older.

The contour of the cheekbones is determined by the structure of the zygomatic arch. This is formed where the zygomatic and temporal bones join. A prominence is created which gives shape to the upper cheek. High cheekbones are generally regarded as being an attractive feature.

The prominence of the cheekbones pushes the superficial blood capillaries nearer the surface of the skin. This makes them more likely to be damaged by lack of protection or incorrect skin care. Dilated capillaries often occur over the cheekbones, particularly on skin which is dry and sensitive.

The skin of the cheeks easily becomes dry and dehydrated if it is not kept soft and well moisturised. Milia often occur above the cheekbones and up towards the temples. The main muscles which move the mouth are located in the cheeks. As the zygomatic and risorius muscles become slack, they cause the nose-to-mouth lines to deepen. The skin above the creases creates the naso-labial folds which are characteristic of ageing. The folds can be produced prematurely by rapid weight loss after illness or strict dieting.

Mouth

The shape of the mouth becomes slightly smaller and less well defined with age. The gums shrink slightly, pulling the skin of the lips inwards and lines develop across the fibres of the orbicularis oris muscle. The deeper these lines get, the more difficult lipstick application becomes. Tension and smoking can also cause lines to appear around the mouth. Deep creases also develop down from the corners of the mouth, as the levator muscles of the upper lip lose their tone and the skin slackens. These lines are exaggerated in people who wear ill-fitting dentures.

Many women become aware of an acceleration in hair growth above the upper lip as they approach middle-age. Dark hair growth in this area is a particular problem in races with a tendency to excessive facial hairiness.

The lips do not contain melanin and burn more easily in the sun: the mouth is a prime site for skin cancer.

Chin and jaw

The front part of the chin is contained in the T-zone and tends to be more greasy than other areas of the face: it is a common site of blocked pores, comedones, pimples and pustules. The area of the lower jaw is similarly affected when acne is present. The horizontal crease in the chin becomes particularly congested if it is not cleansed properly.

The contour of the chin and jawline drops or softens with age. Jowls appear at the angles of the jaw, caused by loss of tone in the masseter muscle. The skin hangs loosely and breaks up the previously sharp, angular shape.

A double chin develops when the deep digastric muscle loses tone. Depending on the severity of the condition, the slackened tissue drops behind the prominence of the chin and fills in the area between it and the upper neck. Although age is the most common cause of a double chin, bad posture is also a factor.

Neck

The neck is often a neglected area in a skin care routine. It is not deep-cleansed and massaged as often and can look sallow and sluggish compared with the face.

The lack of bony support and relatively small amount of fat mean that the skin is attached fairly loosely to the underlying structures. It is pulled and stretched quite easily.

The neck is the first area to lose fat and this will be noticeable in people who have lost a lot of weight through illness or strict dieting. Gradual loss of fat from the neck also occurs during the ageing process. In a very mature person, the front edges of the platysma muscle show through the skin quite clearly. There are very few sebaceous glands in the skin of the neck, so dryness and crepiness are common problems. The necklace lines created over the platysma muscle deepen with age.

Fibrous skin tags often occur on the neck. They are harmless but can become irritating if they are situated where they catch on collars or necklace chains. Sometimes the neck does not receive enough protection in bright sun: rays which catch the neck at a sideways angle can cause damage. Apart from the destructive effects on collagen and elastin, burning by the sun's rays can leave the neck permanently blotchy and discoloured. A patch of brown pigmentation is sometimes evident on each side of the neck when perfume containing a photo-sensitising ingredient (reacting with sun) has been applied directly to the skin from the bottle.

Contra-indications to facial treatments

> Remember
>
> Always examine the skin before treatment and question the client to make sure that there are no contra-indications present which make the treatment unsuitable.

Beauty therapy treatments are designed to improve the appearance and condition of the skin and to help control minor skin problems. They should never be applied to areas of skin which are sore, damaged or infected or where there is a risk of the skin reacting adversely to treatment.

Failure to recognise or respond to a contra-indication could result in:

- cross-infection: an infectious disease could spread to other areas of the face and, also, to other clients or salon staff
- prolonging the condition: disturbing infected or damaged skin could interfere with the natural healing process
- worsening the condition: stimulating treatments could put further strain on damaged blood vessels and also speed up the rate of abnormal activity of diseased skin cells.

The general contra-indications to facial treatments are:

- undiagnosed lumps, bumps and swellings
- cuts and abrasions
- any infectious skin condition
- recent scar tissue (less than six months)
- severe sunburn
- allergic reaction
- malignant tumour.

Most contra-indications are short-term and the client can be reassured that treatment may be given as soon as the skin has recovered. Some contra-indications create a longer-term problem: if there is a serious skin infection or you are suspicious about abnormal changes in the skin, refer the client to their GP for medical advice. In most cases, once the client has been cleared by the doctor, beauty therapy treatment may resume.

Skin types: self-checks

A Fill in the missing words.

1 Skin which is permanently flushed or goes red easily is ____________.

2 Dehydrated skin lacks ______________. It looks _____________ and may feel ________________.

3 Mature skin is no longer _____________ and _______________.

4 Pus is a sign of _____________.

5 Any irregularity in the colour or texture of the skin is called a _____________.

6 A __________ skin is a healthy skin.

7 Dry skin does not have enough ____________.

8 Comedones occur commonly on ____________ skin.

9 Strong sunlight is harmful to the skin because it contains __________.

10 A ____________ skin rarely develops spots and blemishes.

B Answer the following questions.

1 Why is eating a balanced diet essential for healthy skin?

2 How does over-tiredness affect the skin?

3 State two possible causes of permanently dilated capillaries.

4 Give two benefits for the skin of regular exercise.

5 Why is smoking bad for the skin?

6 How do sex hormones affect the skin?

7 Why do our skin and hair suffer when we are ill?

8 Why is greasy skin sallow?

9 What is the significance of the 'T zone'?

10 How is black skin better equipped for being in strong sunshine than white skin?

11 Why do pale skins usually appear more sensitive than darker skins?

12 What advice should be given to a fair-skinned client who is about to go on holiday in a hot sunny climate?

13 Distinguish between UVA and UVB rays.

14 Why must the ozone layer above the earth be preserved?

Skin types: Activities

1 Good product knowledge is essential for you to be able to choose and recommend with confidence the best skin-care preparations for your clients. You must know all about the range of products available in your salon. Make out a treatment chart for each of the basic skin types, referring to products for both salon use and home care. Do not forget to include special treatment preparations, for example for eyes and neck.

2 Practise examining the skin through an illuminated magnifier. You will need to reposition the lamp for examining different areas. Examine as many different 'clients' as you can. Make sure their skin is clean and then go through the full examination procedure. Record your findings and ask a supervisor to check your results.

3 Write out some closed and open questions which would be suitable for asking a client with each of the following:
a) split capillaries over the cheek bones
b) a patch of discoloration on the side of the neck
c) dark shadows underneath the eyes
d) congestion of the skin which is more severe on the chin and forehead
e) excessively dry skin.

Chapter 5

Facial massage and skin care

After working through this chapter you will be able to:

- ▶ understand the importance of basic skin care
- ▶ choose appropriate products for salon treatments
- ▶ sell skin-care products for home use
- ▶ relate the benefits of skin-care products to their contents and methods of use
- ▶ design a skin-care programme for a range of different skin types and conditions
- ▶ state the benefits of facial massage and other skin-care treatments
- ▶ carry out a basic facial treatment.

A beautiful skin is a healthy skin. Good skin care, practised routinely, helps to keep the skin healthy by:

- keeping the outer surface clean, smooth and soft
- ensuring there is enough moisture in the upper layers
- feeding living cells and tissues with a healthy supply of blood
- helping the skin to resist infection and infestation
- providing protection from external damage.

The first step towards good skin care is choosing the right products. It is important for a salon to research the market well before deciding upon which range or ranges to carry. Price is not always the most important factor. A salon which offers a range of specialised facial treatments will need different types of products for both salon use and retail.

A basic skin care programme should include the regular and correct use of cleansers, exfoliants, toning lotions, moisturisers, face masks and products for evening care. Specialised skin care ranges provide for every type of skin and include preparations for treating specific skin problems.

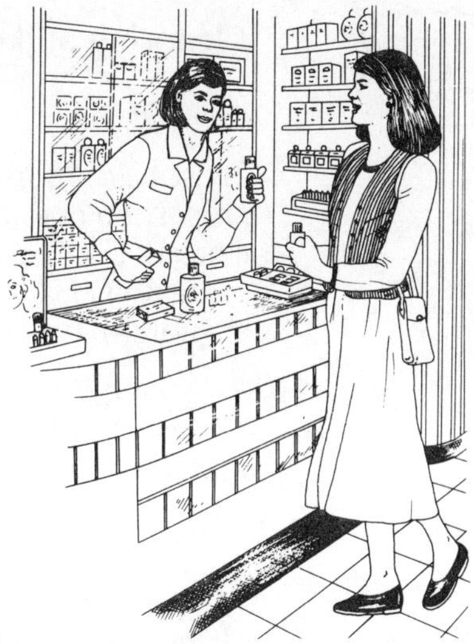

The reception is a good place to display the salon's retail skin care range.

Cleansing

Skin care products and beauty treatments will not be effective if there is make-up or other surface matter presenting a barrier. 'Active' treatments rely on the absorption of substances through the hair follicles and inter-cellular spaces of the epidermis. If these channels are blocked, there is no way through.

Dirt and grime which accumulate on the skin prevent efficient desquamation and block up the pores. Make-up which becomes stale on the skin irritates its surface and blemishes appear. Over the course of the day, the skin's secretions attract dust, parasites and pollution from the atmosphere. These create further congestion which must be dealt with efficiently, or the skin's natural functions become seriously challenged.

Cleansers

> Remember
>
> An emulsifying agent is an ingredient which allows oil and water to mix together instead of separating. Borax is an emulsifying agent which is often contained in skin creams to stabilise the mixture.

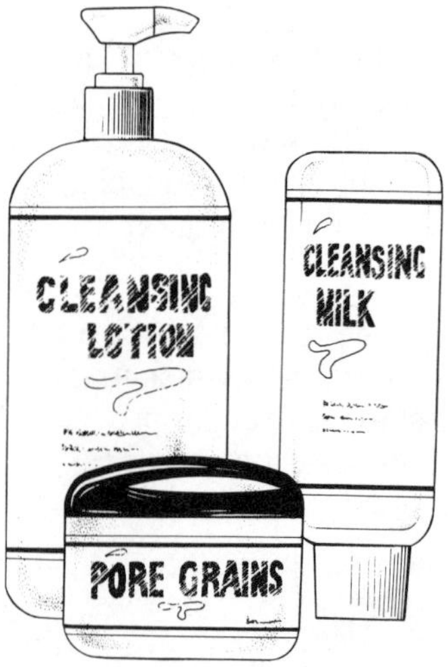

Cleansers are available as creams, milks, oils, lotions, cleansing bars and facial scrubs. Most cleansers are a basic oil and water emulsion with the addition of perfume, and, sometimes, a detergent. Products which contain a higher proportion of oil than water (w/o) have a heavier, creamier texture. Those with a high water content (o/w) are lighter and more fluid.

Cleansing creams

Contents

The mineral oil in a cleansing cream dissolves grease and oil-based products on the skin. A wax such as beeswax or paraffin wax is often added to give the cream a stiffer texture. The water content cools the skin and makes the cream easier to spread.

Uses

Cleansing creams are particularly good for removing make-up and for cleansing balanced and dry types of skin. They melt quickly when applied to the skin but do not soak in, so provide a good medium for the deep-cleanse massage movements.

Cleansing milks

Contents

These have a similar formulation to creams but with a much higher proportion of water and a little detergent added. They are not as efficient as creams for dissolving make-up. The detergent and water content of cleansing milks emulsifies grease on the skin. Because they are water-based, cleansing milks are easier than creams to wipe off the skin.

Some cleansing milks can be worked up into a lather with water to wash the face. Others with a higher oil content will effectively remove a light make-up.

Uses

Clients often prefer the lighter texture of cleansing milks. Their detergent action makes them particularly suitable for younger, greasier skins. More mature clients with a tendency to dryness should only use cleansing milks with a specified high oil content.

Make-up remover

Contents

Water is neither necessary nor effective for removing make-up, whereas oil is absolutely essential. Make-up remover may consist purely of a mineral oil, such as liquid paraffin with a little perfume added, or it may contain a soft wax, for example paraffin wax, to make it more solid. This type of product melts as soon as it is applied and feels just like oil on the skin.

Uses

Special make-up removers are very useful for dissolving stubborn waterproof mascara and heavy wax-based theatrical make-up.

Eye make-up remover pads consist of round pieces of lint soaked in mineral oil.

Cleansing lotions

Contents

These are solutions of detergents in water. Some contain anti-bacterial ingredients (for example hexachlorophene) to medicate a greasy blemished problem skin. Cleansing lotions are not suitable for removing make-up as they do not contain any oil.

Uses

The degreasing action of these products makes them particularly useful for younger blemished skins. They can sometimes be used as a substitute for soap by clients who like to wash their face.

Cleansing bars

Contents

These look and feel like bars of soap, but are actually compressed blocks of cleansing cream containing a soapless detergent. They lather up with water and feel the same as soap, without any of the undesirable side effects. Cleansing bars are usually alkaline-free and have a pH which helps to preserve the natural acid mantle of the skin.

Uses

A cleansing bar may be used to wash the face after removing make-up but it must be rinsed off thoroughly afterwards.

What's wrong with soap?

People with greasy skin are more likely than others to be able to wash their face with soap and water without suffering any ill-effects. The skin stabilises itself quite quickly once the sebaceous glands have produced enough sebum to restore the acid mantle.

People with normal to dry skin run the risk of dehydrating the skin, causing it to become parched, flaky, tight, sore and inflamed. This is because soap is a strong detergent. It strips the skin of grease, thereby removing its protective coating.

Thorough rinsing is not always the answer. Soft water is good for the skin but hard water is lethal! It contains insoluble salts which settle on the skin and dry it out even more. The skin feels very tight after rinsing with hard water.

Soap will not form a lather in hard water. Instead it forms a scum which is also bad for the skin.

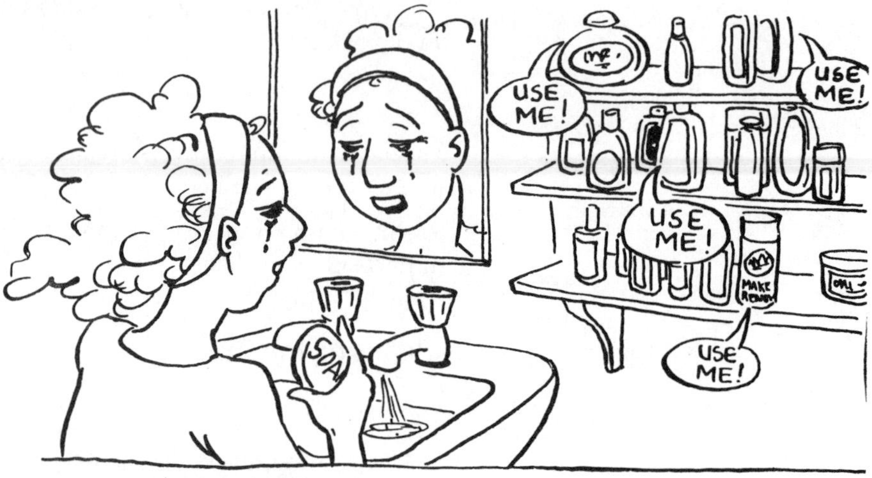

Soap does not remove make-up either!

Cleansing: Self-checks

1 a) What does w/o emulsion mean?
b) Give one example of a skin-care product which is a w/o emulsion.

2 a) Why is a detergent sometimes contained in a cleanser?
b) State one type of cleansing product which contains a detergent.

3 a) Give two advantages of using an 'oily' eye make-up remover.
b) State the type of oil which is usually contained in an eye make-up remover.

4 a) What are 'medicated' skin-care products?
b) Why are medicated skin-care products not suitable for all skin types?

5 a) State three reasons why a client should be advised against using soap for cleansing the face.
b) Give two preferable alternatives to soap.

6 a) List three features of a good cleanser.
b) Why is skin cleansing important?

Exfoliants

To *exfoliate* means to peel off in scales or layers. All types of skin benefit from the weekly use of exfoliating products to brighten up the complexion and refine the skin texture. The rate of skin cell renewal slows down with age and mature skins appear particularly dull as dead skin cells build up on the surface. Special skin treatments are more effective when applied after using an exfoliant.

Facial scrubs

Contents

These products are basically cleansing milks containing a granular material such as ground olive stones, oatmeal or synthetic grains. Facial scrubs have a detergent cleansing action.

Uses

When facial scrubs are massaged over the skin, they have a slightly abrasive effect which loosens dead cells and surface debris and leaves the skin feeling clean, soft and smooth. They should not be used too vigorously or they will over-stimulate the skin and make it sore. Facial scrubs are recommended particularly for greasy skin. The abrasive action helps to loosen surface blockages and improve skin colour.

Peeling creams

Contents

These are usually water-soluble emulsions containing clay for absorbency and natural, biological ingredients to help slough of skin cells and prevent skin irritation.

Uses

Peeling creams are suitable for any skin type but are particularly recommended for dry, mature and sensitive skins which require gentle exfoliation.

Exfoliants: Self-checks

1 a) What is an *exfoliant*?
  b) Explain the benefits of using an exfoliant.

Toning lotions

These have an astringent effect which cools and refreshes the skin. Strong astringents tighten the skin temporarily and make the pores appear smaller. They contain alcohol which dissolves grease and completes the cleansing process.

Toning lotions help to restore the acid balance of the skin after washing or cleansing and are wiped over the skin between different stages of a facial treatment. The strength of a toning lotion depends on the amount of alcohol it contains: skin tonics contain 20–60% alcohol, bracers and fresheners contain 0–20% alcohol.

Skin tonics

Contents

In addition to alcohol, these contain other powerful astringent ingredients such as witch hazel or alum. They dissolve grease and have an anti-bacterial effect on the skin. When the alcohol evaporates off the skin, the superficial blood vessels contract and the skin feels very cold.

Uses

Skin tonics which contain more than 25% alcohol are only suitable for greasy skin. Serious dehydration is likely to occur if a skin tonic containing more than 50% alcohol is used. Milder tonics may be used on a balanced skin to remove the film of grease which remains after cleansing.

Bracers and fresheners

The lower concentration of alcohol in these products makes them less efficient at removing grease. The basic ingredient of bracers is often a flower water such as rose or orange blossom. Bracers containing up to 22.5% alcohol do not usually dry out the skin any more than water would. Fresheners containing 0–10% alcohol often have soothing ingredients added such as azulene, camomile and allantoin.

Uses

Bracers containing alcohol may remove a light film of grease, but those with no alcohol will only remove water-soluble debris from the skin.

> Remember
> Stronger toning lotions are required for removing excess cream from the skin. Milder ones should be used for applying directly to clean skin when there is no greasy barrier.

Recommended % alcohol content in toning lotions for different skin types

Greasy	25–50%
Balanced	10–25%
Dry	0–20%
Sensitive	0–10%

Toning lotions: Self-checks

1 a) Give two reasons why it is important to know the amount of alcohol contained in a toning lotion.
b) Distinguish between a skin tonic and a skin freshener.

Moisturisers

The most important ingredient of a moisturiser is water. Moisture which is lost from the skin needs replacing quickly so that the surface is kept soft and smooth. The living cells in the deeper layers need water so that they will not shrivel and die. If water is splashed onto the skin, it will not stay there. Moisturisers are basically oil and water emulsions which contain a humectant. This ingredient attracts water and helps to 'fix' it in the upper layers of the skin. Tinted moisturisers are available as an alternative to foundation. They sometimes contain UVA and UVB sunscreens to help protect the skin from the damaging effects of sunlight.

> Remember
> Moisturiser should be worn under make-up to:
> - even out skin texture and provide a smooth base for foundation
> - keep the make-up looking nicer for longer by fixing it on to the skin
> - act as a barrier between the skin and make-up so that cleansing is made easier
> - help prevent the penetration of pigmented products into the pores.

Moisturising creams

Contents

These contain approximately 60% water. Their relatively high proportion of oil or wax prevents natural moisture escaping from the deeper layers of skin. Ingredients such as glycerol, glycerine or sorbitol are contained as the humectant.

Uses

Creams are recommended particularly for people with dry skin who benefit from the emollient (softening) effects of the oil and waxes contained in the moisturiser. A cream moisturiser should be worn when the surrounding atmosphere is dry and there is an increased risk of natural moisture loss, for example in central heating and extremes of hot and cold weather.

Moisturising milks

Contents

These have a more fluid consistency because of their higher water content (at least 85%). Apart from increasing the amount of moisture in the upper layers of skin, they attract water from the atmosphere.

> Remember
> A dry atmosphere will take up water from wherever it can. Moisturiser must be replaced frequently to compensate for this. If the water content evaporates, dry air will then draw natural moisture out of the skin.

Uses

Moisturising milks have a lighter texture than creams and soak quickly into the upper layers of a parched dry skin. They are sometimes preferred by clients who do not want a greasy film left on the skin.

Moisturisers: Self-checks

1 a) Why do moisturisers contain a humectant?
  b) Give one example of a humectant which is often contained in a moisturiser.

2 a) Why is it important to keep the skin soft?
  b) What technical word describes the softening effect of a skin-care product?

Cleansing, toning, exfoliants and moisturising: Activities

1 Collect information about all the products available in your salon:
- read the packages and labels to discover the main ingredients
- learn about their specific uses and effects
- note the advice given regarding application and removal of the products
- make sure you know the different sizes available in retail lines and their selling prices.

2 Have a look at some of the record cards at your salon which have been completed for facial clients:
- read the information given about the client's skin and see what recommendations have been made for skin care
- notice the combinations of products which are used for salon treatments and home care.

3 Find out which skin-care products sell particularly well in your salon. Think of ways the salon could promote the sales of slow moving lines.

Evening care

Most people do not have time available to pay attention to their skin during the day. Consequently the effects of the weather, the environment, dust and pollution take their toll. Together with tiredness and, maybe, irregular eating habits, the skin suffers. The evening is usually the best time for treating the skin, when make-up has been removed and the skin has been cleansed and toned.

Clients who come for facials should be encouraged to use special products for evening care which maintain the benefits of their salon treatments.

Night creams

Contents

These are water-in-oil emulsions with special ingredients such as vegetable and plant extracts added for treating particular skin conditions.

Collagen and elastin are sometimes contained in 'anti-wrinkle' creams. It is unlikely that they have any effect on the natural fibrous proteins of the skin but, being humectants, they are useful moisturising ingredients.

Uses

Often described as 'nourishing' creams, these products are emollients. They soften, balance and refine skin texture and help to combat the effects of dehydration and ageing on the skin. Some creams are claimed to improve the elasticity of the skin. This is due to them keeping the surface of the skin soft and pliable so that it does not crack over underlying muscle activity.

Ampoules

Contents

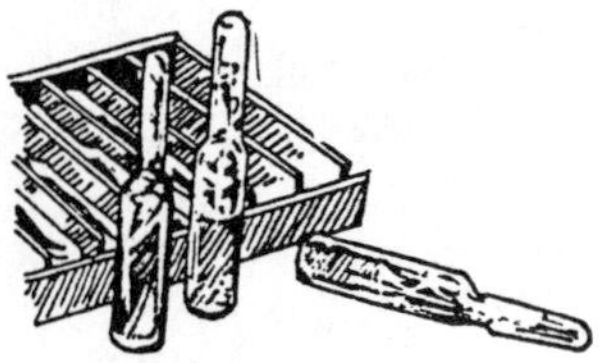

These come packed in hermetically sealed glass phials which keep the ingredients fresh and 'active'. Once the ampoule is opened, the concentrated biological ingredients must be used up to prevent them deteriorating. The 'active' ingredients are selected according to the type and condition of the skin.

Uses

The ampoules are often recommended for use as intensive treatments over a prescribed period. Others may be used regularly, once or twice a week, to complement the regular skin care given with other products from the range. Ampoules are most effective when used after a skin-peeling treatment. They are absorbed by the skin so that they affect it at a deeper level than the surface of the epidermis.

> Remember
> The active ingredients contained in skin care products are most effective during the hours of sleep, when the skin is most receptive.

There is a very wide range of 'active' biological ingredients used in skin care products. You must become familiar with the ones contained in your salon's skin care range. Here are some examples and their uses:

- horse-chestnut, camphor, sage: greasy skin with open pores
- juniper, lemongrass, birch, nettle: acneified skin
- collagen, elastin, patchouli, rosewood: dry skin showing fine lines and signs of premature ageing
- sandalwood, camomile, lavender: mature, dehydrated, sensitive skin
- eucalyptus, lavender: highly coloured, vascular skin.

Eye care

The skin around the eyes is very thin and does not contain many sebaceous glands. It is attached very loosely to the underlying muscles and lacks the fatty supporting tissue which is present in other areas of the face. As a result, the skin in the eye area is the first to show signs of ageing. Dryness, crepiness and wrinkles appear prematurely if the skin is not cared for properly.

Eye creams

Contents

These are basically moisturising creams which contain lightweight fatty materials so that they do not drag and stretch the skin. Very fine oil-in-water emulsions are absorbed easily by the skin and create a good base for eye make-up. Richer water-in-oil emulsions are greasier and are applied at night time.

> Remember
>
> It is important to avoid overloading the eye area with greasy cream at night. The heat of the body during sleep causes a rich cream to melt and invade the eye area. The cream blocks the tear ducts so that fluid becomes retained and the eyes appear puffy in the morning.

Uses

Eye creams used regularly help to prevent the formation of lines and wrinkles around the eyes. The more lightweight products may be used during the day and at night: they are suitable for all skin types.

Richer eye creams are particularly beneficial for dry or mature skins. They are massaged gently into the skin at night time and the excess is blotted off before going to bed.

Eye gels

Contents

These are basically astringents thickened with an ingredient such as methyl cellulose. They work by cooling, soothing, firming and tightening the skin. Witch-hazel is an astringent often used in eye gels. Other ingredients which may be included are plant and herbal extracts, collagen, camomile and azulene.

Uses

The astringent effect of eye gels makes them particularly useful for revitalising tired eyes and reducing the effects of fine lines, puffiness and slackness of the skin.

Eye lotions

Contents

These are similar to eye gels but do not contain a thickening ingredient. A mild astringent such as zinc sulphate is combined with plant extracts to produce a gentle lotion.

Uses

The lotion is usually applied on cotton wool as an eye compress to cool, soothe, tighten and refresh tired eyes.

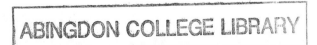

Evening care: Self-checks

1 What are the benefits of applying skin-care products at night?

2 Why should excess cream be removed from around the eyes before going to bed?

3 What are the differences between an eye gel and an eye cream?

Neck care

Many people only start paying attention to their neck when it starts to show signs of ageing. The skin on the neck is thicker than the skin around the eyes but otherwise they have a similar structure and share the same problems.

Neck Creams

Contents

A very rich cream formulation which may contain collagen for moisturising and other ingredients such as plant extracts for softening, tightening and stimulating the skin.

Uses

Neck creams should be used regularly by clients over the age of twenty-five to help soften, tighten and brighten the skin and to aid cellular renewal.

Neck care: Self-check

1 Why does the neck require special skin care?

Selling points

When selling skin care, you should describe the *features* of the products and explain their *benefits* to the client.

Features are the main ingredients and their effects plus any special features of the product, for example:

- fragrance free
- bio-degradable packaging
- not tested on animals
- double-concentrated, so more economical
- contains plant extracts.

Benefits must relate to the client's particular needs, for example:

- particular skin problems
- lifestyle
- ease of use
- reason for buying
- personal preferences.

You will get a better idea of your client's needs by asking questions and listening carefully to the answers.

Face masks

There is a very wide range of ready mixed face masks available for home use. These should be used weekly as part of a regular skin care programme for deep-cleansing the skin and softening and refining its texture.

Non-setting masks cool and refresh the skin. They are easy to apply and can be used for helping to control specific skin problems.

Setting masks dry out on the skin. They usually contain natural earth ingredients which absorb surface matter and draw out impurities. They leave the skin feeling very clean and fresh and some of them help to nourish the skin by stimulating its blood supply.

There are four basic types of face mask which are used for professional beauty treatments: clay-based, peel-off, thermal and biological masks.

Clay-based masks

Contents

A variety of clays and other mineral ingredients are mixed with distilled water, witch hazel or rosewater to produce a creamy textured paste which is painted on the skin and allowed to dry. As the moisture evaporates, the mask contracts and tightens the skin beneath. Impurities are drawn to the surface. The clay content absorbs grease, sweat and loose skin cells and, depending on the ingredients of the mask, the blood supply is either stimulated or soothed. A vegetable oil can be substituted for water to produce a non-setting clay mask.

> Remember
> Use an oil that is not too expensive and does not smell. Arachis (peanut) oil is ideal.

Uses

The client may have a recipe made up which contains the ingredients best suited to her skin. This gives the treatment a personal touch which clients appreciate. Sometimes different masks may be created for treating different areas of the face.

Know your ingredients

Kaolin White (China) clay	Has a 'drawing' effect which is deep cleansing and is useful for bringing spots and skin blockages to a head.
Fuller's Earth Greyish-green clay	Very absorbent and deep cleansing. Has a strong stimulating effect on the circulation, so not suitable for more sensitive skins.
Magnesium Fine, white powder	Mildly astringent. A carbonate gentle refining mask which tightens the pores and softens the skin.
Calamine Pale, pink powder	Mildly astringent. Contains zinc carbonate which soothes the skin and calms down high colouring.

The clays should be mixed with a suitable lubricant, depending on skin type:

- Greasy: witch hazel
- Balanced: distilled water or rose water
- Dry: rosewater or vegetable oil
- Sensitive: vegetable oil.

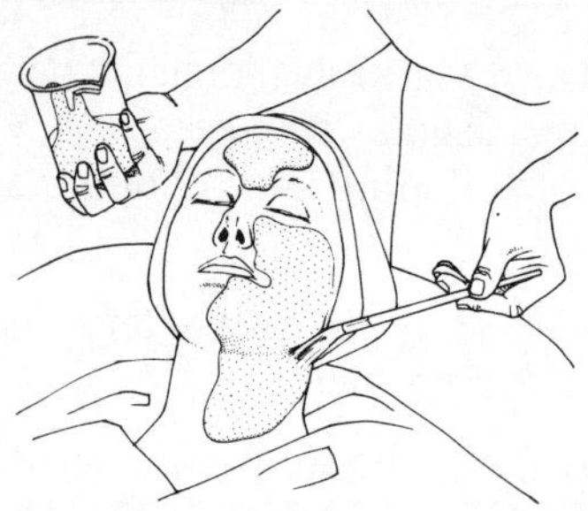

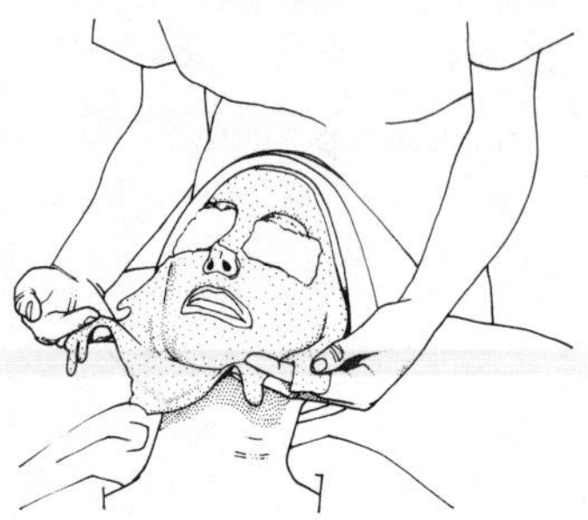

Peel-off masks

Contents

These are based on waxes (for example paraffin), gums (for example tragacanth, acacia), latex or plastic resins which are applied wet but dry out on the skin. They have a milder effect than clay-based masks because they are not absorbent.

Gel masks have a mildly astringent effect and cool the skin. Latex, wax and plastic masks produce an occlusive film which promotes sweating and increases the amount of surface moisture. They are very deep-cleansing and stimulate the blood supply, causing the skin to go slightly pink. Peel-off masks are designed to be eased off the skin in one piece, taking with them loose skin cells which have been softened.

Uses

Gel masks are particularly suitable for mature skins because of their tightening, soothing effects. Latex, wax and plastic masks are suitable for all skins except those which are sensitive and prone to high colouring.

Thermal masks

The ingredients of these masks either generate heat or rely on a heat source for their effectiveness.

Contents (i)

A paste is mixed which is applied to the skin over a special skin cream. After a few minutes the paste begins to harden and a chemical reaction occurs between the ingredients which creates heat and warms the surface tissues. The heat disperses after twenty minutes, after which time the mask becomes rigid and can be eased away from the skin.

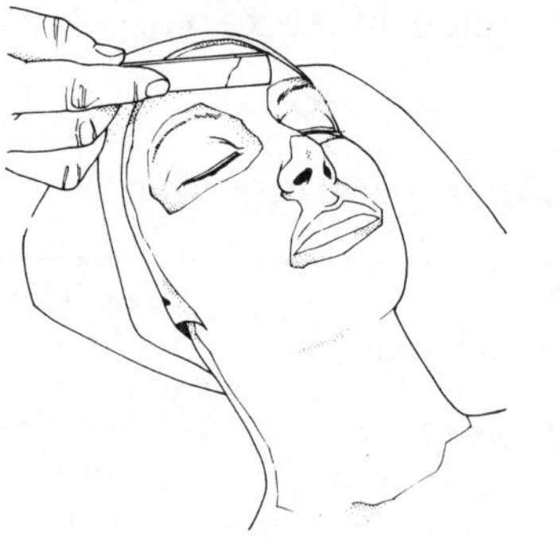

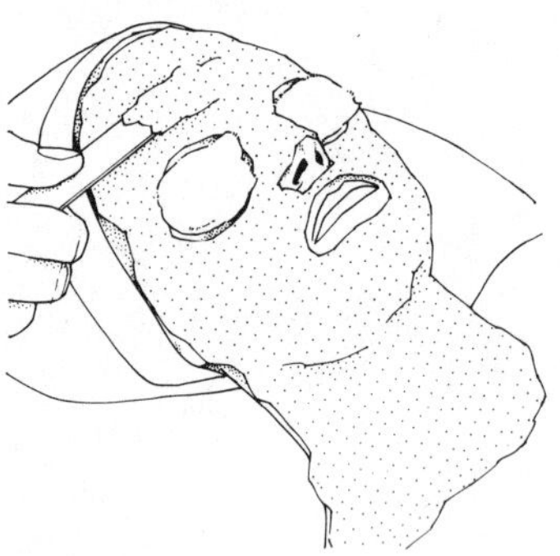

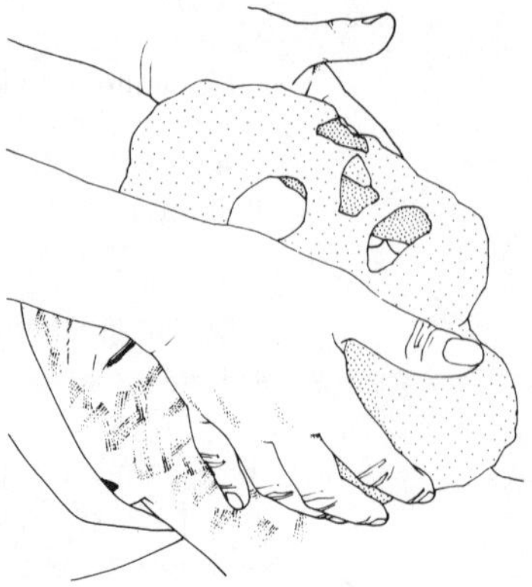

Uses

This mask has powerful deep-cleansing, tightening and stimulating effects. The heat produced encourages absorption of the cream applied underneath. Clients with a nervous disposition or who have sensitive skin are not suitable for treatment.

Contents (ii)

Vegetable oils such as arachis, olive and almond are particularly beneficial when they become absorbed by the upper layers of skin. Warm oils penetrate more readily on a warm skin. An infra-red lamp is used during the treatment to keep oil which has been applied to the face on gauze at a comfortable temperature. The oil which remains on the skin after treatment is used to perform a facial massage.

Uses

Warm oil treatments are particularly beneficial for dry, crepey, mature skins. They are not suitable for clients with very sensitive skin who have an extremely vascular complexion.

Biological masks

Contents

These products have a gentle but effective action on the skin. They are based on natural ingredients such as flower, plant, herbal and vegetable extracts. Available as creams, gels or emulsions, they form a light film on the skin which becomes firm and dry but does not tighten. The biologically active ingredients have different effects on the skin depending on their source.

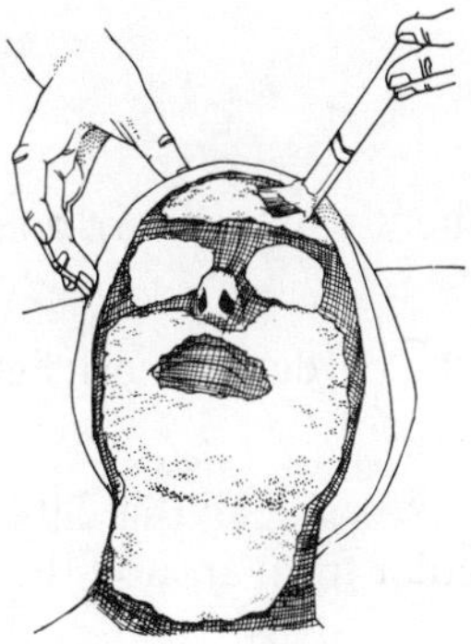

Uses

Biological face masks can be made up in a variety of recipes to treat any skin combination of skin problems. The following is a very general guide:

- Soft fruits: correct the pH balance of a dry skin and increase its moisture level
- Plants: stimulate the circulation and increase cell metabolism
- Herbs and vegetables: tone, stimulate, balance and regenerate a problem skin

Manufacturers provide instructions on the most effective ways of using their products.

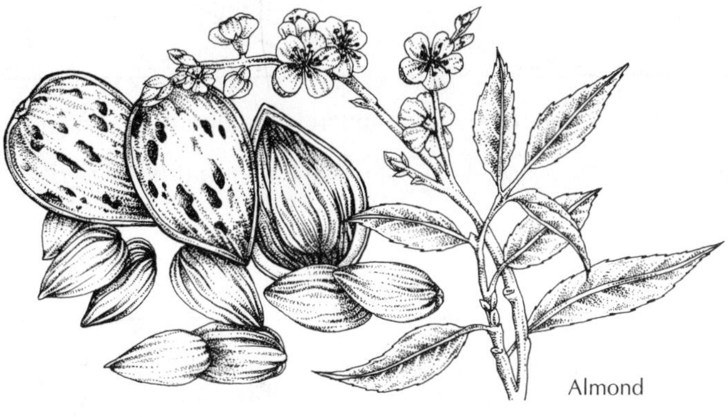

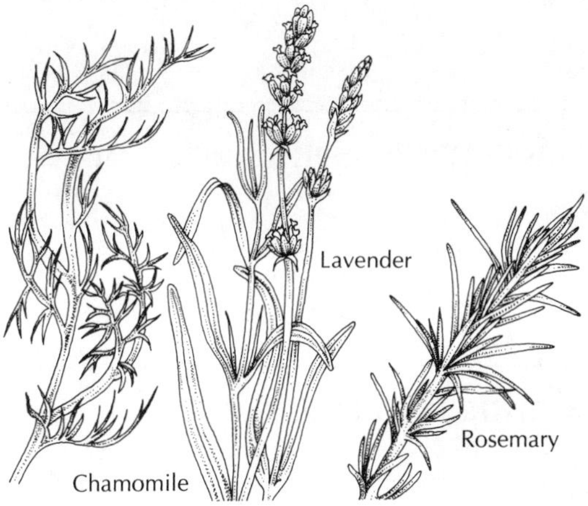

Applying a face mask

Information will be provided by the manufacturer regarding the mixing, application and removal of specialised face masks. Make sure you have a good knowledge of the products used in your salon and follow the manufacturer's instructions.

The following method is for applying a clay-based mask. This type of mask is more time-consuming to prepare and remove than a ready-mixed mask, but the basic treatment techniques are the same.

> *Remember*
> Do not use your mask brush to do the mixing otherwise clay will collect at the base of the bristles and will discolour or damage them.

Preparation

1 Tuck a facial tissue under the edge of the headband to prevent it from becoming soiled.

2 Decide upon the basic mask ingredients required. These may be different for treating different areas of the face and neck.

3 Use a spatula to mix the clay and lubricant to a smooth, creamy consistency.

> *Remember*
> Do not apply the mask very thickly. The effects of the treatment occur where the skin is in contact with the mask, so building it up thickly is both uneconomical and a waste of time.

Application

1 Apply the mixture neatly and quickly with a mask brush, ensuring even coverage of the face and neck but avoiding the area immediately around the eyes and mouth.

2 Apply mask to the centre panel first if this area is being treated separately from the rest of the face.

3 Make sure the mask is applied right down to the base of the neck.

4 When application is complete, apply cool, soothing eye pads and lift the front towel up over the client's shoulders.

> *Remember*
> The resting period during the mask treatment is very important for continuing the relaxing effects of the massage. Make sure the client is kept warm and undisturbed during the treatment.

Removal

1 Discard the eye pads and explain to the client what you are going to do.

2 Use clean warm damp sponges to soften the hardened mask before wiping it away with firm upward movements.

3 Repeat the removal procedures until you are satisfied that all traces of the mask have been removed, in particular from around the hairline, eyebrows and nostrils.

4 Finally, tone and blot the skin and apply moisturiser.

> *Remember*
> Clay which has not been removed from the skin dries and forms a fine film. This is particularly noticeable on black skins.

Face masks: Self-checks

1 Why is skin peeling beneficial before applying an ampoule?

2 Why is a clay-based mask not always suitable for a mature skin?

3 What are the general features of biological face masks?

Caring for black skin

It would be very wrong to generalise about the treatment of black skins. Many of the blemishes and abnormalities which are obvious on a white skin become much harder to diagnose when they are obscured by

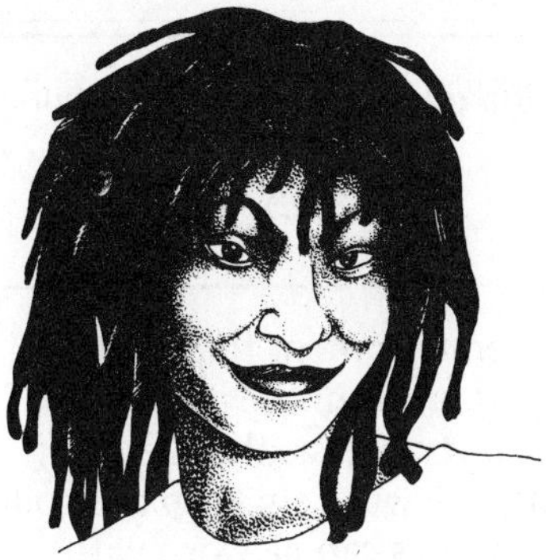

skin colour. The Wood's light is an invaluable aid to analysing black skin. Very careful questioning of the client is required in order to make the best recommendations for skin care.

It is true that black skin has more sweat and sebaceous glands than white skin but this very often leads to an assumption that all black skins are greasy. Black skins do tend to be shiny, but this is a normal characteristic. Some black skins are greasy, of course, but not all of them. A wrong assumption can result in the use of products which are too harsh and may irritate the skin and cause more problems.

Cleansing

This is probably the most important part of the skin care programme. Black skin is thick and desquamates more than white skin. Dead cells build up on the skin surface, attracting dust and grime from the atmosphere. Skin which is not cleansed thoroughly morning and evening looks dull. It develops skin blockages and an uneven texture.

Cleanser

Cleansing milks are usually preferred for the deep cleanse. These are particularly beneficial when combined with a brush cleanse. The friction of the brush helps to loosen the accumulated surface matter and improve the texture of the skin.

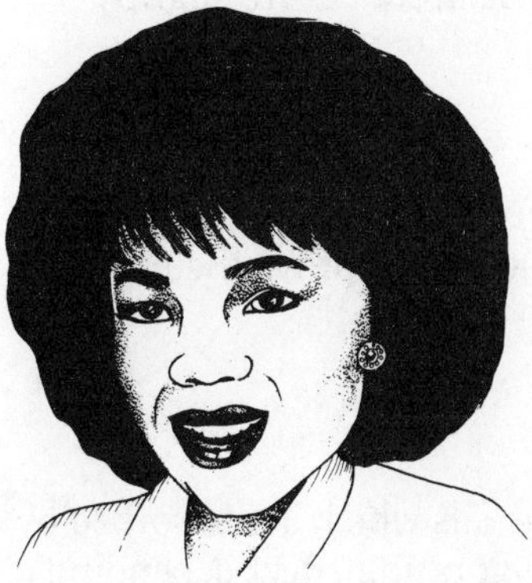

Toning lotion

Mild tonics or flower waters are more suitable than stronger preparations. Alcohol may act as an irritant on black skin.

Exfoliants

These should be used at least once or twice a week to control the effects of desquamation. Greasy skins benefit from the abrasive effects of a facial scrub; otherwise peeling creams may be used.

Moisturising

Oil-in-water emulsions which have a matte finish are preferable to greasy creams which leave a shine.

Evening care

Clients with black skin do not need to worry so much about the use of rich, 'anti-ageing' skin care preparations. Their skin has very strong protein fibres which keep wrinkles and crepiness at bay, usually until they are well into their late fifties. Evening care should concentrate on the prevention of moisture loss and the use of creams for the eyes and neck, where the skin is thinner and less protected.

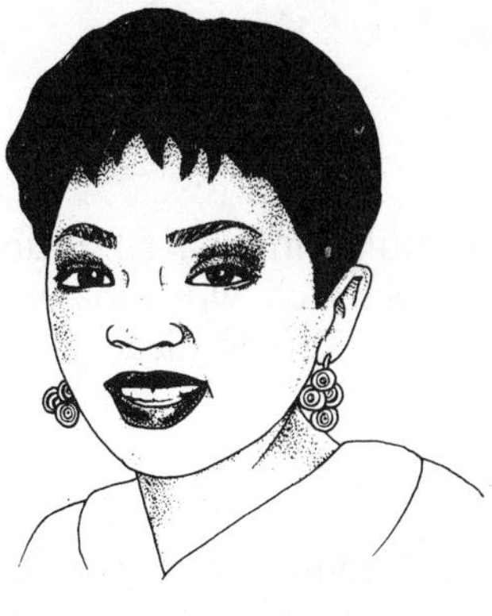

Biological skin care preparations containing plant extracts have a stimulating effect and help to refine skin texture.

Face masks

These should be used weekly as part of a regular skin care routine. Clay-based face masks are particularly beneficial due to their absorbent and astringent effects. Great care must be taken to remove all traces of the clay so that a fine film is not left on the skin and in the pores.

Caring for black skin: Self-check

1 Why is the regular use if an exfoliant particularly beneficial for a client with a black skin?

Body care

The skin of the body is less exposed to the environment than the face and hands. It does not suffer to the same extent from the effects of sunlight, pollution and external damage. Nevertheless, the effects of ageing are the same and preventative skin care will help keep the body in good condition so that more revealing clothes can be worn with confidence. Products are also available for treating specific problems which affect the skin of the body.

Body lotions

Contents

These are lightweight, non-greasy oil-in-water emulsions which contain moisturising ingredients such as glycerol, collagen or plant extracts to soften and smooth the skin. The products are slightly perfumed.

Uses

Body lotions replace moisture which is lost from the skin during bathing or when having a shower. They help to improve the tone and texture of the skin.

Body oils

These products contain vegetable or plant oils which are absorbed by the skin and have either a relaxing or invigorating effect depending on their base. Other ingredients may be added to help treat particular problems.

Uses

The oils are most effective when massaged in to warm skin, for example after a bath or shower. They prevent dehydration and make the skin soft and smooth. Depending on their active ingredients, body oils can help in the treatment of problems such as cellulite (a condition which produces dimpling of the skin on the thighs and bottom) and acne which often occurs on the upper back.

Body scrubs

Contents

These are exfoliants which have a similar formulation to facial scrubs. The abrasive ingredient is often polished grains which, when massaged over the skin, stimulate the blood circulation and remove dead cells and impurities from the surface.

Uses

Body scrubs are deep cleansing. They help to decongest areas which are prone to blocked pores and blackheads, such as the upper back. Rough areas such as the knees and elbows benefit from the increased desquamation. Body oils and lotions are more effective when applied to skin after a body scrub. The product is massaged into the skin and then rinsed off.

Firming creams

Contents

Different products are available for treating different areas of the body. They are basically moisturising creams which contain an astringent to tighten and tone the skin.

Uses

The creams are massaged into the skin daily to help firm body contours. Products are available for different areas of the body, for example bust, upper arms and thighs.

Body care: Self-check

1 When is the best time to apply body cream or body oil?

Sun care

> *Remember*
> Fair skins are more at risk in the sun than dark skins but all skins need protecting from the ravaging effects of UV.

The damaging effects of the sun's rays upon the skin are well known. Despite this, there are many people who feel more confident and attractive when they have a sun tan. It is essential to advise your client about a sensible approach to sunbathing and to recommend the appropriate skin care products.

The incidence of skin cancer is increasing. Over the last decade, cases in America, Australia and Scandinavia have doubled. In Scotland, during the same period, there was an 80% increase in the number of patients suffering from malignant melanoma. Research into the environment has shown that there will be a sustained annual 10% decrease in ozone, leading to an increase of over 300 000 cases of non-melanoma skin cancers per year.

> *Remember*
> The salt in sea water intensifies the effects of the sun. Burning is a serious threat if the skin is not protected when swimming or relaxing in the sea.

Sunscreens

Contents

A chemical sunscreen ingredient is contained in the formulation for a basic skin cream, milk or oil. The greasier the product, the more effective is the sun screening effect. Moisturising ingredients help prevent the skin from drying out.

Uses

Sunscreens filter out harmful UVA and UVB rays so that they do not penetrate and damage the deeper layers of the skin. They are smoothed over the skin before exposure to sun and are replaced regularly, particularly before and after swimming.

The effectiveness of a sunscreen product is measured by its Sun Protection Factor (SPF). The SPF number is identified on the product and usually falls within the range 2–30. It indicates how much longer a person wearing the sunscreen may stay out in the sun before getting burned.

> Remember
> SPF numbers relate only to UVB. They do not indicate the amount of protection provided against long UVA rays which cause premature ageing of the skin. A star system is currently being developed for giving sunscreen products a UVA protection rating in addition to an SPF.

Skin Type	SPF	Effect
Fair-skinned person who normally goes pink after 15 min	Uses SPF 10	Skin will take 10 times longer (150 min) before it burns
Person with skin which tans easily but tends to get sore during initial stages of sunbathing	Uses SPF 2	May stay out in the sun up to twice as long before burning
Person with pale skin which burns very easily, particularly over bony prominences	Uses SPF 25+	This is a total sun block which gives complete protection if applied regularly

After-sun care

Contents

These are moisturisers which contain an astringent such as zinc carbonate to cool the skin and an ingredient such as calamine to soothe.

Uses

After-sun lotions prevent the skin from drying out and peeling. They make the skin feel more comfortable after sunbathing and prolong the effects of a tan.

> Remember
> The effects of a self-tanning cream will be more natural if it is applied after using an exfoliant. This will ensure that the skin texture is smooth and even. Care should be taken to wash the cream off the hands immediately after application so that the palms do not turn orange!

Self-tanning creams

Contents

The active ingredient is a harmless cold tar derivative called dihydroxyacetone. This chemical reacts with the keratin in the skin and then gradually oxidises to produce a yellowish brown colour.

Uses

Self-tanning creams are particularly useful for fair-skinned people who want to look tanned without being exposed to the sun. They can be used to even out patchy skin colouring and to top up a natural tan which has started to fade. This type of fake tan lasts for a few days and fades as the surface skin cells desquamate.

Sun care: Self-check

1 What is the significance of the SPF number on a sunscreen product?

General skin care: Activities

1 Referring to your product information, write out a list of the features and benefits of each of the items in your salon's retail range. Try learning what you have written so that you are well prepared for your next sale!

2 Design a skin-care chart for each of the basic skin types which can be referred to when giving home-care advice. Recommend 'special' products for problems associated with each skin type.

Your chart should specify products from your salon's retail range and should recommend a morning and evening skin-care routine. Where there is a choice of suitable products available, indicate the benefits of each.

Facial treatments

With such an extensive range of skin care products available, a new client may wonder why they need come for professional facial treatments! The answers are simple: apart being able to enjoy the benefits of a pleasant and relaxing salon environment, the client will be treated by a trained therapist who has:

- specialised knowledge which is necessary for correctly diagnosing and advising on skin problems
- technical knowledge of the treatments and products available so that reliable advice can be given
- professional skills which ensure that each client gets maximum benefits from the treatments
- the use of professional tools and equipment which make treatments more effective and, sometimes, more comfortable for a client
- the knowledge and skills to treat the skin safely and hygienically
- the ability to monitor a client's progress and adapt the treatments when necessary
- the confidence of having a professional qualification
- up-to-date information about new treatments and products.

> *Remember*
> Not all clients have serious problems with their skin. Many clients have regular facials simply because they enjoy them and their skin feels good afterwards. There is nothing wrong with that! The psychological benefits of professional treatments are just as important for many clients as the physical ones.

Salon facials allow the client to benefit from specialised equipment and treatments which would otherwise be unavailable to them. They also provide the opportunity for discussing progress with home care and receiving qualified advice on other beauty problems.

Preparing for a facial

As usual, the area must be well organised to avoid wasting time during the treatment. Consult the client's record card for details of previous treatments and products used. Get a new record card to fill in for a client who has not already had a consultation. Make sure you have a range of products available so that you can adapt the treatment to suit the client.

Preparing the treatment area

A facial is always given with the client lying down, or in a semi-reclining position, and the therapist working from behind. This helps to promote total relaxation which is important for the success of the treatment. Other ways of creating a relaxing atmosphere are by making sure that:

- there is no unnecessary noise
- the room is warm and there are no draughts
- the lighting is subdued (the illuminated magnifier will be used for close work)
- there are pillows and bedding for the client's comfort; the client may need extra support under the back and knees
- everything needed is readily available to avoid interrupting the treatment.

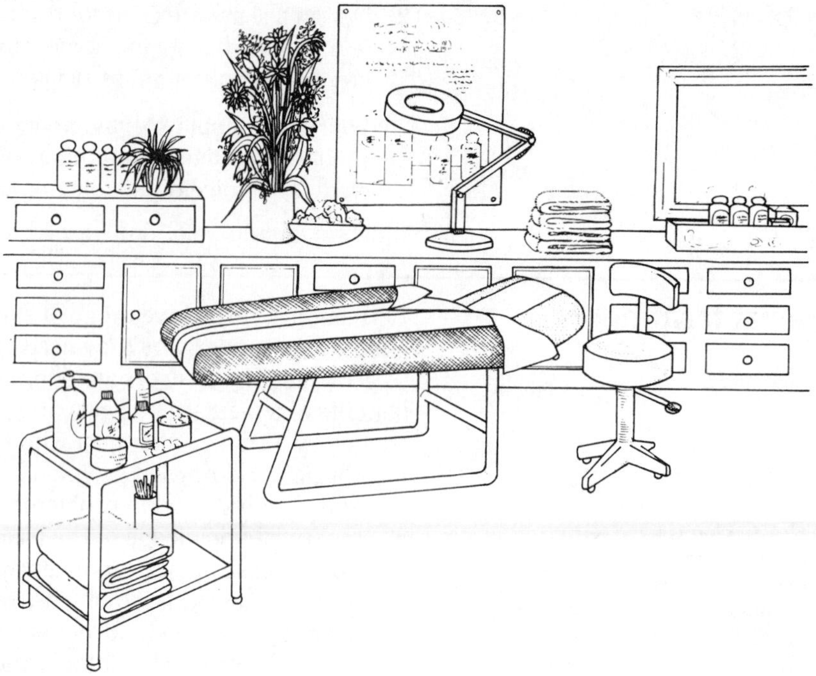

The treatment area

Preparing the trolley

The trolley should be clean, tidy and well stocked. The products should be arranged in a logical order so that you can go straight to them without searching. Arrange your products attractively so that they catch your client's attention. Remember, creating an interest usually leads to sales!

You will also need:

- selection of skin care products
- jar of prepared sterilising fluid
- comedone extractor
- clean spatulas
- cotton buds
- cotton wool pads
- tissues
- 4 bowls: for waste, for client's jewellery, for cotton wool and for mixing/removing face mask
- 1 headband
- 1 hand towel
- 1 mask brush
- 2 mask sponges
- record card and pen
- hand mirror.

You may also need a complexion brush, a facial steamer, a mechanical brush cleanse unit and tweezers.

Preparing the client

A new client will be unfamiliar with salon procedures and may even be a little embarrassed or nervous on the first visit. Give clear instructions

> Remember
> The client should not wear any clothes which are tight or which may restrict access to areas of the body included in the facial. The fewer clothes that are worn, the more comfortable and relaxed the client is likely to be.

> Remember
> Clients wearing contact lenses should be advised to take them out before treatment and keep them safely in soaking solution. This will prevent irritating the eyes when massaging and wiping over the eyelids.

> Remember
> A full facial treatment lasts over an hour. You must check your working position to avoid developing backache and tension in the neck and shoulders.

and explain which items of clothing should be removed. Respect the client's privacy and offer a gown or bathsheet for cover which can be removed before getting on the couch.

Having settled the client comfortably on the couch, ensure that the shoulders are free from straps and that earrings and necklaces are removed.

Allow the clients to choose between keeping their arms inside or outside the bedding and place a towel over the chest, tucked into underwear straps if they are being worn.

Finally, adjust the height of the couch (and your stool if you prefer to be seated) so that both you and the client are comfortable.

The client's head should be raised slightly to take the strain off the neck and to prevent dizziness when getting up after the treatment.

Now, you are ready to begin, but first, remember:

- always use a clean spatula for removing cream from its container
- transfer cream to the client from the back of your hand
- pour runny creams in to the palm of your hand before using them
- put tops back on bottles and jars immediately to prevent their contents from becoming spoiled or spilled
- wash your hands immediately before and during the treatment as required.

> Remember
> The cleansing products work by either dissolving grease or by using a detergent action which suspends dirt and make-up so that they can be wiped off the skin.

> Remember
> The skin of the eyes and lips is cleansed later. This is more hygienic and prevents spreading heavily pigmented make-up products over the face.

> Remember
> The superficial cleanse may have to be repeated if a heavy make-up is being worn.

Superficial cleanse

Even if the client claims not to be wearing make-up, always give a superficial cleanse. This will help you to make an accurate assessment of the skin. It will also help the other skin treatments to be more effective.

1 Apply the appropriate cleansing product to the neck and main facial areas, omitting the eyes and lips.

2 Use gentle upward stroking and rotary massage movements to spread the cleanser and work it well into the skin creases (for example above the chin and at the sides of the nose) where grease and make-up tend to build up.

3 Remove the cleanser with firm upward and outward movements:

- use good quality, soft facial tissues to absorb the greasy film left by an oil-based cleansing cream or make-up remover, or
- use slightly dampened cotton wool pads to remove cleansing milk and water-soluble debris from the skin.

Effective cleansing has taken place only when the tissues or cotton-wool pads used for removing the cleanser appear clean when wiped over the face.

4 Instruct the client to keep eyes closed. Apply a small amount of cleansing milk or non-oily eye make-up remover to the eyelids. Spread the cleanser over the upper eyelids with small gentle rotary massage movements. Use the pads of the 'ring' fingers (the ones next to the little fingers) and avoid applying pressure on the eyeball.

> Remember
> The ring fingers exert the least pressure. They are the best ones to use when working over the very thin and delicate skin around the eyes.

5 Stroke a little cleanser underneath the eyes, working towards the nose. Ensure that cleanser does not penetrate the eyes.

6 Use damp cotton wool pads to wipe away cleanser from around the eyes. Treat one eye at a time. Stroke outwards over the upper eyelid and then keep the skin supported while cleaning underneath with a second pad.

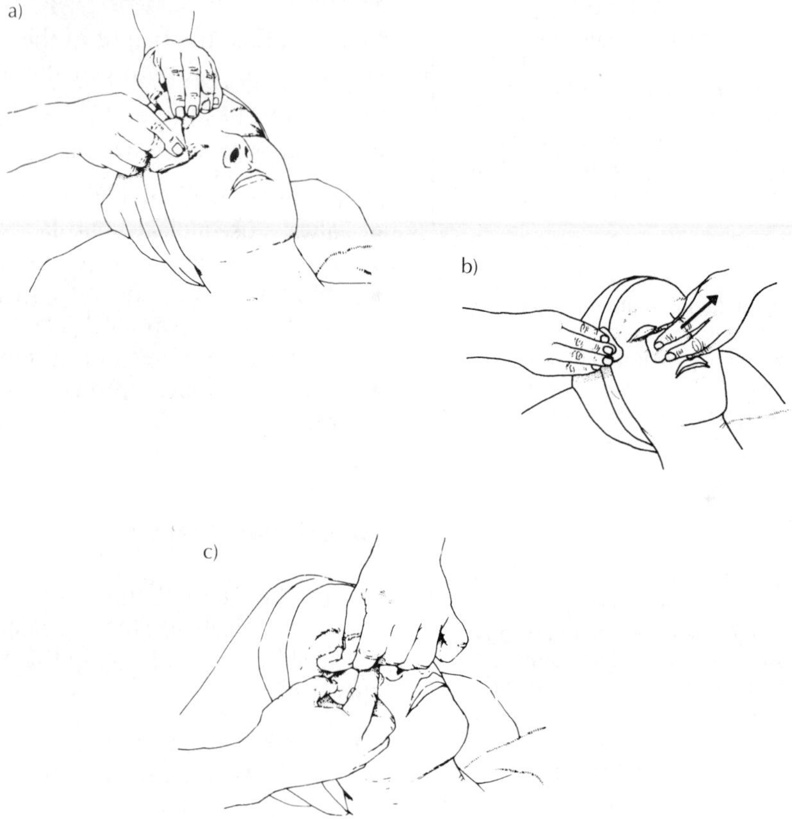

Supporting the skin helps to prevent it from becoming pulled and stretched.

> Remember
> Use an oily eye make-up remover to remove stubborn waterproof mascara.

7 For removing mascara, place damp cotton-wool pads beneath the lashes and dissolve mascara with a suitable eye make-up remover. A tipped orange stick or cotton bud is useful for this.

8 Remove make-up from the lips with small, rotary massage movements and wipe away cleanser and dissolved make-up with damp cotton wool pads

> Remember
> Be gentle and use the right products: if you are heavy handed or use products which are too strong, the skin will become over-stimulated and will not show its normal characteristics for the skin analysis.

9 Wipe over the skin with a mild toner (low alcohol content) on damp cotton wool pads. This should remove the greasy film remaining after the cleanse without disturbing the skin's surface.

10 Blot excess moisture on the skin. Split a tissue into single ply and create a hole in the centre for placing over the nose. Lay the tissue over the face and gently press it against the skin. Gradually roll the tissue down the face and onto the neck.

Deep Cleanse

Once the type and condition of the skin has been assessed, choose a suitable deep-cleansing product and apply it to the face and neck.

The deep cleanse involves the use of special massage movements which:

- stimulate the flow of blood and lymph through the skin
- assist the penetration of cleanser into the hair follicles, dissolving make-up or dirt which has penetrated them
- help soften and loosen surface blockages
- aid desquamation (shedding of surface cells)
- are relaxing.

Procedure for deep cleanse

The following sequence ensures that all areas of the face and neck are treated thoroughly, and that the movements flow smoothly into one another so that a relaxing rhythm is maintained.

Whichever procedure you use, make sure that:

- your hands are clean, smooth and relaxed. Stiff hands put extra pressure on the face which is less comfortable for the client.
- the movements are adapted to the size and shape of the area being treated, for example over the cheeks and forehead.
- pressure is reduced when working over bony prominences and sensitive skin.

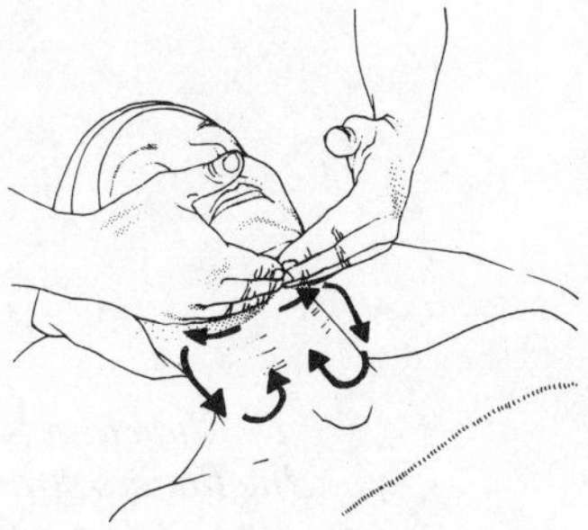

1 *With hands resting on the jawline, stroke them towards the angles of the jaw, then down the sides of neck and firmly upwards from the base, avoiding pressure over the trachea (wind pipe); repeat 6 times.*

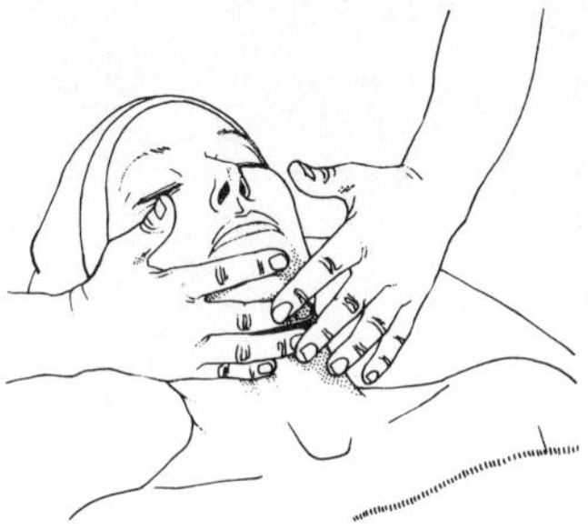

2 *Slide hands up over the chin and work in to the crease with the index fingers, one after another, sliding them back under the chin to repeat the movements; repeat 6 times for each hand.*

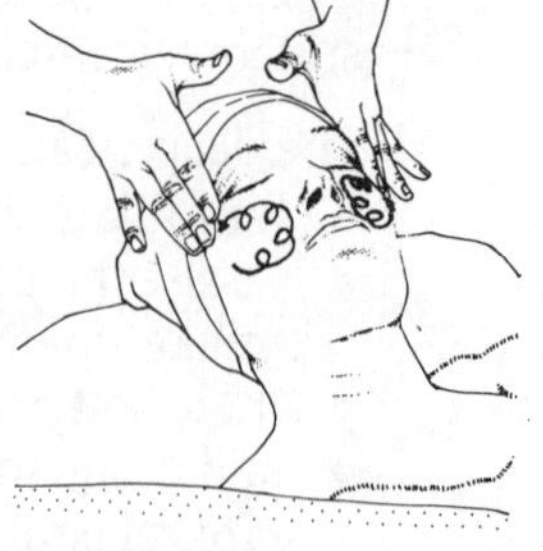

3 Perform small circular movements with the pads of the fingers, covering the cheeks from the corners of the mouth to the sides of the nose and carrying on up to the temples. Slide hands back gently to the corners of the mouth to repeat the movements (6 times).

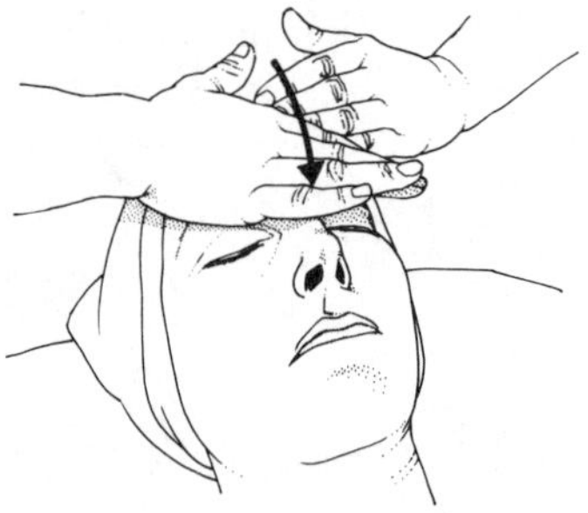

4 Slide hands from the temples to the centre of the forehead and, keeping the fingers straight but relaxed, stroke them down the nose, one after the other, 6 times for each hand.

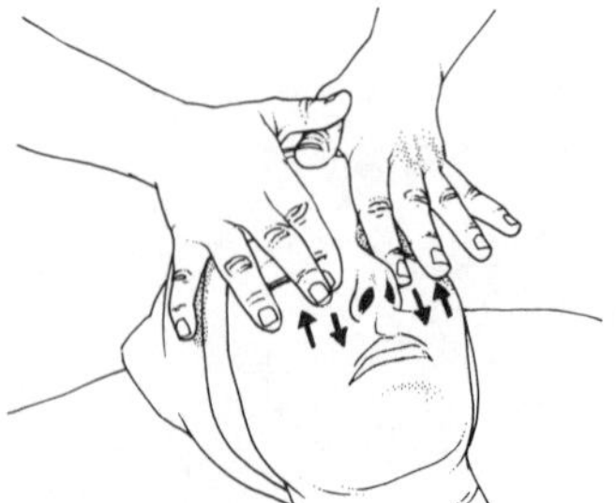

5 Use the pads of the ring fingers to work thoroughly, upwards and downwards, into the creases at the sides of the nose; repeat 6 times in each direction.

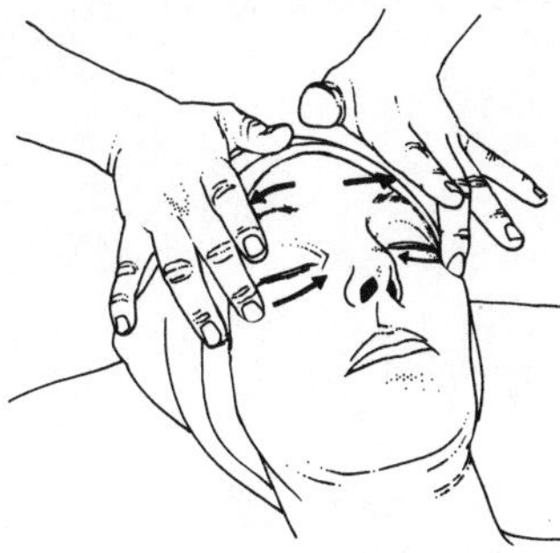

6 Slide the hands back up the sides of the nose. Stroke out over the eyebrows and then inwards, underneath the eyes, producing a big circular movement; repeat 6 times.

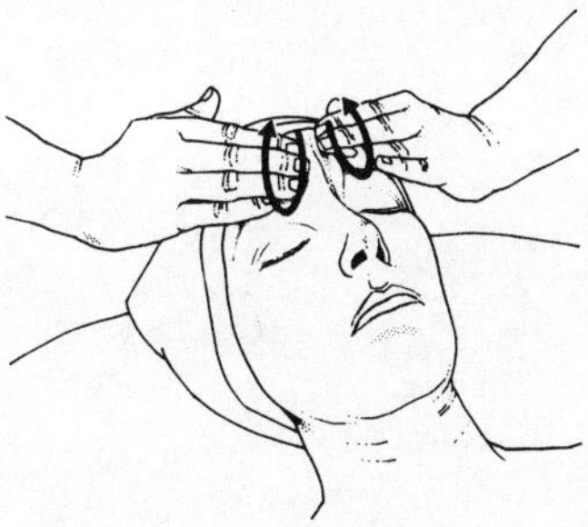

7 Perform circular movements over the forehead with the pads of the fingers. Work from temple to temple, one hand following the other, so that the forehead is covered (6 times), finishing in the centre.

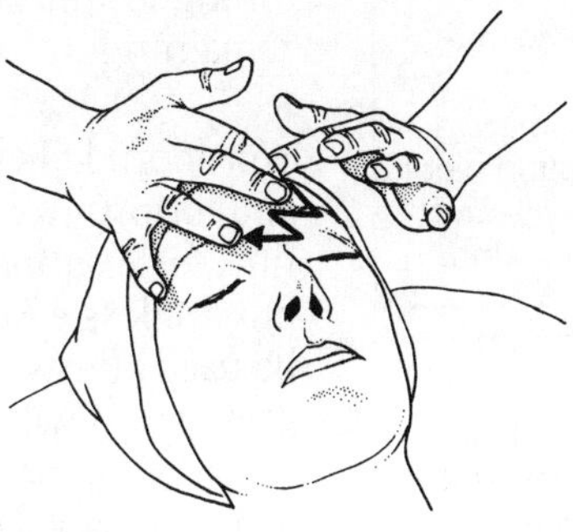

8 Still using the pads of the fingers, work from temple to temple across the forehead, with small interlocking zig zag movements. Cover the forehead (6 times), finishing in the centre.

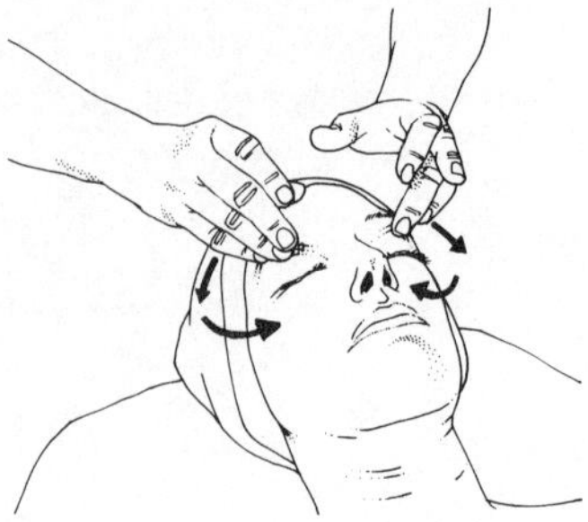

9 *Stroke the ring fingers out over the eyebrows and then in underneath. As a circle is completed, gently perform three very light lifting movements beneath the brow, starting with the index finger. The ring finger should then be correctly positioned for repeating the whole movement: 6 times.*

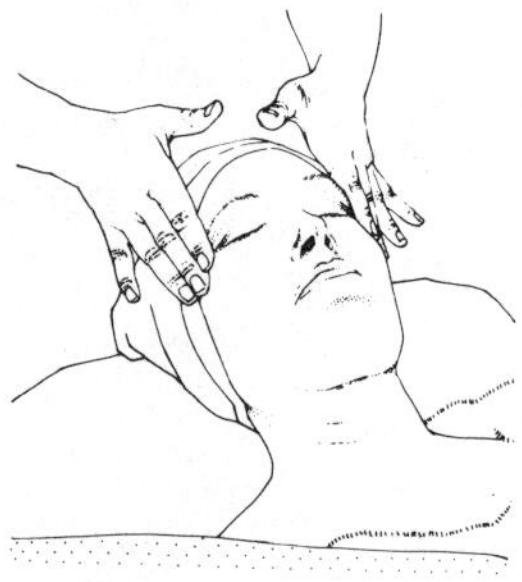

10 *Finally, slide the fingers up the sides of the nose, over the forehead and apply a little pressure at the temples to let your client know the routine has finished.*

Remember
Use only the best quality of tissues and cotton wool when treating the face. Poor quality materials have a rough texture which is uncomfortable when wiped over the skin. Sometimes they contain small hard fragments which may damage a sensitive skin. Cheap cotton wool does not hold together well and is a false economy in the salon.

Remember
Do not worry if the deep cleanse procedure you learn is different from the one described here. As with most beauty therapy treatments, there are different correct ways of giving the treatment.

After the deep cleanse

Remove all traces of cleanser and wipe over the skin with a suitable toning lotion. Blot the skin dry and check that there is no grease remaining in the skin creases, eyebrows, eyelashes and hairline.

You should always use damp cotton-wool pads for removing creams and lotions from skin which is dry, sensitive, mature or particularly fine, for example the eyes and lips. These are more gentle than tissues but are less efficient for absorbing oil-based preparations. A toner must be used afterwards which contains just enough alcohol to remove the greasy film without stripping the skin of its natural sebum.

Although the deep cleanse should be relaxing, its main aim is to rid the skin of impurities and prepare it for the next stage of the treatment. The whole cleansing procedure should take no longer than 5 minutes. This does not include the extra time needed for analysing the skin of a new client during a consultation.

Removal of skin blockages

> Remember
>
> Damp hot cotton-wool pads are pressed over the area to be treated to help dilate the pores and loosen skin blockages. They may need re-applying as the skin cools down.

The deep-cleansing procedure helps to soften comedones (blackheads) and excess sebum which has collected in the pores. Warming the skin with hot damp cotton-wool pads or by steaming also makes it easier to remove them without damaging the surrounding skin.

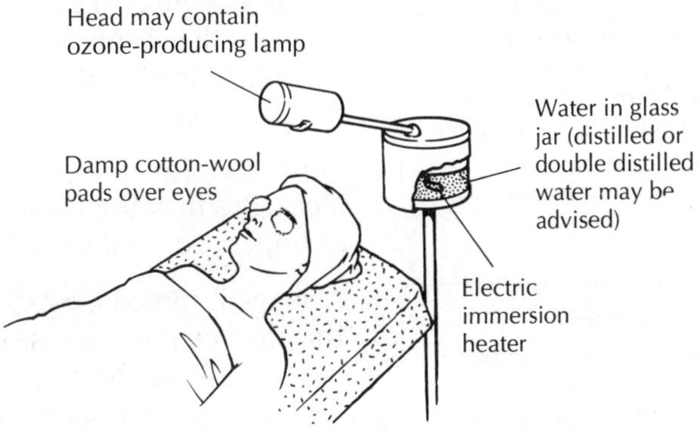

Steaming is done for between 3–20 minutes, depending on the type and condition of the skin and keeps the skin warm so that sebum is softened not only at the surface, but also deeper down the hair follicles.

Remember that heating the skin stimulates its blood supply to the surface. Do not steam very sensitive skin or over areas of dilated capillaries. Fair skin should appear only slightly pink after steaming. Do not over-stimulate the blood supply or you will limit the other treatments which may be given.

Adjust the distance of the steam outlet from the face according to skin type: 40 cm. (about 15 in.) for dry, mature skin, 30 cm. (12 in.) for balanced skin and 25 cm. (10 in.) for greasy skin.

> Remember
>
> Even though ozone is very unstable, there is some evidence that it can be damaging to health if inhaled in high concentrations over water vapour. Given the normal amount of use of ozone therapy equipment, it is unlikely that dangerous concentrations could build up in a room which is well ventilated.

Most facial steamers are designed so that the steam can be produced on its own or combined with ozone for helping to heal greasy, blemished skin. Ozone is drying and has an anti-bacterial effect.

However, the salon should seek the approval of the local health authority before offering ozone steaming treatments. They are restricted in some areas.

Ozone is not necessary for loosening skin blockages. Steaming alone benefits the skin by:

- warming and softening sebaceous blockages dilating the pores
- stimulating the sweat and sebaceous glands
- softening and hydrating the skin
- increasing the rate of blood and lymph flow through the skin
- increasing desquamation.

Take care

The treatment involves the use of electrical equipment and boiling water. Precautions must be taken to avoid injuring the client, yourself and anyone else in the area:

- make sure steamer has a stable base
- check the plug, lead and machine head for safety before use
- do not position steamer where it is likely to get knocked
- make sure that the lead to the machine is not trailing where it could cause someone to trip up

> Remember
> By cleaning and maintaining the machine regularly, a light, even flow of steam is produced rather than an erratic discharge of boiling water which could burn the client. Make sure you read and follow the manufacturer's instructions on how to look after the steamer.

> Remember
> Using an illuminated magnifier helps you to be accurate when looking for and removing skin blockages.

> Remember
> Do not risk damaging the skin by trying to force out stubborn blockages. Comedones which have been present for some time may need more steaming and skin softening treatments before they can be released.

- follow the manufacturer's instructions when filling and heating up the water vessel
- keep the steam outlet directed away from the body while the water is heating
- check that a light, even vapour is produced before applying to the face
- keep a check on the client's skin reaction during treatment
- turn the steam outlet away from the client before turning the machine off and moving it to a safe place immediately after treatment.

After steaming, the face should be blotted with a tissue. The loosened blockages may then be removed by using either a comedone extractor or fingers covered with tissues or a soft fine towel.

A 'looped' comedone extractor is used to apply light pressure around the blocked pore to ease out the contents. Blockages may be treated individually or the extractor may be stroked along a crease in the skin to remove accumulated matter.

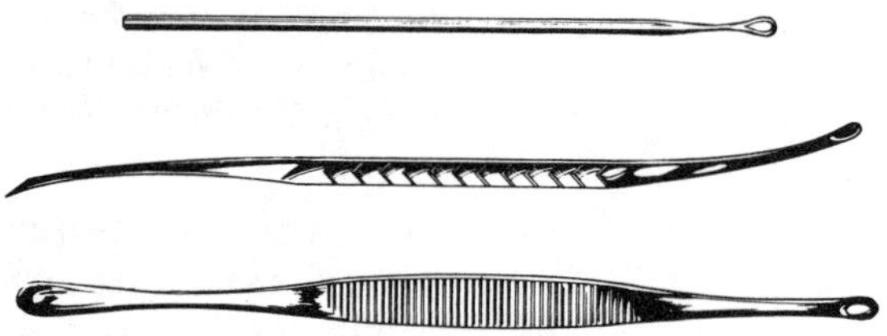

The looped end of the extractor is rounded to avoid damaging the skin.

The area around the blockage is rolled and squeezed between the fingers so that the contents are forced gently out of the follicle without breaking the skin. A clean tissue takes up the waste.

Brush cleansing

This may be done after removing skin blockages using a gentle soapless lathering cleanser and a soft complexion brush. The dampened brush is used in small circular movements over the face and neck to distribute the cleanser and work it into the pores.

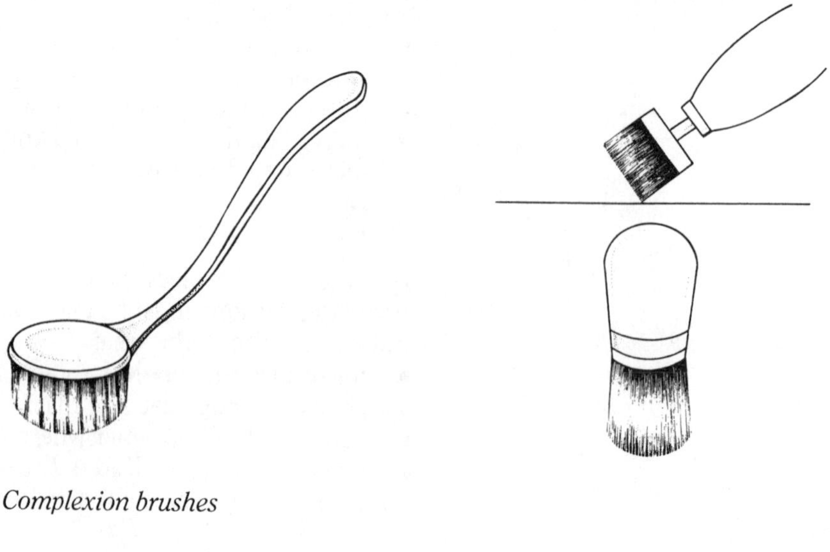

Complexion brushes

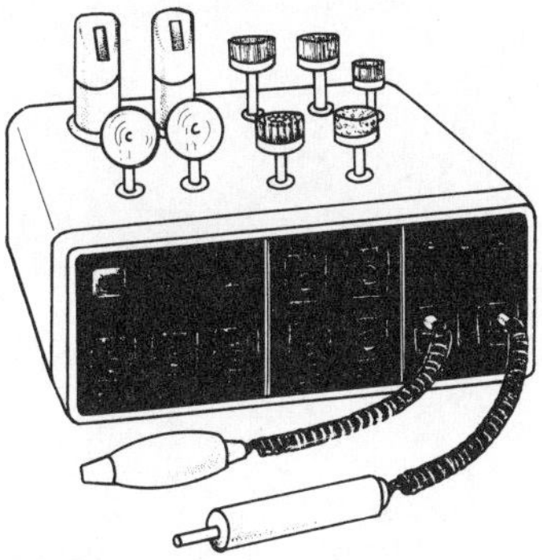

Mechanical brush cleansing

This piece of electrically powered equipment has a variety of applicator heads which may be used as alternatives or in addition to manual cleansing and massage treatments.

Treatment with a mechanical brush system is adapted by using different applicator heads and by varying the speed and directional controls:

- sponge head: used dampened with a foaming deep-cleansing product

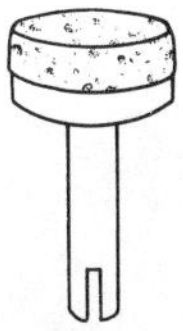

- soft brush heads: available in a range of shapes and sizes for deep cleansing and massaging different facial and body areas

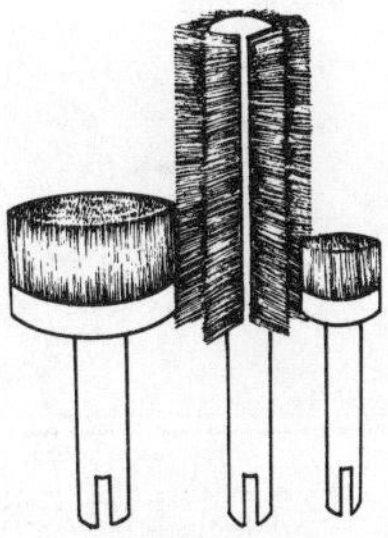

- bristle brush head: particularly good for male clients. Used to deep cleanse, desquamate and stimulate strong firm skin

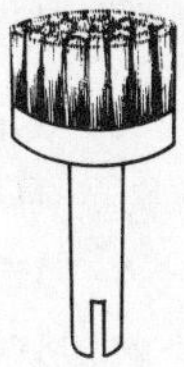

- pumice head: used as a peeling stone for increasing desquamation and refining a coarse skin texture.

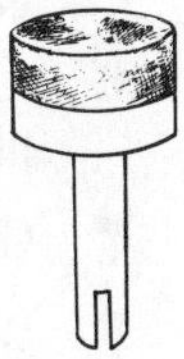

Pressure should not be applied with the brush but strokes should be directed upwards to avoid dragging and stretching the skin.

Contra-indications to mechanical brush cleansing are:
- broken skin
- infected skin
- dilated capillaries
- very loose skin
- inflamed or irritated skin
- very sensitive skin.

The cleanser is removed from the face with clean warm water and facial sponges and the skin blotted in readiness for the next stage of treatment.

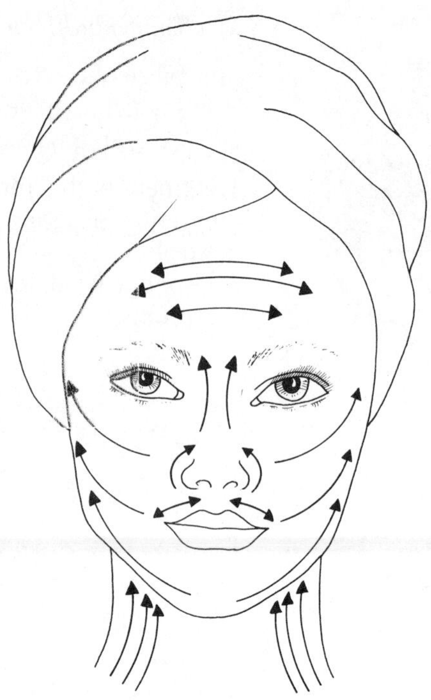

Direction of strokes for brush cleansing

Facial treatments: Self-checks

1. List 5 advantages in being treated by a professional beauty therapist.
2. What advice should be given to a client with contact lenses when booking her in for a facial?
3. Give four ways of helping a client to relax during a facial treatment.
4. Why should the client's head be raised slightly during a facial treatment?
5. Give four hygiene precautions which should be taken when applying skin-care products.
6. At what stage in a facial treatment should the skin analysis take place?
7. Give five beneficial effects of a deep-cleansing massage.
8. What special care is required when removing cleanser from the face of a client with dry mature skin?
9. Why should skin blockages be softened before being removed?
10. Why is a facial steamer more efficient than hot cotton wool pads for softening skin blockages?
11. State six safety precautions which should be taken when using a facial steamer.
12. Why is using a looped comedone extractor preferable to using the fingers when removing skin blockages?
13. Give four contra-indications to mechanical brush cleansing.
14. What should the skin look like and how should it feel after a deep cleanse treatment?

Facial massage

> Remember
> One of the best compliments your client can pay you is falling asleep while you are giving them a massage. You can't get much more relaxed than that!

> Remember
> Look after your hands and train them to work well for you. Keep them smooth and soft and practise hand and finger exercises regularly to keep the joints supple.

Effective massage requires extreme sensitivity and an expert touch. The cream or oil used to perform the massage helps to improve the appearance and texture of the skin. It also, provides 'slip' so that the massage movements are performed smoothly without causing discomfort.

The benefits of facial massage are that the process:
- increases supply of oxygen and nutrients to skin and muscles
- stimulates removal of waste products from the tissues
- improves cellular activity
- relieves tension and fatigue
- improves the texture of the skin
- promotes total relaxation

Classifications of massage movements

There are many different types of massage movements and routines used for treating the face. The combination of movements used depends on the main reason for the massage (for example lymphatic drainage, relaxation), the condition of the skin and underlying tissues and client preference.

Effleurage

Light, even, stroking movements which prepare the tissues for deeper massage and link up other movements in the facial sequence. The pressure of effleurage strokes may be increased over less bony areas.

The effects of effleurage are:
- relaxation from lightly applied effleurage movements
- an aid to desquamation and loosening of surface adhesions
- stimulation of an increased rate of blood flowing through the superficial circulation causing a slight increase in skin temperature.

Deep effleurage movements are also relaxing: they increase the rate of blood and lymph flow through the deeper skin tissue and muscles.

Petrissage

Compression (pressure) movements using either the whole of the palmar surface of the hand or just the pads of the thumbs and fingers. Kneading, knuckling, rolling and pinching are examples of petrissage movements which may be included in a facial sequence. Small, deep petrissage movements are more stimulating than larger, more superficial ones.

The effects of petrissage are:
- an increase in the rate at which blood and lymph flow through the area, due to the rhythmical filling and emptying of vessels and ducts which occurs with petrissage (this improves cellular nutrition and aids the removal of waste products)
- the skin appear smooth, clear and refreshed as a result of desquamation
- muscle fibres become relaxed and their tone is improved.

The trapezius covers the upper back and shoulders and the back and sides of the neck. The muscle becomes hard and develops tension nodules which can be felt along the upper fibres of the back in clients who are tired or stressed.

Thumb kneading to the trapezius helps to release the knotted muscle fibres and restore their parallel formation. This breaks up tension nodules and increases the supply of blood to the muscle.

Tapotement

> Remember
> Tapotement massage movements are very stimulating. They should not be applied over dilated capillaries or to a nervous highly strung client.

Percussion movements, for example tapping and slapping, which are performed lightly and briskly without compressing the skin.

The effects of tapotement are:
- stimulation of the superficial nerve endings causing temporary toning and tightening of the skin.
- improved blood flow resulting from alternate constriction and relaxation of blood vessels.
- removal of static lymph from tissues, e.g. from beneath the chin in a client with sluggish circulation.

Vibrations

These are quite difficult movements to perform. The muscles of the lower arms and hands are rapidly contracted and relaxed so that a mild shaking or trembling movement is produced by the fingers or thumbs. The vibrations run through a nerve centre or along a nerve path. There is very little surface stimulation.

> Remember
> Regular massage helps to nourish and revitalise ageing skin and muscles. It also relaxes the client, reducing the effects of stress, tension and fatigue.

The effects of vibrations are:
- relaxation
- gentle stimulation of the deeper skin layers
- relief from fatigue and muscular pain.

The following massage sequence combines variations of each of the basic massage movements to produce a treatment which stimulates the tissues, but also relaxes the client.

Massage movement		Main muscle(s) affected
1	Effleurage to shoulders (6 times)	Deltoid

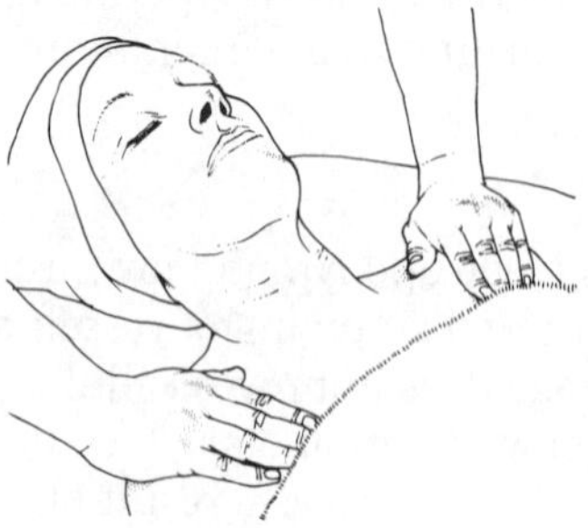

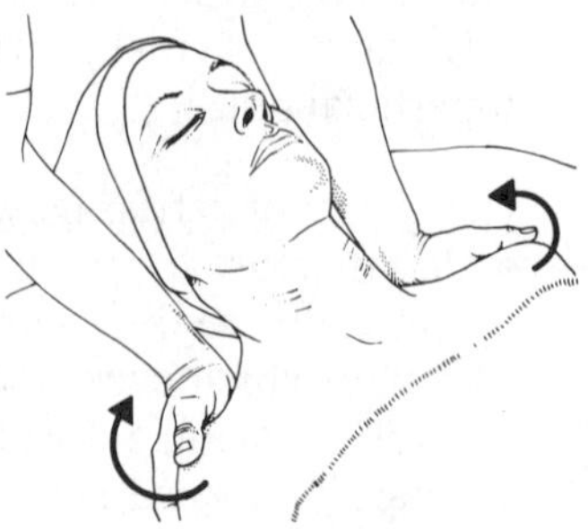

Massage movement	Main muscle(s) affected
2 a) Thumb kneading shoulders, upper back	Trapezius
b) Thumb stroking up neck to occipital cavity	Trapezius
c) Link effleurage over upper chest	
d) Repeat whole movement (6 times)	

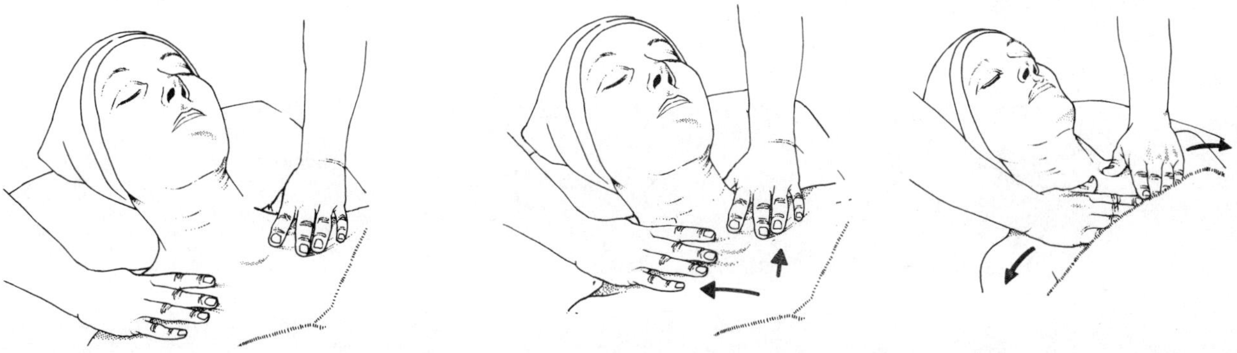

3 a) Finger kneading shoulders	Trapezius
b) Light vibrations, occipital cavity	

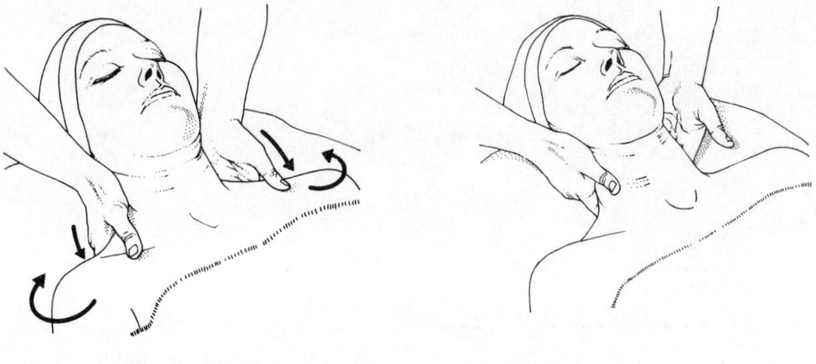

4 a) Finger kneading to neck	Platysma/sterno-mastoid

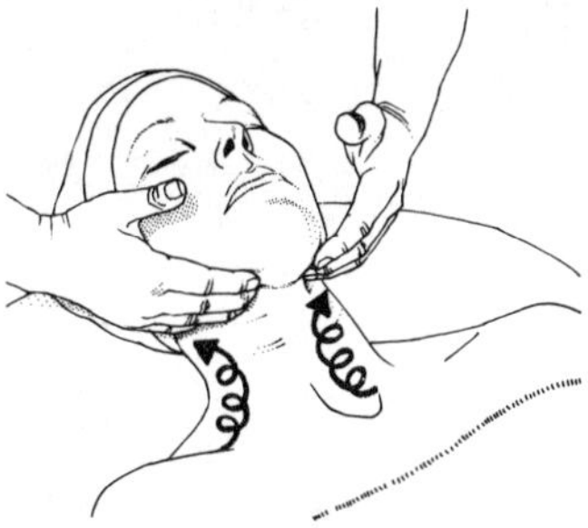

	Massage movement	Main muscle(s) affected
5	a) Firm, reinforced effleurage to neck	platysma/sternomastoid
	b) Link effleurage to other side of neck	
	c) As 5a	platysma/sterno-mastoid
	d) Repeat whole movement (6 times)	

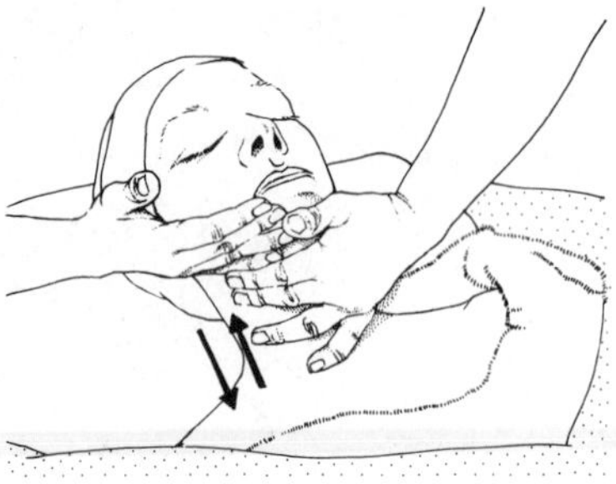

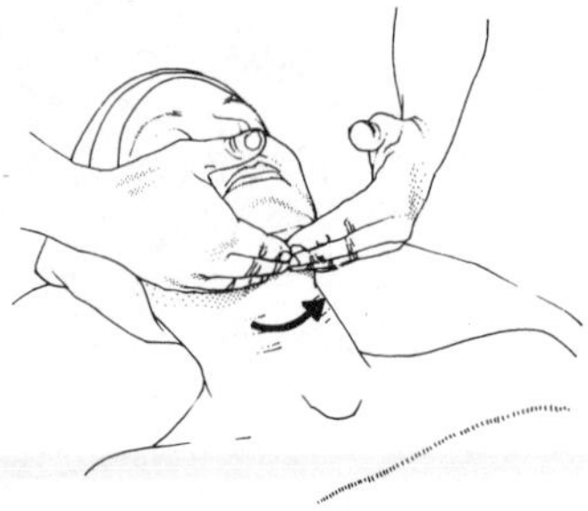

	Massage movement	Main muscle(s) affected
6	a) Knuckling to neck	platysma/sterno-mastoid

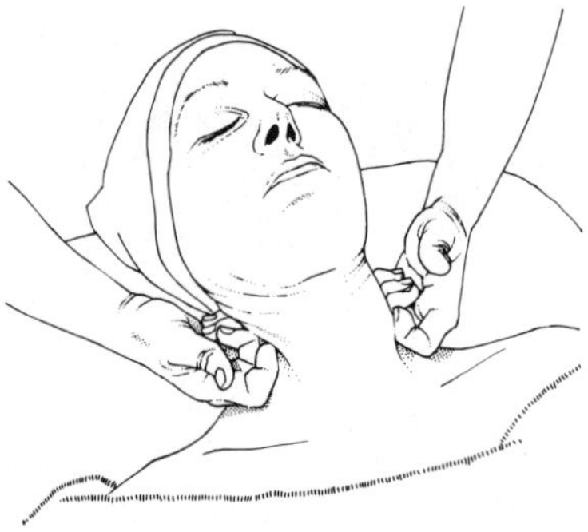

	Massage movement	Main muscle(s) affected
7	a) Chin brace of lips/masseter	depressors and levators
	b) Link effleurage	
	c) Repeat whole movement (6 times)	

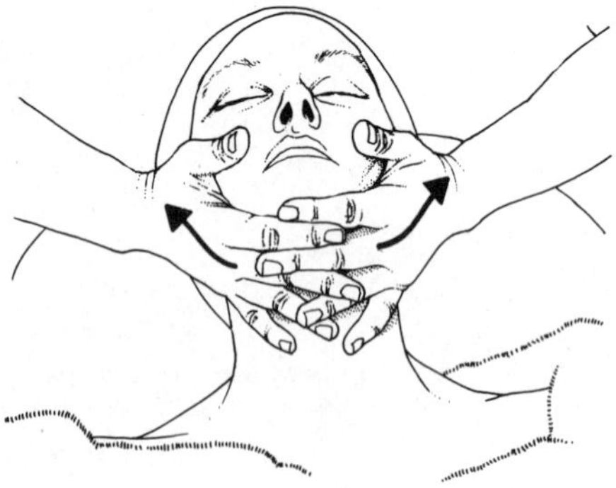

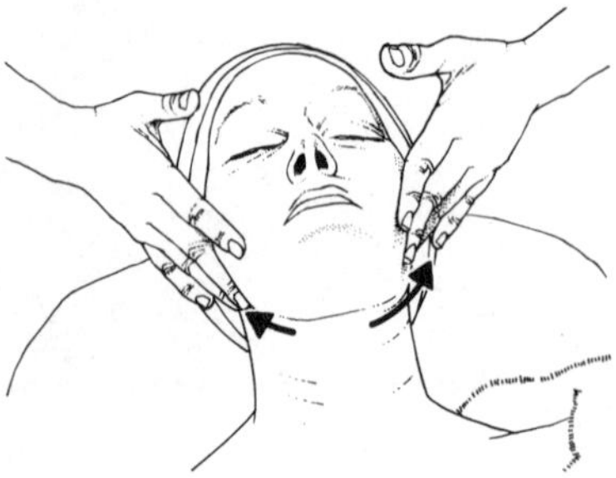

Massage movement	Main muscle(s) affected
8 a) Thumb kneading above chin and lower jaw b) Treat each side there and back (3 times) finishing on chin	depressors and levators of lips/masseter

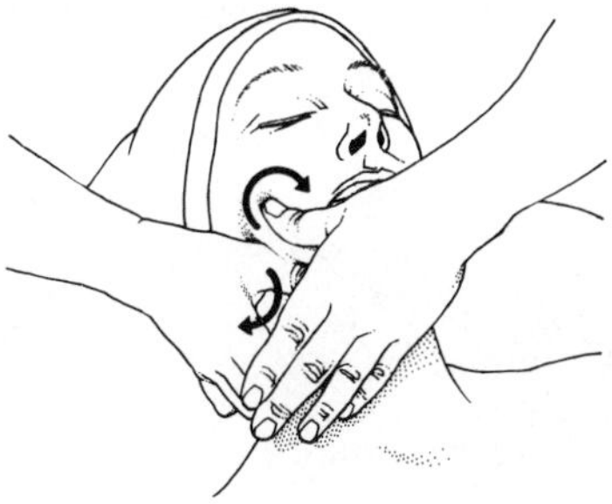

Massage movement	Main muscle(s) affected
9 a) Swift flick-ups to corners of mouth	orbicularis oris/risorius/buccinator

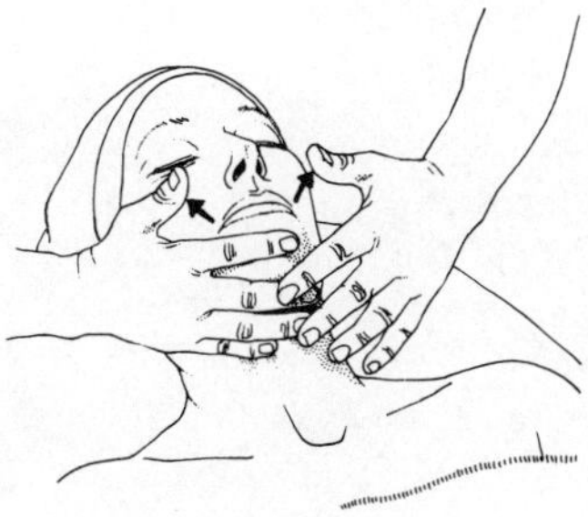

Massage movement	Main muscle(s) affected
10 a) Full face brace b) Link effleurage c) Repeat whole movement (6 times)	platysma/masseter/depressor and levators of lip/zygomaticus/buccinator/risorius/pyramidalis/frontalis

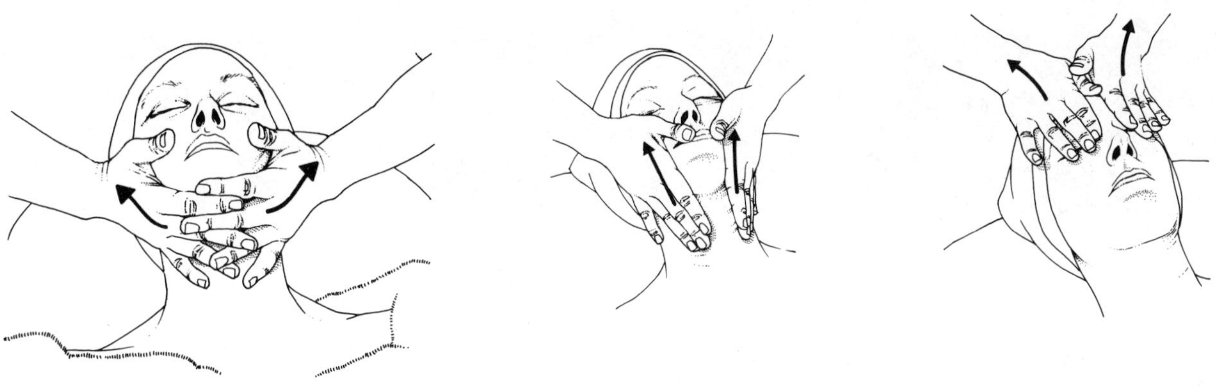

Massage movement	Main muscle(s) affected
11 a) Upward stroking eyebrow lifting frontalis/pyramidalis/temporalis b) Repeat whole movement (3 times)	

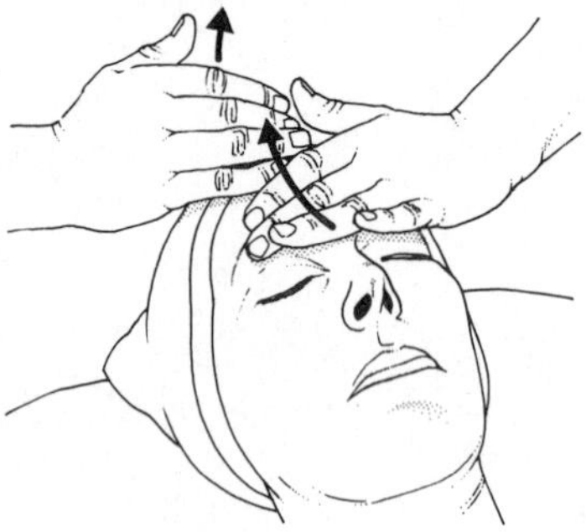

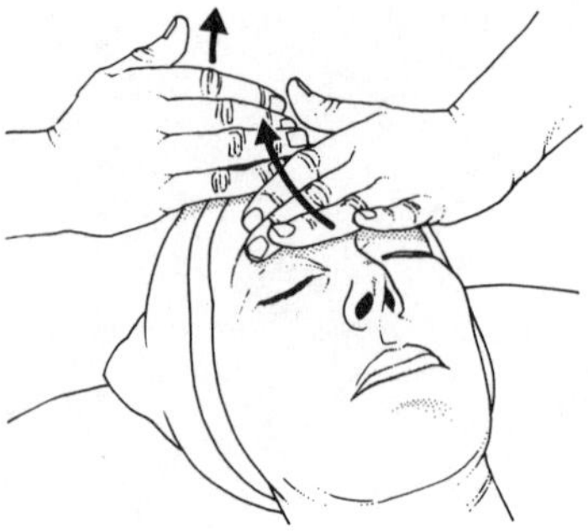

12 a) Stroking to temples (3 times), under eyes (3 times) and temples (3 times) b) Repeat other side and complete whole movement (3 times)	temporalis/orbicularis oculi/temporalis

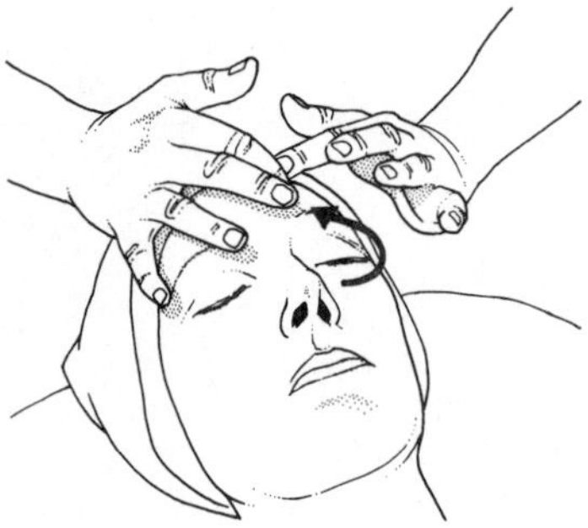

13 a) Half face brace b) Link effleurage c) Repeat whole movement (6 times)	mentalis/depressors and levators of lips/orbicularis oris/ zygomaticus/risorius/buccinator

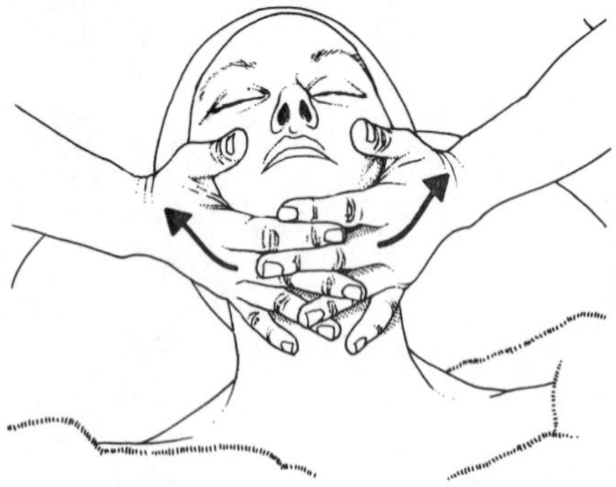

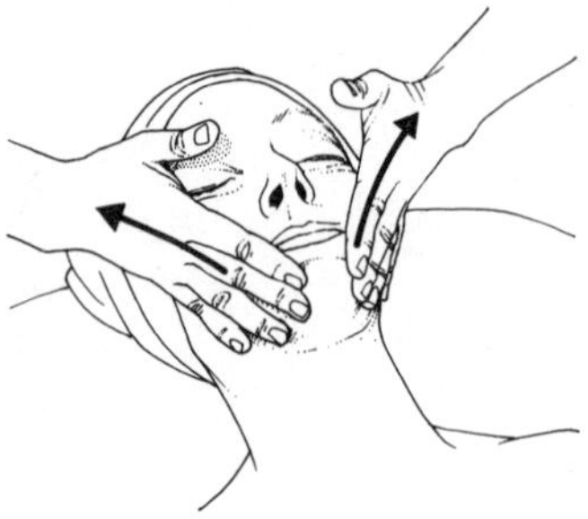

Massage movement	Main muscle(s) affected
14 a) Finger kneading chin, mouth, nose, temples b) Link effleurage c) Repeat whole movement (6 times)	mentalis/triangularis/depressors and levator of upper and lower lips/orbicularis oris/buccinator/zygomaticus/masseter/temporalis

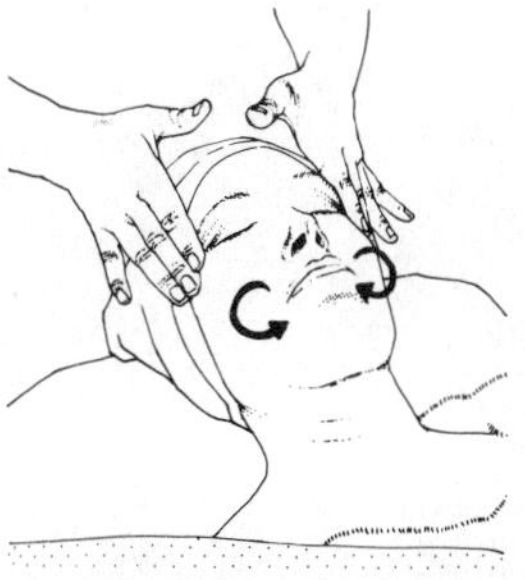

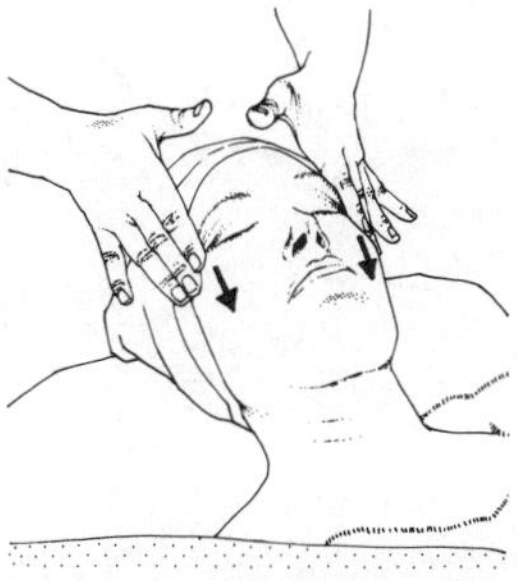

15 a) Thumb kneading to cheeks	buccinator/risorius/masseter/zygomaticus

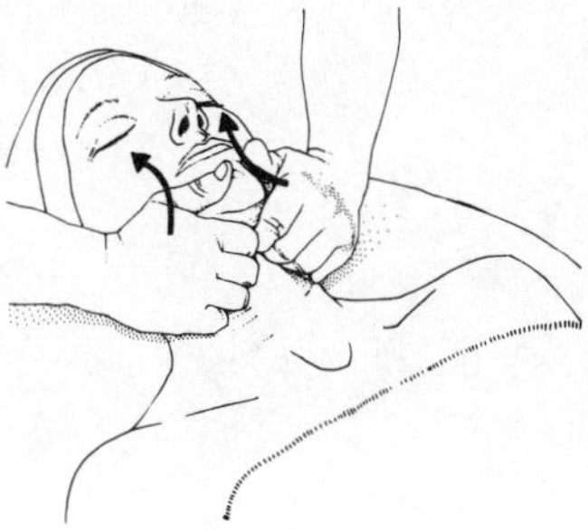

16 a) Tapotement beneath chin and mandible b) Cover length of jawline (6 times)	digastric/platysma

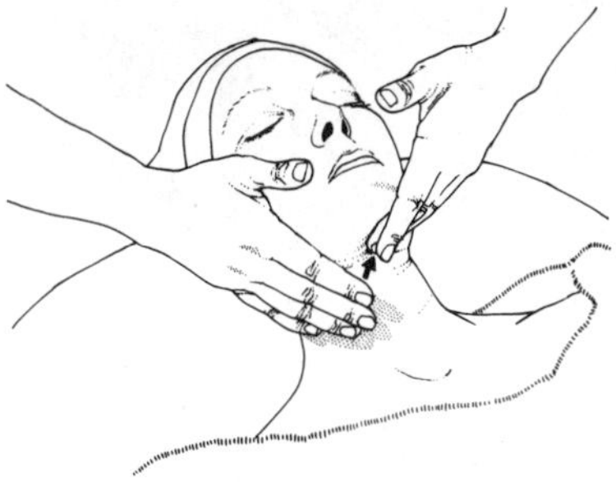

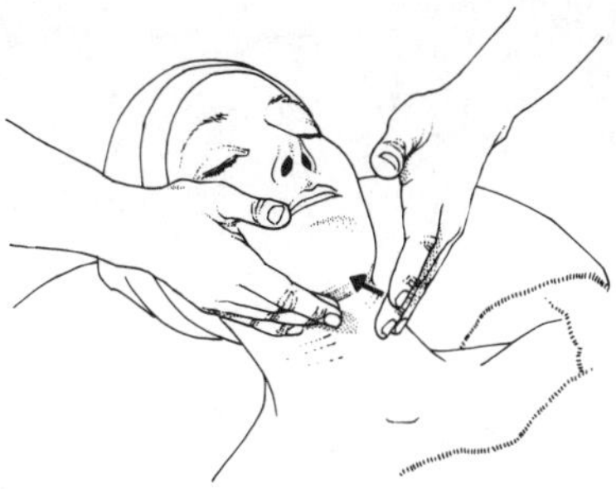

Massage movement	Main muscle(s) affected
17 a) Lifting masseter alternately each side b) Repeat whole movement (6 times)	masseter

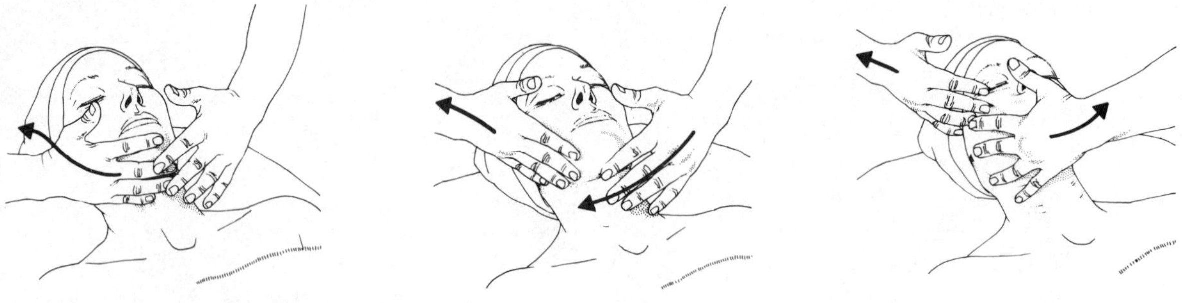

18 a) Rolling and pinching cheeks	buccinator/risorius/ zygomaticus/masseter

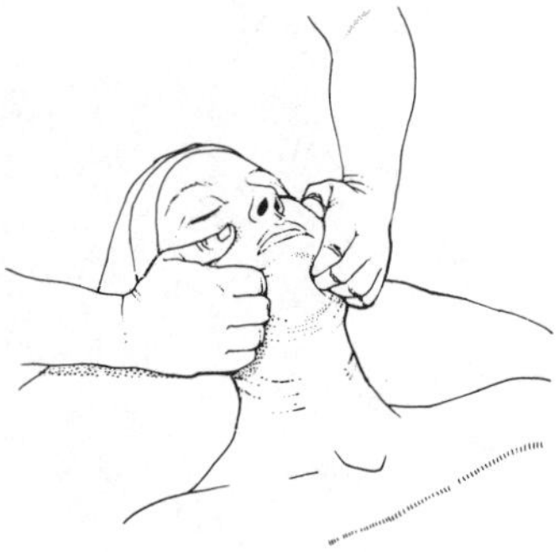

19 a) Lifting mandible b) Link effleurage c) Repeat whole movement (6 times)	platysma/digastric

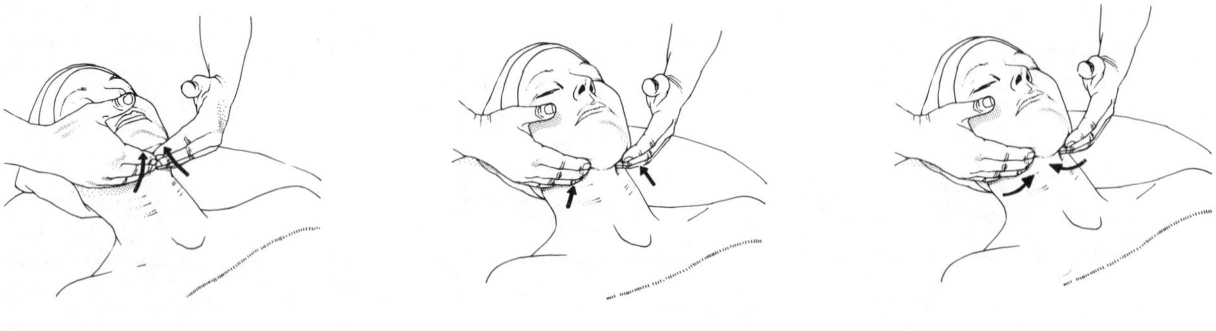

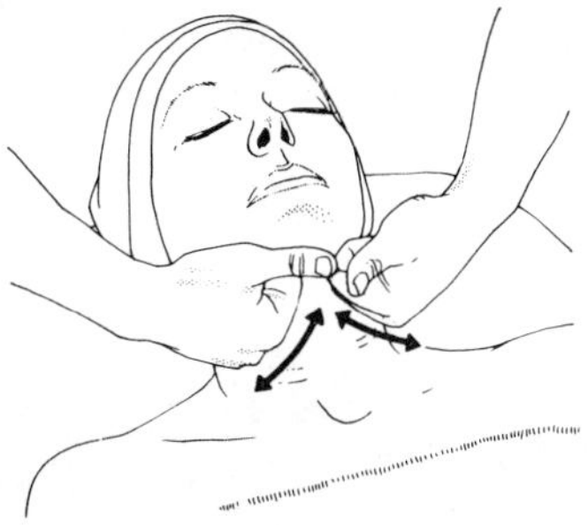

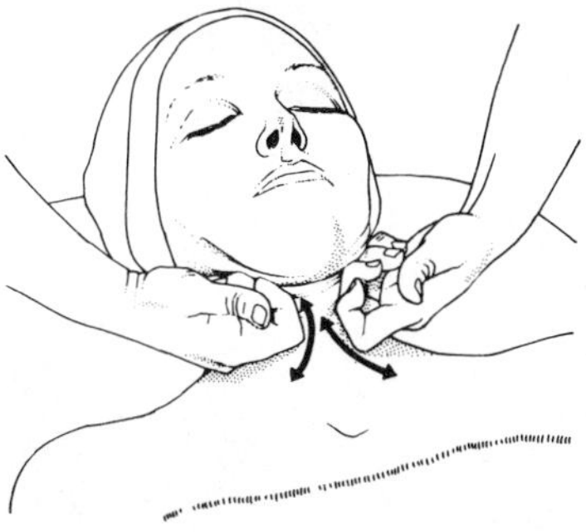

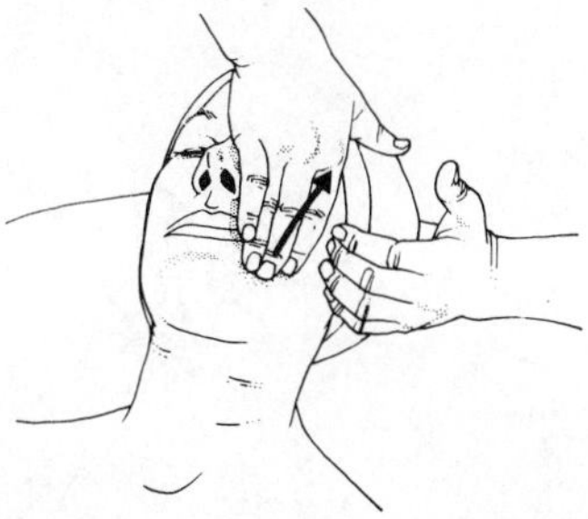

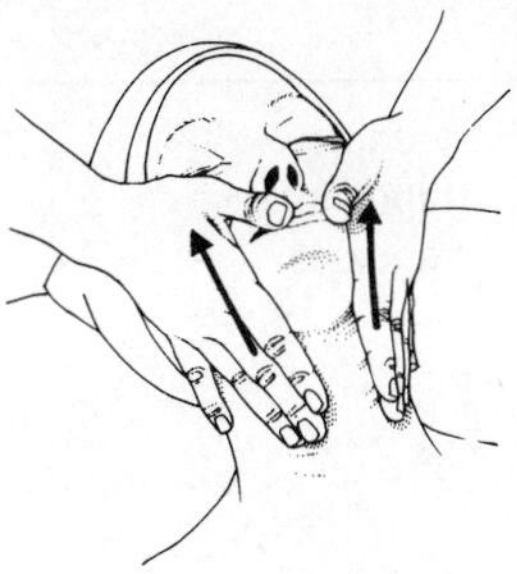

Massage movement	Main muscle(s) affected
20 a) Knuckling above and below jawline	mentalis/triangularis/masseter/ depressors of lower lip

21 a) Lifting tapotement to cheeks b) Repeat movement each side of the face (6 times) each hand	zygomaticus/buccinator/risorius

22 Full face brace as 10(a)-(c)

23 a) Scissor movement to eyebrows b) Link effleuage c) Repeat whole movement (6 times)	frontalis/orbicularis/oculi/levator palpebrae orbicularis oculi

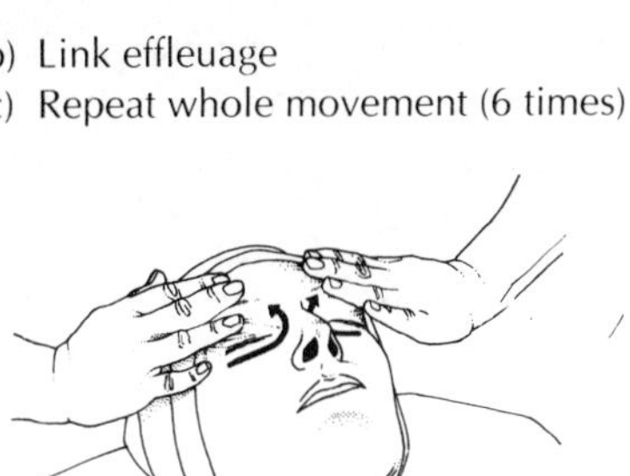

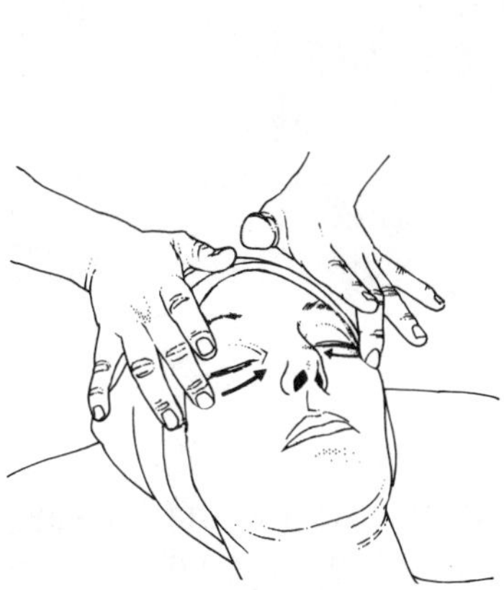

Massage movement	Main muscle(s) affected
24 a) Light tapotement around eyes b) Repeat whole movement (6 times)	orbicularis oculi/frontalis

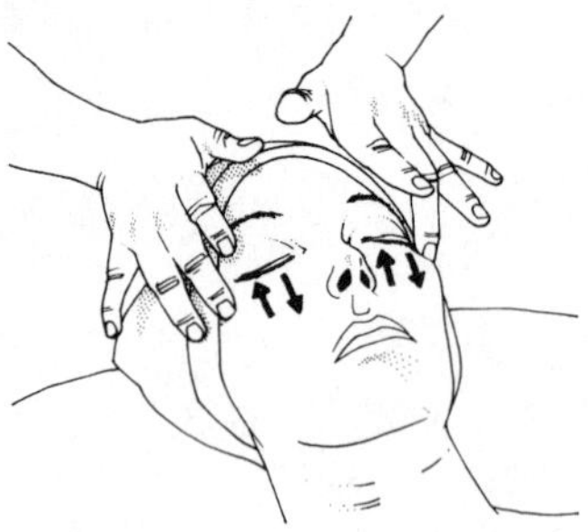

25 a) Stroking around eyes b) Repeat movement (6 times)	orbicularis oculi

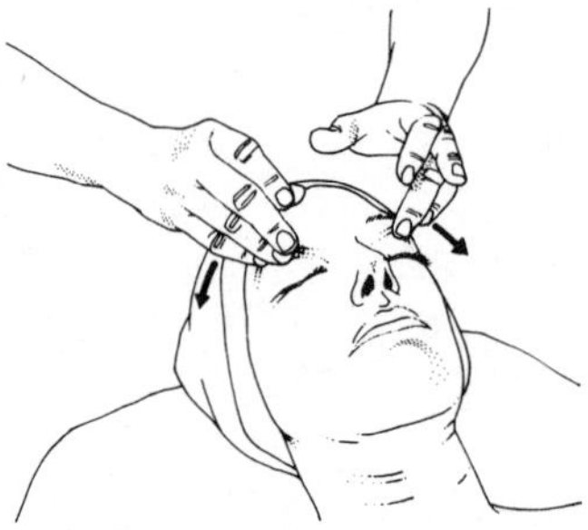

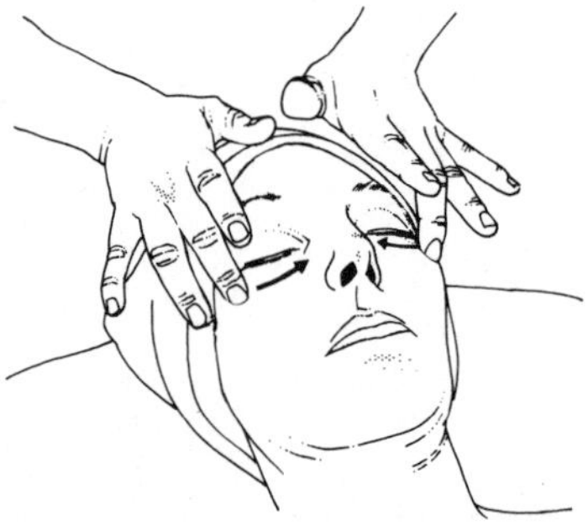

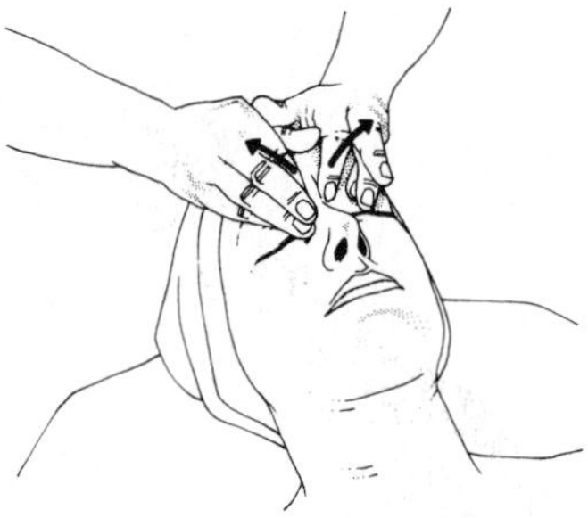

26 a) Repeat movement 1 b) Link effleurage c) Repeat movement 3b	deltoid trapezius trapezius

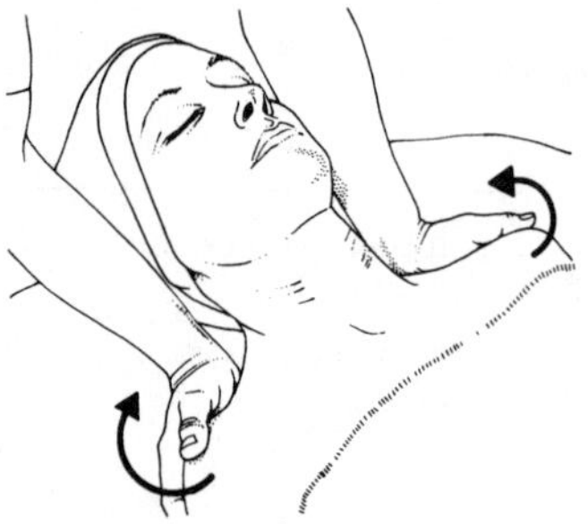

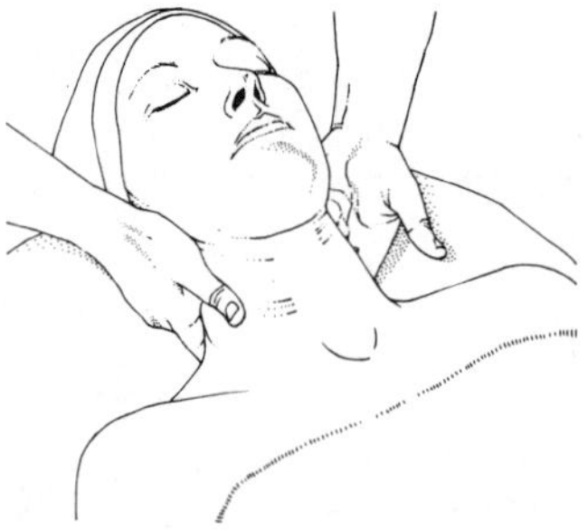

By this stage of the massage, the skin should feel slightly warm and appear clean, smooth and refreshed. Remove excess cream and tone and blot the skin in preparation for the face mask.

The stimulating effects of the massage continue for up to 48 hours after the massage. During this time, the skin throws off waste and toxins which may cause blotchiness and minor blemishes. The client should be warned in advance that these reactions are likely to occur and that they are due to the deep cleansing effects of the treatment. A soothing lotion will help to calm down any unwanted redness.

The skin should look at its best two to three days after a facial massage.

Completing the treatment

> *Remember*
>
> A heavy make-up is not suitable immediately after a facial treatment. Clients should be warned of this when making their appointment.
>
> Do not be talked in to applying any more than a light covering of face powder, basic eye-make-up and lipstick after a facial treatment.

Clients who arrive at the salon wearing make-up sometimes expect to be wearing it when they leave. Others prefer the feeling of clean fresh skin which may be spoiled if make-up is applied.

Whatever the personal preferences, the last few minutes of the treatment should be spent preparing the client for their departure and giving after-care advice.

This is a good time for encouraging the client to try special electrical treatments offered by the salon. Apart from their specific benefits, electrical treatments add variety and interest to a regular salon programme.

Treatment	Features	Benefits
High Frequency	Uses an electrical current and special applicators to heat the skin gently and stimulate the blood supply	Greasy skin: has a drying, healing effect which is particularly beneficial for mild acne
	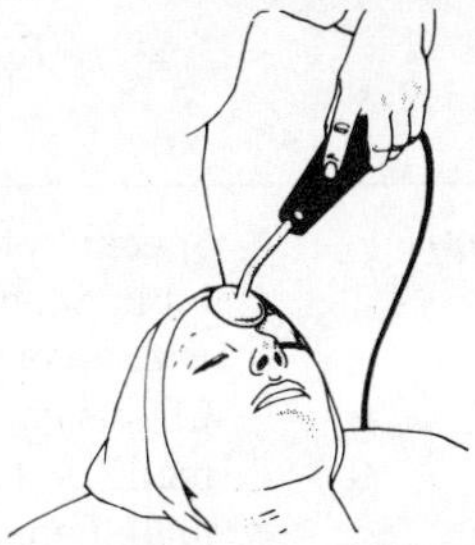	Balanced, dry, mature skin: increases the beneficial effects of the manual massage and aids the absorption of treatment creams
Vacuum suction	A type of mechanical massage which drains the lymphatic vessels using specially shaped cups and ventouse applicators	Deep-cleansing, loosens and removes skin blockages. Especially good for treating a greasy skin
	Stimulates the blood supply and aids desquamation	Nourishes, softens and smoothes a dry skin
	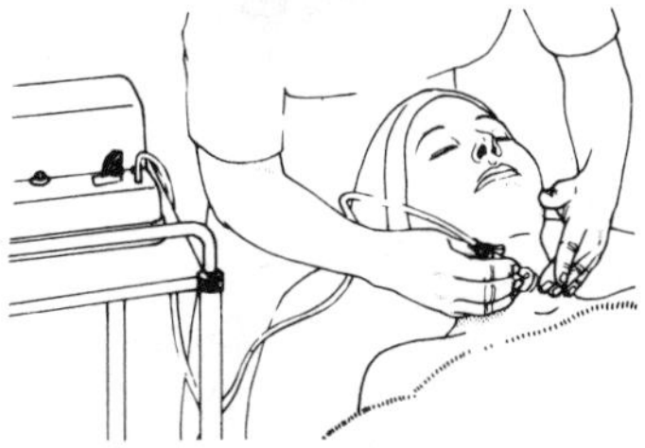	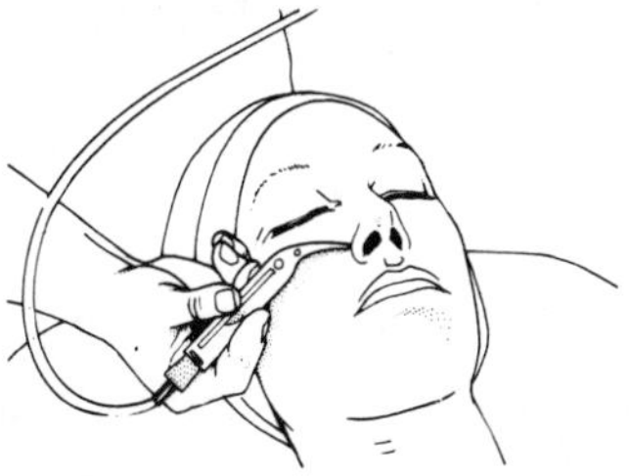

Treatment	Features	Benefits
Faradism	Form of 'passive exercise'. Client relaxes and machine does the work!	Regular treatments help to tone up loose muscles and firm facial contours. Helps reduce or prevent the effects of ageing.

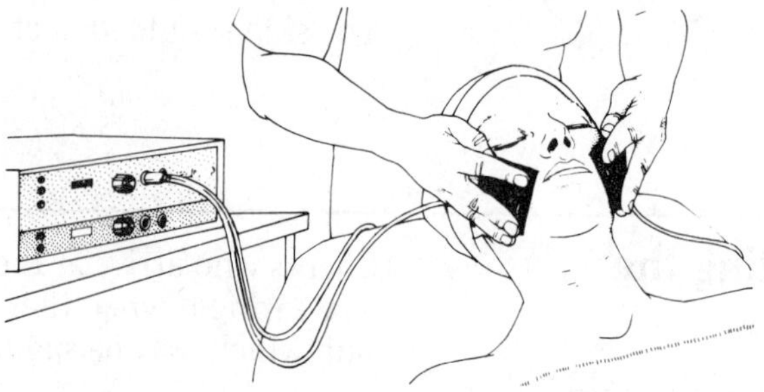

Treatment	Features	Benefits
Audio-sound	Machine produces sound waves which are absorbed by skin and muscles. Treatment does not produce surface stimulation	Very good for relieving stress in the upper back and across the shoulders. Particularly beneficial for clients with very sensitive skin who cannot have stimulating forms of massage.

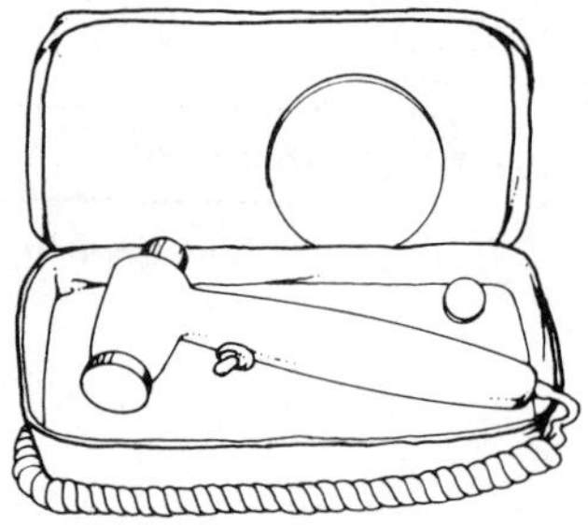

Treatment	Features	Benefits
Galvanism	Special substances are introduced into the skin with an electric current. Clients can have recipes made up from biological ingredients suitable for their skin type or problem.	Desincrustation: a special product is used to form a type of soap on the skin. A very deep-cleansing treatment which is particularly beneficial for greasy skin. Iontophoresis: there are 'active' ingredients available for treating a wide variety of skin conditions. The improvements can be seen immediately after treatment.

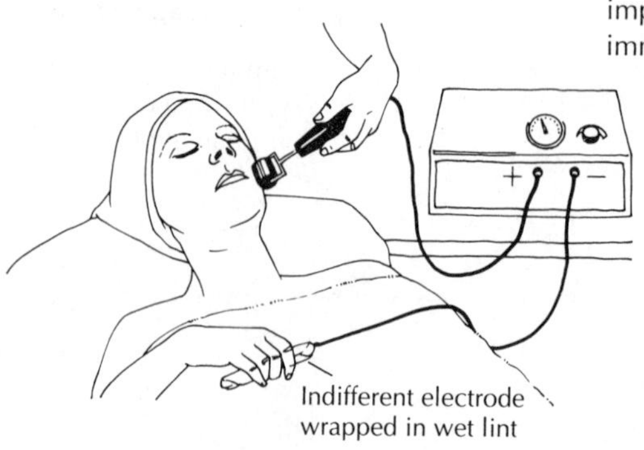

> *Remember*
> If the client gets up too quickly, there will be a sudden rush of blood away from the head, causing dizziness.

When the treatment is finished, ask if the client is happy with the results and then slowly raise the head of the couch to an upright position.

Check if the client will shortly run out of any home-care products and advise accordingly. Enter final details of treatment and purchases on the client's record card and assist with arranging the next appointment.

> *Remember*
> Do not rush your client once the treatment is over. The last few minutes are invaluable for reinforcing important aspects of home-care advice and selling products from the salon's retail range.

To summarise facial procedure:

- remove make-up (superficial cleanse)
- analyse skin....ask questions....discuss
- deep cleanse. steam, exfoliate, pore cleanse
- shape eyebrows
- massage
- apply face mask
- moisturise, apply a light make-up
- give home care advice
- check the client's retail requirements
- advise about further salon treatments
- complete the record card.

Facial massage: Self-checks

1. Name the four main classifications of massage movements and describe their effects.
2. How should massage movements be adapted for different areas of the face?
3. Why should a client be advised against having a facial massage on the day of a special event?
4. Why are eye pads applied during the face mask treatment?
5. What particular care is required when removing a clay-based mask from a client with a black skin?
6. Why is moisturiser required after a clay mask treatment?

Facial massage: Activities

1. Find out which electrical treatments are offered in your salon. Read any information leaflets which are available and ask your supervisor if you may watch the treatments being given. Try describing the treatments in your own words as if you were advising a client.
2. With a friend, discuss all the different ways in which you could promote retail sales during a facial treatment. Set yourself a target of selling at least one skin-care product to each of the next six clients you treat: good luck!

Chapter 6

Make-up

After working through this chapter you will be able to:

- appreciate the benefits of a range of make-up services
- recognise particular problems associated with different make-up services
- know the basic ingredients contained in make-up products
- choose and use the correct make-up products, tools and equipment
- carry out appropriate hygiene procedures
- adapt the make-up application for a range of different clients and services
- understand the need for *hypo-allergenic* cosmetics
- appreciate the effects of colour and texture when designing a make-up
- complete a make-up chart for a client.

> Remember
>
> All make-up treatments provide ideal opportunities for retail sales. Have confidence in the products you sell in your salon by using the products yourself. Clients will often make a purchase as a direct result of admiring the make-up you are wearing when they come for treatment.

The salon may offer a wide range of services to promote make-up treatments. Some of these create exciting challenges for the creative beauty therapist who has a particular interest in developing specialised make-up skills.

Offering a make-up service

The range of make-up services offered by a salon depends very much on the nature of the business and the expertise of the staff who are employed there. Here are some ways in which you could be expected to use your make-up skills:

- basic after-facial make-up
- make-up lessons for day and evening wear
- weddings
- make-up for evening and special occasions
- portrait photography
- demonstrations
- fashion shows
- remedial camouflage.

Basic after-facial make-up

> Remember
>
> Clients really appreciate how clean, smooth and soft their skin feels after a facial. They do not usually want make-up applied straight afterwards and they are happy to leave the salon with just a light application of moisturiser to protect the skin.

Some of the effects of a full facial continue for a short time once the treatment has finished. A stimulating massage speeds up the rate at which waste products are removed from the deeper layers of the skin and this can temporarily upset its acid balance. The skin may react with the foundation, turning it an orange colour. The foundation may also go blotchy, making it difficult to achieve a smooth finish. The skin is usually at its best 48 hours after a facial and, once it has calmed down, the make-up problems are solved.

> Remember
>
> If the client is not going home straight after the treatment, she may appreciate a light application of loose face powder, eye make-up and lipstick.

Make-up lessons

Many clients do not realise how attractive they are until they have had their make-up applied by a professional. Not surprisingly, once they have seen the possibilities, they want to be able to achieve the same effects for themselves.

Most lessons commence with creating a make-up for day wear which is then adapted for evening wear. The lessons take place with the client seated in front of a large mirror so that she can watch the demonstration of techniques on her own face and then copy them under the scrutiny of the therapist!

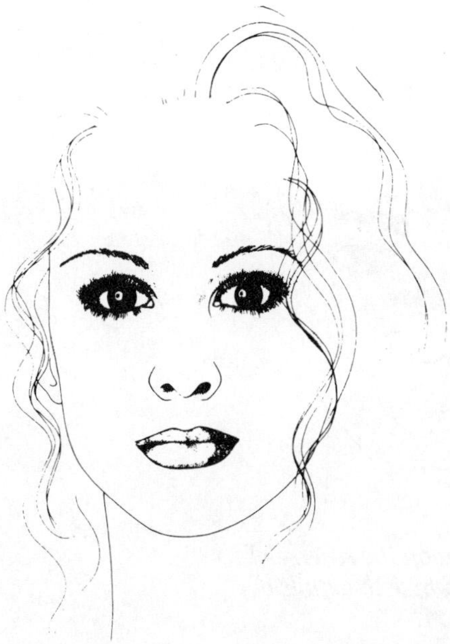

> Remember
>
> You need not worry about losing clients by sharing your make-up secrets with them. If your lesson is linked with sales of products from the salon's retail range, the client will keep returning to replace and build up her collection.

> Remember
>
> You will have to adapt your advice for people who wear spectacles or contact lenses.

> Remember
>
> Clients who do not have much experience of applying make-up often prefer to use pencils and sponge applicators rather than brushes which are a bit harder to control. Be patient with your client. Techniques which are easy for you may be very difficult for a client who is not used to applying make-up. You must encourage the client, not demoralise her.

The client participates in the facial analysis and the relevance of structure and colour is explained at each stage. Particular emphasis is placed on:

- preparing the skin for make-up: advising on the importance of a clean 'canvas' and recommending the most appropriate cleanser, toner and under-make-up base
- choosing and applying the cosmetics: matching the colour, texture and types of products to the client's features and the effects required.
- handling the skin correctly to avoid stretching or over-stimulating the skin
- supporting the hand, keeping control of the applicator to ensure a good finish when making up the eyes and lips
- using make-up and equipment effectively and hygienically: matching client's abilities with the types of products and applicators used and stressing the importance of keeping them clean
- keeping the make-up looking fresh: touching up with pressed powder, using a fine mineral water spray or damp cotton wool and refreshing lipstick application
- removing make-up from the skin: choosing and applying cosmetic cleansers and appropriate after-care.

> **Remember**
> Once the client has become confident with applying her own make-up, she will become more adventurous and will want to try out new products. Make sure you keep accurate records of the products which a client has purchased and keep her informed of new colours and additions to the make-up range.

At the end of the lesson, the client is issued with a make-up chart, filled in by the therapist, which identifies the most suitable products and how they should be applied.

It is important that the client looks and feels wonderful after the make-up lesson, but it is even more important that they are able to re-create the effect themselves, using products purchased from the salon. Most clients are more aware of their bad points than their good points. A make-up lesson should make the client feel good about herself and help to build up her confidence.

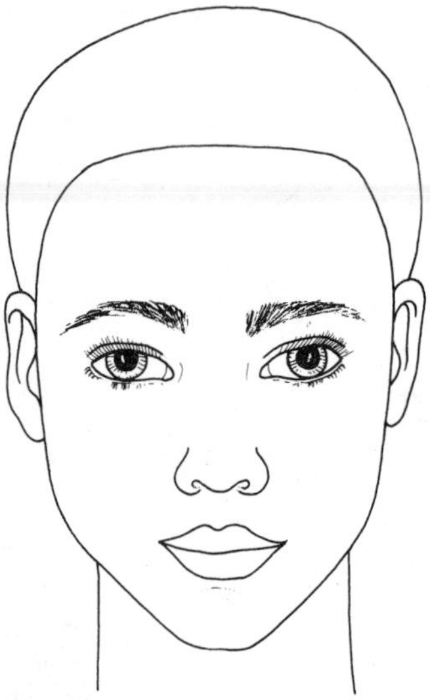

A facial diagram on the reverse of the card is filled in with details of the products used

MAKE-UP RECORD CARD

Surname: First Names: Address: Tel no:	Date of Birth: Client requirements:
Date of Consultation:	Consultant:

	Colour:	ADVICE	AM	PM
Skin	Type:	Under make-up base		
	Problems:	Colour correction		
		Foundation		
		Powder		
Bone Structure	Face shape:	Blusher		
	Problems:	Highlighter		
		Shader		
Eyes	Colour: Shape/size:	Eye shadow		
	Problems:	Eye liner		
		Mascara		
		Eyebrow pencil		
Lips	Shape/size:	Lip pencil		
	Problems:	Lipstick		

Offering a make-up service: Self-checks

1 Why is it advisable *not* to have a facial massage immediately before a special make-up treatment?

2 State three benefits to a client of having a professional make-up lesson.

3 State two products which you could 'link-sell with a lipstick purchase.

Make-up for weddings

> **Remember**
> Stimulating skin treatments should be given at least 48 hours before the wedding day to give time for the skin to calm down.
>
> The eyebrows should be shaped and individual false lashes applied one or two days before the wedding. This saves time on the day and reduces the risk of the eye area being sensitive when the wedding make-up is applied.

There are enough things which can go wrong on a wedding day without the bride's make-up being one of them! Many brides prefer to have their make-up applied professionally so that they can be confident of looking their best on their very special day.

Spring is traditionally the season of the white wedding and this is a particularly good time for promoting special offers for the bride and, sometimes, for the bridesmaids and the bride's mother too!

Of course, not all weddings are white. They do not necessarily take place in a church and the bride can be any age between sixteen and ninety! It is, therefore, impossible to generalise on specific wedding make up techniques: the make-up must, as usual, be adapted to suit the individual. The features of a make-up service which are common to all weddings are more to do with designing the overall effect of the make-up and organising events leading up to the wedding.

A preliminary consultation with the bride is essential. Apart from providing important information, this will give you an opportunity to get to know your client better and gain her confidence.

You will need to find out:

- the date and time of the wedding: this will help you to schedule pre-wedding appointments for carrying out a facial assessment, applying beauty therapy treatments and practising the make-up

The final make-up appointment will have to be scheduled within the overall wedding preparations and enough time must be allowed for the bride to be able to relax and enjoy the treatment.

Ideally the make-up should be applied just before the hair is dressed and the wedding gown is put on. Some brides prefer to have their make-up applied in the relative calm of the beauty salon. Others may request that you visit their home, in which case there will be a charge for the extra time that you are not available at the salon.

- details of the wedding dress: the design, colour and material of the dress will influence the make-up design. Make-up colours will look stronger in contrast with a pale, traditional wedding gown than with a more colourful outfit. The make-up look will have to be softer for lightweight materials than for heavier or embossed fabrics
- hair style and head dress: the bride's choice of head dress may require her hair to be styled in a different way, which may affect the appearance of her face and the balance of her features. Corrective make-up work may be necessary to compensate for this
- flowers: lipstick and nail enamel colours must tone in with the colour scheme of the bouquet and any other flowers which are being carried or worn
- the client's own experience with make-up: all brides want to look beautiful on their wedding day, but they also want to feel comfortable with how they look. Importantly, they want to be recognised! A wedding day is not the right time to go for dramatic change. The bride must feel confident that the make-up is enhancing the way she likes to look

> **Remember**
> False tanning or sunbed treatments may be recommended in preference to body make-up for evening out skin colour if the dress has a low back or scooped neckline which reveals pale areas of the body.

> **Remember**
> It is helpful if you can see a sample of the wedding dress material and, also, that of the bridesmaids, so that you can co-ordinate your make-up scheme with them.

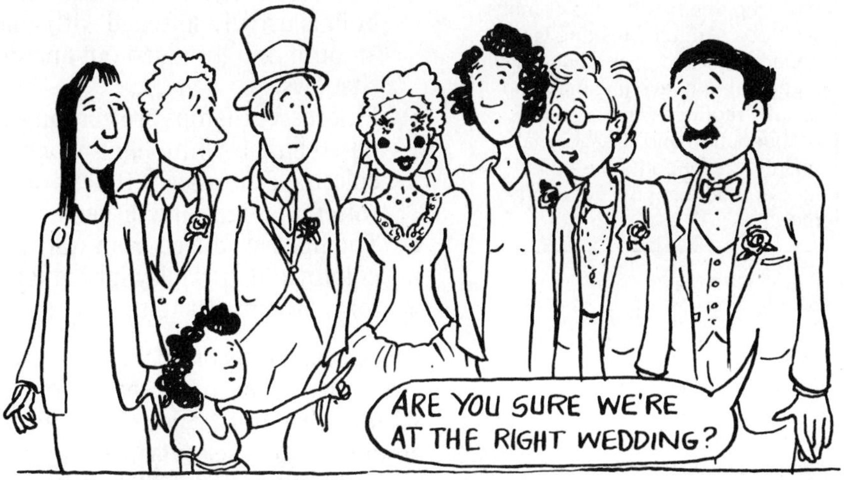
ARE YOU SURE WE'RE AT THE RIGHT WEDDING?

> **Remember**
> To cool down the skin and prevent the foundation from becoming shiny, press a cotton wool pad dampened with eau-de-cologne or witch hazel over the face. The pad can be kept moist in a waterproof wrapping. If the bride is not carrying a bag, the pad can be tucked conveniently inside her dress until it is required.
>
> A compact of pressed powder slips easily into a small bag and is ideal for touching up make-up during the day. The powder helps to absorb excess grease and reset the foundation. This is important for minimising the effects of shiny skin on the photographs.

- after-wedding arrangements: make-up applied in the morning may be expected to survive not only the marriage ceremony and formal reception, but, also, an evening party when the bride may be meeting some of the guests for the first time. Your client will need advice on keeping her make-up refreshed throughout the celebrations. She will be photographed throughout the events and will need to replenish her lipstick regularly to maintain colour balance.

The make-up contributes greatly to the image of the bride captured for the wedding album on film, and probably also on video. A make-up which is applied well and subtly blended will look good close up and will also withstand the discerning eye of the camera lens.

Make-up for weddings: Self-checks

1 List four points which should be taken into consideration when planning the make-up for a bride.

Make-up for evening and special occasions

Whatever the event, if the client wants to look special, then the occasion is special. Most special occasions are evening events and the effects of artificial lighting have to be taken into account when choosing make-up colours. Basic techniques also have to be adapted to produce extra definition to the make-up.

The effects of lighting on make-up

Natural daylight is pure white light which shows up the true colours of make-up. Although it is produced from the sun, daylight does not just fall on the face from above. It is reflected onto the face from any light-coloured surface it hits, including walls and floors. If the client wants a natural looking make-up, then subtle shades must be used which are blended well without any hard demarcation lines.

The effects of artificial lighting on make-up depend on the source and type of lighting.

- Filament lamps contained in standard light bulbs produce a yellowish light which dulls the effect of blue-toned colours and makes red tones appear darker. The bright glare produced from a bulb is usually softened with a lampshade which reduces the amount of light given out and directs it downwards, creating sharp shadows.
- Fluorescent lamps are contained in tubes. White tubes give out a harsh bluish-white light which takes the warmth out of make-up colours. Fluorescent tubes are usually covered with diffusers which soften the light and disperse it so that very little shadow is created.
- The light produced from warm white fluorescent tubes is closest in colour to natural daylight and is the best type of artificial lighting for matching make-up colours.

> *Remember*
> The whiter the light falling on the make-up, the brighter the colours will look. Artificial lighting is not generally as strong as daylight. As a general rule, evening make-up usually requires warmer shades of foundation and stronger make-up colours for contouring the face and defining the eyes and mouth.

The special occasion make-up must complement the outfit that will probably have been purchased for the event so that a total look is achieved. Exciting colour combinations, high gloss and pearlised products and false eyelashes may be used where appropriate for helping to achieve the desired effect. Ultimately, the make-up may not be suitable for normal day wear, but it will make the client feel extra glamorous for her special occasion.

Portrait photography

It is not only royalty who have portrait photographs taken! There are significant events in many people's lives which prompt them to have a special sitting for a photographer and a professionally applied make-up can help to ensure that the camera catches them at their best.

If you are involved with work of this type, you will be fascinated by the range of effects which a photographer can create by adjusting camera angles and lighting schemes and by using special lenses. Here are some general considerations which you will have to bear in mind when applying make up for photographs:

- Photographic lighting can get very hot and the make-up may begin to melt, particularly during a long sitting. Do not apply a heavy make-up and keep the skin as cool as possible during application.
- Grease on the face produces an unattractive shine and emphasises creases and open pores. Do not use a greasy under-make-up base. Avoid using cream textured products. Re-apply loose translucent face powder throughout the make-up procedure to achieve a matte finish.
- Pearlised make-up products can look attractive on photograph but they reflect light and can cause glare. Keep the use of pearlised products to a minimum: they will look more effective when contrasted with matte textures. An eye make-up comprising of a number of pearlised products will lose definition. Pearlised products used on the face will emphasise flaws and defects.
- The camera will pick up patches of discoloration and natural shadows created by skin folds. You will need to even out the skin colour and lighten areas such as under the eyes and the creases at the sides of the nostrils and above the chin before you apply the foundation.
- Photographic lighting wipes out the natural highlights and shadows created by facial contour. You will have to use highlighting and shading techniques to define the bone structure and balance the features. The foundation colour should be as light as possible to enhance the effects of the contour cosmetics.

> Remember
> A satisfied client may be persuaded to let you have a copy of her portrait to display in the salon as an advertisement for your make-up!

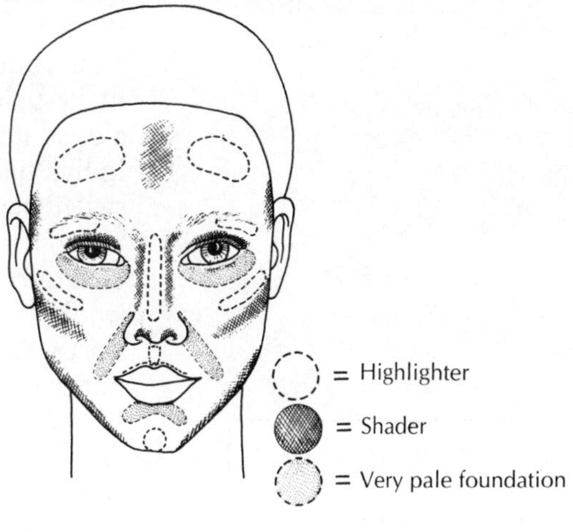

Specialised contouring techniques for photographic work

- Hard lines are emphasised on camera: all make-up products must be blended well, ensuring that there are no hard demarcation lines. This is particularly important when applying contour cosmetics and blending foundation down the neck and into the hairline.

Make-up for evening and special occasions: Self-checks

1. Which type of artificial lighting is closest in colour to natural daylight?
2. Give three ways in which a make-up for evening is different from a make-up for day wear.
3. State three make-up problems which can be created by the effects of artificial lighting.

Demonstrations

> *Remember*
> Always take plenty of price lists with you to a demonstration and make sure you understand enough about the full range of treatments to be able to explain their benefits and give general advice.

> *Remember*
> Demonstrations run more smoothly when the work is divided between two people. One person applies the make-up and the other provides the commentary. If the demonstration is being carried out in a hall or large room with a high ceiling, sound will not carry very well and you may need to use a microphone.

> *Remember*
> Promote the products and treatments offered at your salon when you are answering questions from the audience.

Make-up demonstrations are an excellent way of attracting new clients to the business. They have good entertainment value because they are visual and the effects are immediate. Local community groups are usually very pleased to schedule demonstration evenings in their social calendar and these provide opportunities for promoting the salon and the range of services offered. Special discount arrangements for people attending the demonstration often prompt an initial visit to the salon which results in them having regular treatments.

A good make-up demonstration needs organising well. Here is some advice to help you with the planning.

- Find out as much about your audience as possible: you will need to know approximately how many people will be attending and their age range. This is useful for preparing your talk and selecting the most appropriate products.
- Try to visit the venue beforehand: once you have seen the room you will have a better idea about the lighting and acoustics. You may wish to liaise with the organisers about seating arrangements, organising a display area and accessing facilities.
- Find out when the demonstration is due to finish: the premises may have to be vacated by a particular time and you will need to plan your talk accordingly, allowing extra time for answering questions from the audience.
- Make a list beforehand of everything you need to take: the demonstration may be taking place at the end of a working day. If you plan well, you can use the interval before the event to have a break and freshen yourself up for the evening. This is much better than rushing about at the last minute.
- Pack your products and equipment neatly and in logical order: make-up display stands are useful for transporting, as they provide a good range of colours and minimise the number of small individual items that you need to take. Make sure that drawers are sealed before you leave so that they do not get damaged in transit. Try to use as many unbreakable containers as possible for carrying cleansers, toners and moisturisers. Take prepared pads of cotton wool in a plastic bowl with a sealed lid and provide disposal bags for waste. You may need to take a container of water if the room does not have a supply of running water.
- Plan to arrive at the venue at least half an hour before the demonstration is due to start: you will need to set up the area and prepare your equipment in peace. It is more difficult to do this once the audience starts to arrive, as your display will probably attract a lot of attention and you may be distracted by having to answer questions.

The first demonstration you are involved in will probably be quite a nerve wracking experience! Don't worry: the time passes very quickly once you have started and you will probably surprise yourself at how knowledgeable you are! Confidence grows with experience and each demonstration is good practice for the next one. Here are some guidelines to help you through your first demonstration.

- Starting proceedings: begin on time, smile and welcome the guests. Make sure that everyone knows your name (and your colleague's) and which salon you represent. If anyone looks puzzled, describe the actual location of the salon.
- Inviting a volunteer from the audience to model: if you have a choice, do not select the youngest and most attractive person who applies their own make-up well. Choose someone who will look significantly different at the end of the demonstration.
- Instructing on skin care and make-up: at each stage of the demonstration, explain about the products you are using and the best way of applying and removing them. Tell the audience what you intend to do and how you are going to do it. When you have finished, invite them to confirm that you have done it!
- Keeping the audience interested: make sure you do not block the view of the audience when applying the make-up: involve the audience in what you are doing. Invite them to help you choose colours and then explain your final choice. Always talk to the audience and project your voice so that people at the back can hear you. Maintain good eye contact and keep smiling!
- Maintaining the flow: if you are providing a running commentary and someone else is demonstrating the make-up, do not read a prepared speech. Reading shows lack of confidence and encourages you to talk to the floor; your voice will become monotonous and will not be heard by most of the audience. If necessary, use small prompt cards in the order of the talk. These will have key words written on them as a quick reminder of where you should be up to.
- Seeking approval: invite the audience to acknowledge how lovely your model looks before you show her the final effect. The approval of other people will give her the confidence to accept her new look.
- Finishing the demonstration: ask the audience to join you in thanking the model and, if possible, offer her a small gift. This could be a lipstick or a gift voucher for the salon. Invite the audience to have a closer look at the finished make-up and make yourself available for answering questions.

> *Remember*
>
> Although you want to be helpful, some of the questions you are asked may be better answered in the salon when the skin can be inspected properly during a consultation. Make sure that people who show particular interest leave the demonstration with a business card and price list.

Demonstrations: Self-checks

1 What information is it useful to have before planning a make-up demonstration?

Demonstrations: Activities

1 You can pick up lots of useful tips by watching experienced demonstrators at work. If you have an opportunity, watch the professionals who often demonstrate in the cosmetic departments of large stores. If a more senior member of staff in your salon is due to give an outside demonstration, ask if you can go and watch and keep notes on things that seem to work really well.

2 Find out which are the most common problems experienced by people applying their own make-up. Talk to friends, colleagues and clients. Prepare some good advice and make-up tips for your next make-up lesson.

Fashion shows

A customer who shops regularly at a local boutique is a potential client for your salon and may be tempted to visit you if she comes across your business cards when she is buying clothes. Likewise, your salon can provide a similar service for neighbouring shops and hairdressing salons who are not your competitors. It makes good sense for local businesses to support each other and attract extra customers to the area: fashion shows are a very effective way of involving different businesses in a joint promotional venture. Besides sharing the work and costs of putting on the show, they also share the publicity and the likelihood of extra business.

> *Remember*
>
> Stage lighting can produce a lot of heat, particularly if spotlights are used. Do not apply face make-up thickly: it will make the face perspire even more, the foundation will melt and there is a greater risk of the clothes becoming damaged in between costume changes.
>
> Define the make-up by using strong colours with a greater contrast of highlighted and shaded areas.

The techniques used for evening, special occasion and photographic make-up are adapted for the catwalk or stage: the strong, artificial lighting which floods the stage drains a lot of colour out of the make-up and this has to be compensated for with warmer shades of foundation and bolder colours for eyes and lips. The make-up will be less obvious to people sitting near the back of a large hall or theatre, so extra definition is required when contouring the face and shaping the eyebrows and lips.

Look after your models during the show. Help them to keep cool so that the make-up is not spoiled. Use a fine mineral water spray over the face or press over the make-up with damp cotton wool pads. Re-apply face powder to keep the surface of the make-up dry.

Fashion shows: Self-checks

1 What steps can be taken to prevent a model's make-up melting during a fashion show?

Remedial camouflage

Special training is required for learning remedial camouflage techniques. This type of work is concerned mainly with concealing disfiguring birthmarks, pigmentary disorders and bad scarring resulting from skin injury or plastic surgery. The clients for remedial camouflage are often psychologically disturbed by their skin problem and include men and children who have to be taught how to apply the make-up for themselves. Remedial camouflage is often carried out by a qualified therapist in a hospital out-patient's department. The work is also offered as a private service which is usually appreciated by clients who are reluctant to visit a beauty salon with their problem.

The products used for remedial camouflage are different from the standard ones: they usually combine very dense pigments in a light textured base so that they can even out the skin colour in an area without creating too much of a contrast with the texture of surrounding skin. The make-up is designed to be resilient and some of the products are waterproof.

Different colours may have to be mixed to match up a skin tone and this may mean adding yellow, green, black or white pigments from the range.

Remedial camouflage: Self-checks

1 Why are special make-up products required for remedial camouflage?

Hygiene precautions

The main sources of infection during a make-up treatment could be: infected skin, dirty tools and equipment or contaminated make-up products. A high standard of personal and treatment hygiene protects against the risk of infection and builds client confidence.

Personal hygiene

- Wash your hands immediately before the treatment and keep them clean throughout the make-up procedure.

Treatment hygiene

- Do not apply make-up over infected skin.
- Use only clean tools and equipment.
- Maintain a clean working area.
- Remove creams from pots and jars with a clean spatula, not your fingers.
- Where possible, transfer products to a clean make-up palette or your free hand before applying them to the face.
- Replace lids and caps on make-up containers immediately after use.
- Protect the applied make-up with a clean tissue when supporting your hand on the face.
- Dispose of waste immediately in an appropriate container.

> *Remember*
> An ultra-violet cabinet is ideal for keeping small items in once they have been disinfected.

Tools and equipment

It is important to prevent make-up applicators from becoming contaminated. This is achieved by cleaning and disinfecting them after use and storing them hygienically between treatments.

Cleaning

This is done with hot, soapy water. Liquid detergent should be worked well into the fibres of brushes and sponges before rinsing them thoroughly under running water. Make-up palettes may need scrubbing gently with a brush before rinsing.

Disinfecting

Sponges and brushes are more difficult to disinfect than solid items of equipment.

- Sponges: soak these in a solution of hypochlorite for at least an hour and then rinse them thoroughly in clean water.
- Brushes: give the fibres a final cleaning with alcohol or a solution of suitable disinfectant (e.g. Cetrimide) before allowing them to dry.

> *Remember*
> Never store damp sponges and brushes in an enclosed container. If you do, they will grow bacteria or mould on them and start to smell.

Make-up products

There is very little risk of make-up products becoming contaminated if normal hygiene procedures are followed during the treatment and if containers are kept clean and in good condition.

Particular care must be taken to avoid contaminating products which are normally applied directly to the face.

- Pencils: sharpen pencils before using them to expose a clean surface.

> *Remember*
> Apart from looking very unprofessional, broken lids and cracked containers collect germs. Make sure you store make-up products properly and handle them with care.

- Sticks: transfer a small amount of the stick to a clean spatula before applying it to the face.
- Pressed powders: keep a good supply of clean make-up brushes available to avoid contaminating blushers and eye shadows.
- Mascaras: automatic mascaras cause a particular problem because the brushes are designed to be fitted back into the tube container after use. You can overcome this by using a different spiral brush to apply the mascara which can be cleaned and disinfected in the normal way.

> Remember
> Don't throw away the brush with an empty mascara container: clean it thoroughly and add it to your collection!

Hygiene precautions: Self-checks

1 List five precautions which should be taken during a make-up treatment.

2 Describe how make-up brushes and sponges should be cleaned and stored after use.

3 What action should be taken if a cosmetic sponge smells bad?

Hygiene precautions: Activity

1 Salons are becoming increasingly aware of the need for high standards of hygiene and safety: as a result, some manufacturers have started producing disposable make-up items. Visit your wholesaler and find out what is available. Compare the costs of these products with standard lines.

Preparing for make-up

It is important to have the make-up area well organised before the client arrives. A wide range of cosmetics should be available to suit a variety of clients.

The following are the standard requirements for a make-up treatment.

- Tools and equipment: clean headband, cape or gown and tissues for protecting the client's hair and clothing; selection of clean make-up brushes, an eyebrow brush, a pair of manual tweezers, cosmetic sponges, cotton buds, spatulas and a make-up palette; cotton wool pads, soft facial tissues and paper towels; small jar of prepared sterilising fluid; bowl of clean, warm water; client record card and make-up chart; hand mirror.
- Skin care preparations: eye make-up remover, cleansers, toner and bracer, moisturiser, under make-up base.
- Make-up for the face: colour corrective creams, concealer sticks, selection of foundations, blushers, shaders, highlighters and translucent face powder.
- Eye make-up: eyebrow pencils, selection of matte and pearlised eye shadows, eye liners, eye pencils and mascaras.
- Lip make-up: selection of lipsticks and lip gloss.

> Remember
> With experience, you will learn which products and colours are the most popular. Keep a particularly close eye on the stock levels of these items and make sure you always have some available for retail sales

> Remember
> A display of colour always attracts attention. This helps to promote interest in the products and increase sales. When preparing your make-up area, arrange the products attractively so that they catch the eye.

Preparing the client

A client who is comfortable will relax and enjoy the treatment. Make sure your client will be comfortable by:

- asking them to loosen or remove restrictive clothing before placing protection around the neck

> *Remember*
> Most make-up treatments will take place with the client seated in front of a mirror. Light should fall directly onto the face without casting shadows. Warm white fluorescent lighting is nearest in colour to natural daylight.

- removing their ear-rings and neck chains which could be caught or pulled during make-up application
- securing their hair off the face
- ensuring their head is supported well to prevent straining the neck
- advising the client to remove contact lenses if appropriate .

Once the client is settled, the treatment may proceed.

Procedure of treatment

Prepare skin	Make sure the skin and eyelashes are left clean, dry and fee from grease
Assess client	Identify contra-indications Advise client Note skin characteristics, colouring and structural features
Discuss client's requirements	Question client Chose make-up products Agree a make-up plan
Apply under make-up base	Use a light moisturiser or matt gel to suit skin type Apply concealer and colour corrective creams
Apply foundation	If in doubt, patch test foundation first: apply small samples of selected products to the forehead and leave for a minute to assess colour reactions. Choose foundation which gives desired colour effect
Apply face powder and contour cosmetics	Apply products which need setting *before* the face powder. Pearlised and powder-based products are applied afterwards. Remember to brush off excess powder
Apply eye make-up	Apply each of the products to both eyes in the order of: eye shadows eyeliner mascara eyebrow pencil
Apply lip make-up	Outline the shape of the mouth Fill in with colour Blot with tissue Apply second coat of colour and gloss if required
Make final checks	Examine blending around hairline Confirm symmetry of application Check overall balance of colour } Rectify if necessary
Seek approval by the client	Offer the client a hand mirror for closer inspection Ask if the client is pleased with the make-up } Adapt if necessary
Fill in make-up chart	Provide client with chart and revise make-up procedure Interest client in retail purchases
Fill in record card	Enter details of treatment and purchases
Assist client	Remove headband and protective clothing Ensure possession of all personal belongings Accompany to reception for processing payment

continues overleaf

Tidy up!	Dispose of waste materials and remove soiled linen Wipe over make-up containers and return to store Wash and sterilise tools and equipment Prepare the area hygienically for the next client

Choosing and using make-up products

Cosmetics are not selected purely on the basis of colour. When it comes to making the best choice for a client, the textures of products and their contents make some more suitable than others.

Colour corrective creams

These are pigmented creams which are applied after the moisturiser and before the tinted foundation:

- Green: counteracts redness in areas of high colouring, for example the cheeks and nose
- Pink/lilac: brightens a sallow complexion

Application

Do	Don't
Restrict the use of green cream to the pink or red areas of the face. (You could make your client look quite ill otherwise!)	Disturb the green cream when you apply the rest of the make-up. Stipple the foundation over it to prevent the green from spreading.

Concealer sticks

These combine powder and pigments in a wax base and are particularly useful for disguising the vivid red colour of individual dilated capillaries and dark shadows under the eyes. They are usually produced in fair, medium and dark shades to blend in with the tinted foundation.

Medicated sticks are available for applying to spots and blemishes. These should never be used directly on the skin.

Application

Do	Don't
Scrape a little of the concealer off the stick with a spatula before applying it to the face with a clean brush or fingers.	Use concealer stick under the eyes on loose, crepey skin. It is too heavy and will emphasise the creases there.

Foundations

These provide the background colour to the facial make-up and enhance the appearance of the skin. Most foundations are an emulsion of oil and water with pigments and other ingredients added to change the texture and effect of the product.

- Cream: wax, powder and a humectant such as glycerol are added to the basic emulsion. Cream foundations are recommended for normal/dry skins and usually require setting with powder.

All-in-one creams are available which contain a greater proportion of powder and leave a matte finish.

- Liquid: this is a thinner version of a cream foundation and contains a higher proportion of water.

Sometimes the oil is replaced by alcohol which evaporates, leaving a residue of powder and pigments on the skin.

Liquid foundations are suitable for greasy skins. The ones containing oil may also be used on smooth, unblemished skin to provide colour without being too heavy.

Medicated liquid foundations contain antiseptic ingredients which make them suitable for applying over acne.

- Cake: most modern cake foundations are compressed creams with extra powder added for good cover. This type of foundation is popular for home use because of its convenient compact form.

More solid cake foundations, which consist mainly of powder and a binding agent such as wax or gum, are available for greasy skins.

Cake foundations are usually applied with a damp sponge. They can be applied as thinly or thickly as required by adjusting the amount of water used. This makes them very useful for covering minor blemishes.

- Gel: sometimes the client may not want or need the covering properties of a standard foundation. A gel product will provide a thin translucent film of colour which looks quite natural. Gels which produce a tanned effect are very popular during the summer and some contain sun-screens. The jelly-like consistency is produced by adding an ingredient such as gum tragacanth to a liquid foundation formulation.

Foundations will deteriorate if they are not stored properly:

- Keep them in a cool place, away from sunlight. Clean round the tops of tubes and bottles before replacing the lids.
- Always finish off using one tube or jar of foundation before opening another one of the same colour.
- Throw away all empty containers.

Application

Do	Don't
Apply the foundation with clean hands or a clean damp cosmetic sponge. Make-up wedges help to blend foundation over awkward areas such as around the nose and the eyes. Make-up wedges are designed so that varying amounts of pressure may be used to match the different facial areas.	Dot foundation over the face and neck before you blend it in. It will start to dry out as soon as it touches the skin and may go blotchy.
Work quickly when applying foundation. If you don't, the make-up will streak where wet foundation meets make-up that has already dried.	Over work the foundation: you will start lifting it off the skin and it will streak.
Blend foundation outwards from the centre of the face towards the hairline. This helps to prevent a build-up of make-up in the hairline.	Be heavy-handed when applying foundation: you will not get a good finish and you will over-stimulate the skin.
Mix a little moisturiser with the foundation under the eyes and over the neck if the skin is crepey.	
Cover the eyelids and lips with foundation	
Check the application afterwards. Make sure that foundation has not built up in the eyebrows, hairline and facial creases and that there is no demarcation present line on the neck.	

Face powder

All cream based make-up products which have been applied to the skin are set with powder. Face powder absorbs grease and helps to conceal minor blemishes. It also prevents the make-up from melting when the skin gets warm.

'Heavy' powders contain a high proportion of kaolin and chalk and an ingredient such as titanium dioxide for giving extra cover. They are often pigmented to complement a foundation shade.

'Fine' powders are based on talc. Most fine powders are translucent. They allow the colour of the skin or foundation to show through.

Chalk, starch and powdered silk are often added to powders to give the skin an attractive, smooth finish. Some powders contain finely ground metallic particles which create a pearlised effect, suitable for high fashion and evening wear.

- Loose powder is used for all professional applications.
- Pressed powder is produced in a block which fits in to a compact. A binding agent, usually gum or wax, holds the particles of powder together. Compact powders are very useful for touching up make-up during the day.

Pressed powder is not used in the salon for two reasons: it is not fine enough to produce an even finish over freshly applied foundation, and it is not as hygienic to use as loose powder

Application

Do	Don't
Make sure the client's eyes and mouth are shut before applying powder. Always use a pad of clean cotton wool for applying loose powder and press it firmly into the foundation. Powder does not set the make-up as effectively if it is applied with a brush. Apply powder over the eyelids and lips. Remove excess powder from the skin with a clean brush. Brush up the face first, against the direction of hair growth, to loosen excess particles. Finally brush down the face to smooth down the facial hairs and produce an even finish. Use a clean brush to remove any powder which has settled in the eyebrows or eyelashes.	Apply powder over infected skin, areas with excessive hair growth or very dry, flaking skin.

Contour cosmetics

These consist of blushers, highlighters and shaders which are similar to foundations and face powders but with different pigments added. The pressed powder type are the most popular. Liquid, cream and gel products are more difficult to control and mistakes with stronger colours are not easily rectified.

Good quality powder products have a creamy texture which makes them easy to blend and produces an attractive finish.

- Blushers: these add warmth to the make-up and help define facial contour. They are produced in a wide range of colours from palest pink to deep burgundy. The paler colours 'soften' the features. The brighter ones accentuate them . Blushers balance the make-up once the eye and lip cosmetics have been applied.

- Shaders: the brown pigments contained in shaders produce colours which range from medium beige to dark brown. Shaders are used to create artificial shadows which define bone structure or reduce the size of an area.
- Highlighters: the very pale colours of highlighters reflect light and, depending on how they are applied, emphasise features and create the illusions of extra width or length. Pearlised products are even more effective as highlighters.

Application

Do	Don't
Use clean sterilised brushes for applying contour cosmetics.	Apply blusher and highlighter over skin which is infected, crepey, lined or excessively hairy.
Apply powder blusher with a soft, rounded brush. Flat, square ended brushes often produce a demarcation line which is difficult to blend in with the surrounding make-up.	Apply blusher too near the nose or eyes.
Apply liquid and cream blushers with a rolling action of the pads of the fingers to prevent spreading the colour too far.	Create hard demarcation lines. The products should blend imperceptibly with the rest of the make-up.
Tap excess blusher off the brush onto a tissue before applying it to the face.	
Use upward movements when blending blusher along the cheekbones.	
Regularly check that you are achieving a balanced effect when applying contour cosmetics.	
Keep contouring effects subtle for day wear, when clients usually prefer a more natural look.	

Corrective techniques using contour cosmetics

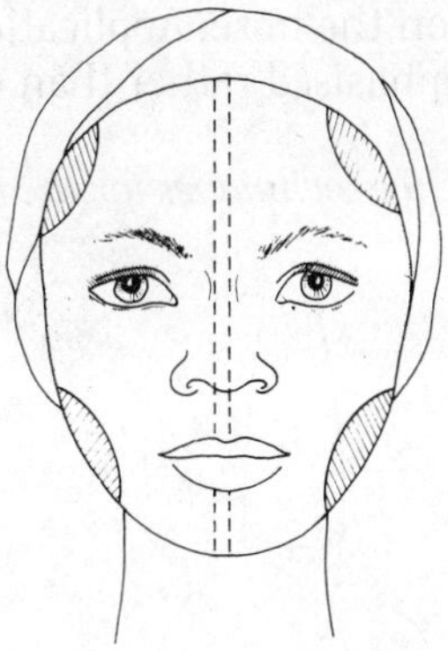
1. Round face

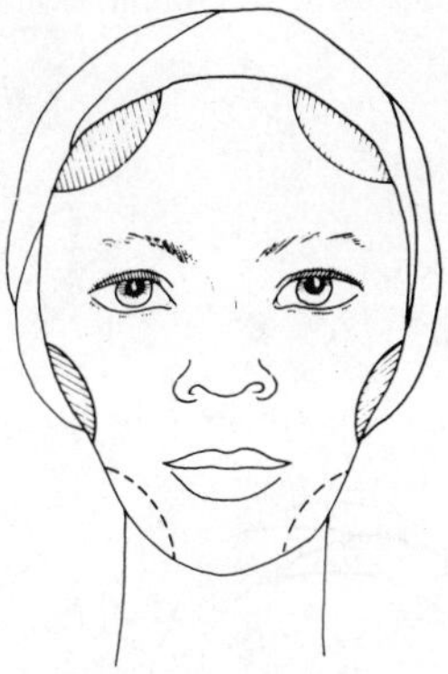
2. Heart-shaped face

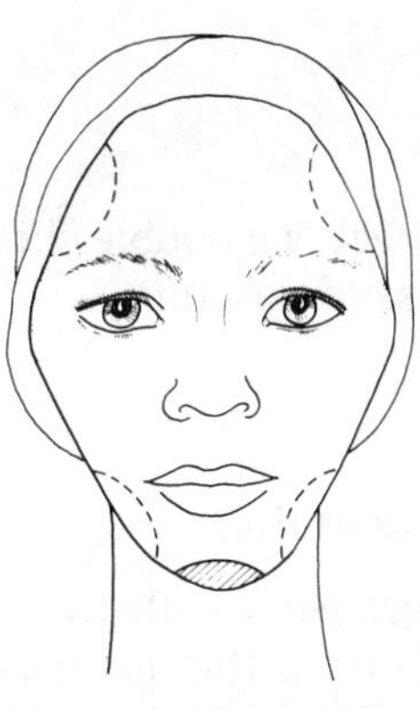
3. Diamond-shaped face

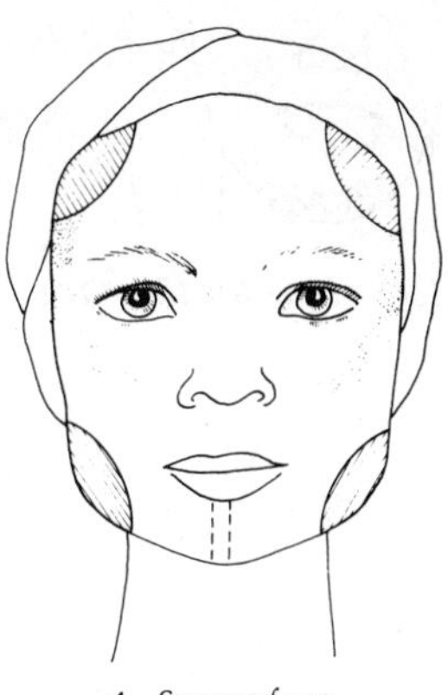
4. Square face

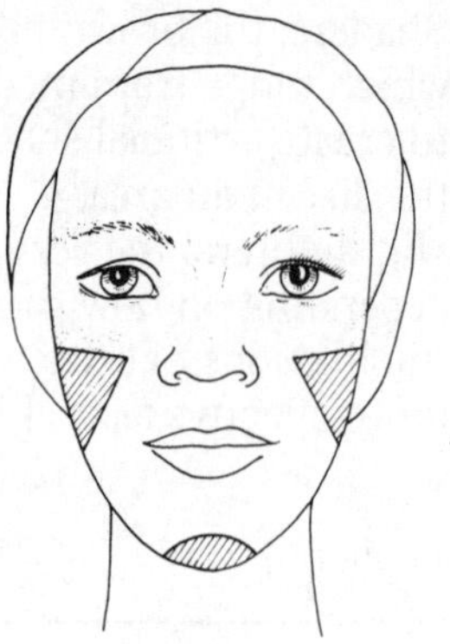

5. Long face

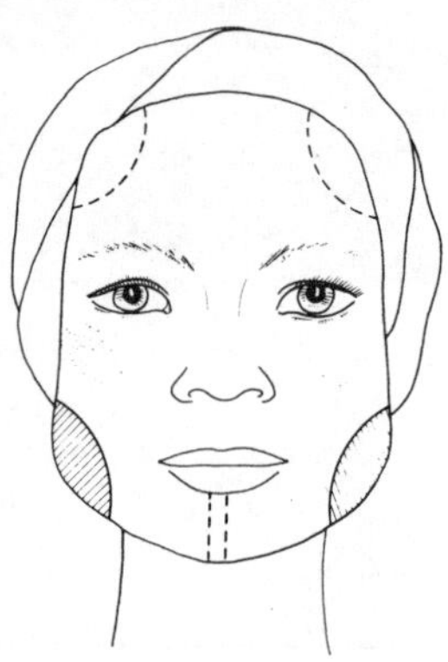

6. Pear-shaped face

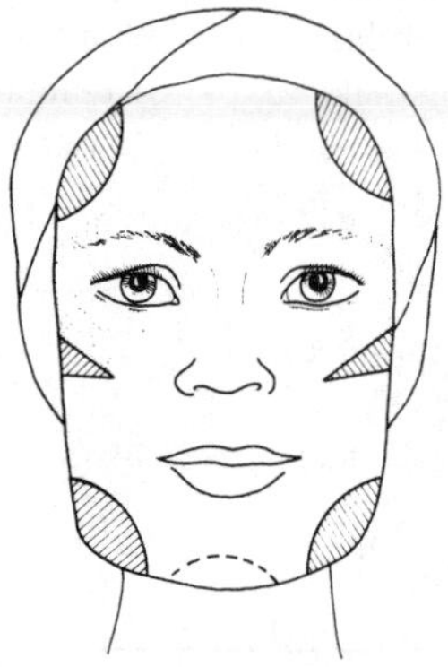

7. Rectangular face

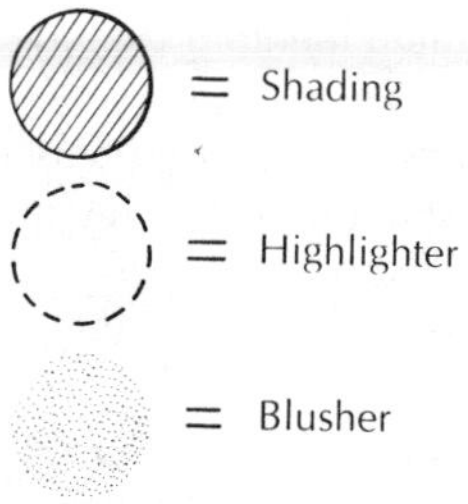

Shaders and highlighters must be used with discretion for corrective work on the nose. Application must be very accurate, or problems may be emphasised rather than disguised.

Corrective techniques for the nose

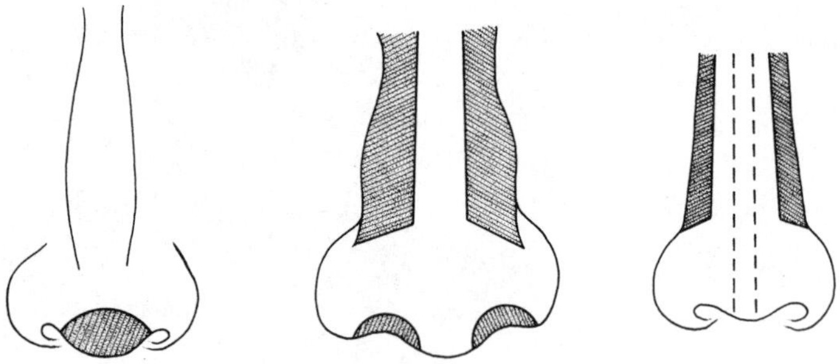

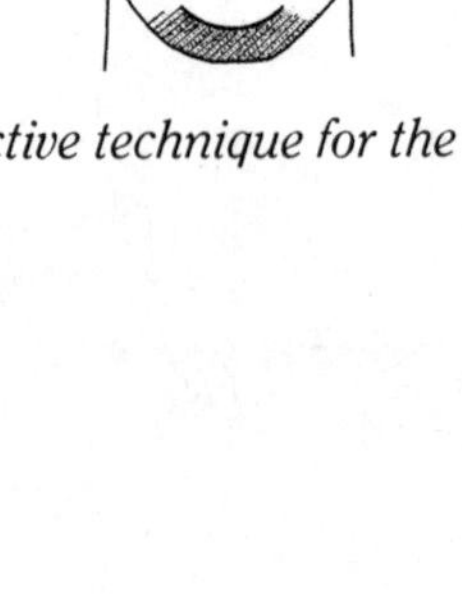

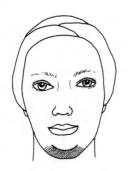

Corrective technique for the chin

The effect of a double chin may be reduced by applying shader to the fullness of the chin.

Eye cosmetics

The eyes are usually the main focus for the make-up: this is not surprising as they are used extensively for communicating and expressing our personalities.

There is virtually no limit to the effects that can be achieved with the extensive range of products and colours available. It is sometimes possible to change the whole character of a person with expertly applied eye make-up.

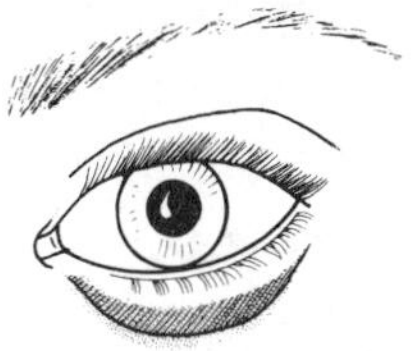

Corrective technique for puffy eyes: shader applied to fullness under the eyes

Great care is needed when using eye cosmetics. The skin around the eyes is very thin and is easily stretched. Make-up entering the eye can set up an irritation and cause the eyes to water and become inflamed.

The EC Cosmetics Directive of 1976 limits the ingredients which may be contained in eye make-up products. Only pigments which are known to be non-toxic and non-irritant are allowed. These include ultramarine (blue), chromium oxide (green), iron oxide (red/brown), yellow ochre and carbon black.

Eye shadows

Eye shadows are used to emphasise the eyes and to co-ordinate the colour of the make-up with clothing. They are available as powders, creams, gels and liquids. Creamy textured pressed powders are the most popular.

Ingredients such as bismuth oxychloride or mica produce a frosted or pearlised effect.

Corrective techniques make use of contrasting colours and textures of eye shadows for helping to change the shape of the eye.

Corrective techniques for the eyes using eye shadow

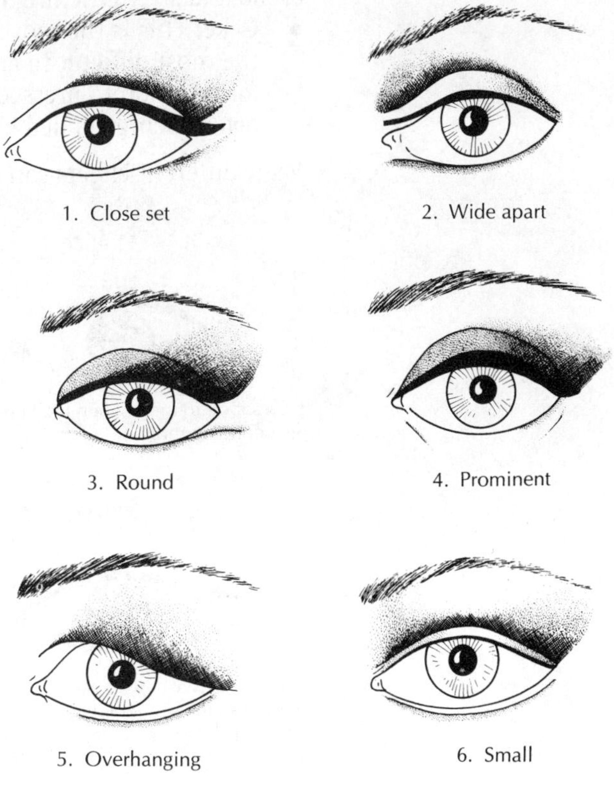

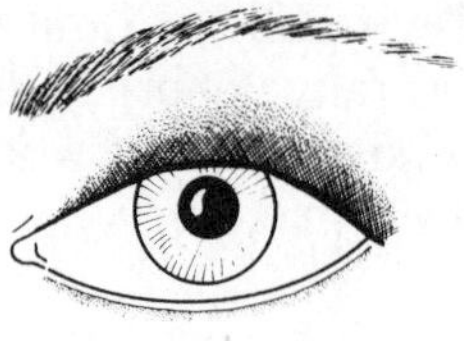
7. Deep-set

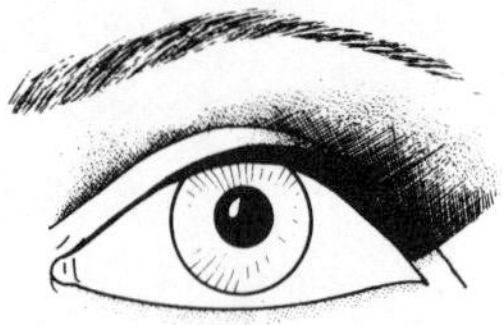
8. Downward tilting

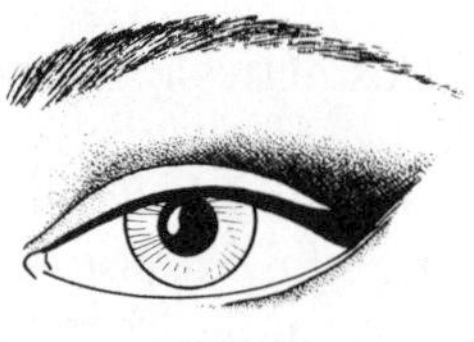
9. Narrow

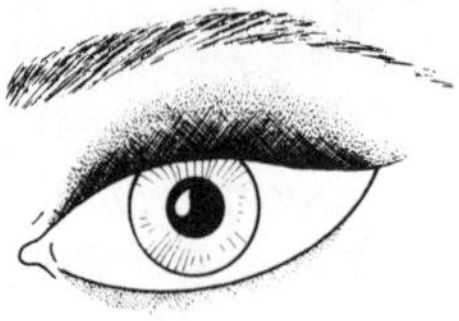
10. Oriental

Application

Do	Don't
Support the skin when applying eye shadow and protect the surrounding make-up with a tissue. Use clean, sterilised brushes or sponge applicators. Blend the products well so that no hard demarcation lines are produced. Make sure that the client's eyes are kept closed or that she is not looking directly at a bright light when applying the eye shadow.	Overload the applicator with eye shadow. Excess powder could enter the eye or fall onto the face and spoil the rest of the make-up. You could cause discomfort to the client and overstretch the skin. Apply eye shadow if there is an infection present or if the eyes are feeling sensitive.

Eyeliner

Eyeliner is used for emphasising the shape of the eye by framing the eyelid and strengthening the colour of the lash line.

- Cake: This is the most versatile of the eyelining products but is also the most difficult to apply. Cake eyeliners have a similar formulation to pressed powder eye shadows but they are wetted before being applied to the eyelids with a fine tapered brush.

Many different effects can be achieved with eyeliner.

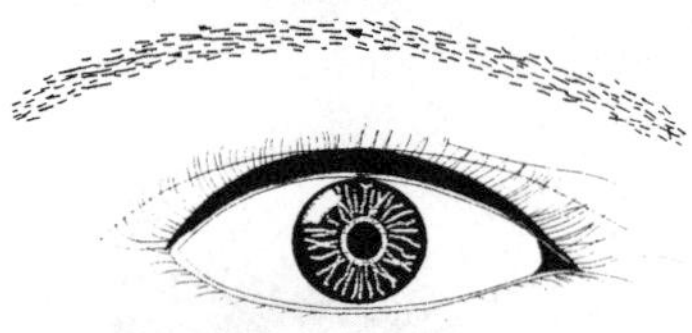
1 Eyes look rounder when the line is deeper in the middle

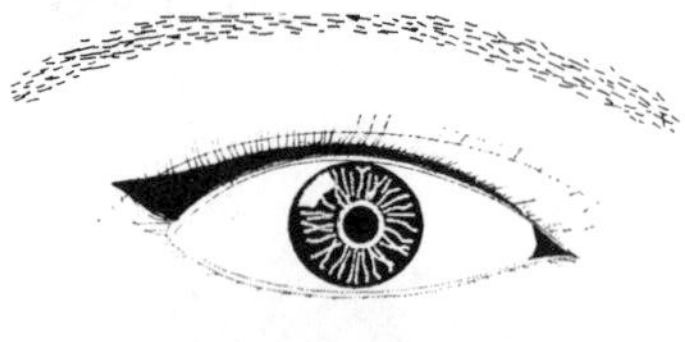
2 A softened upwardly tapered line provides a more youthful 'lift' to the eye

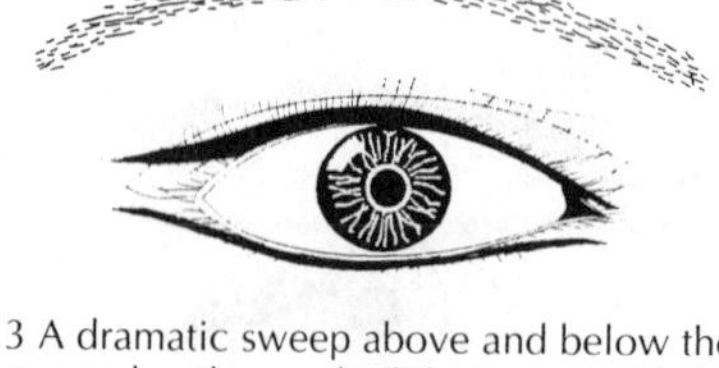
3 A dramatic sweep above and below the eye makes the eye look larger, provided that the lines do not meet and 'close up' the eye

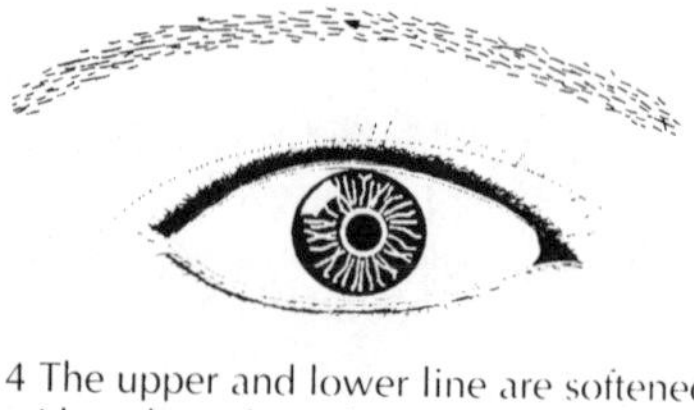
4 The upper and lower line are softened with a clean damp brush – providing more subtle emphasis

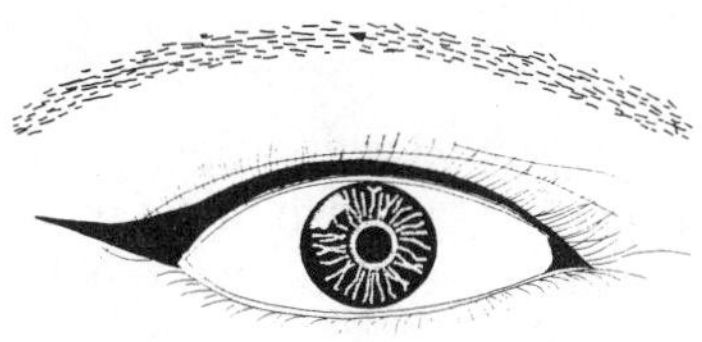

5 Fifties 'flick' for a fashionable effect

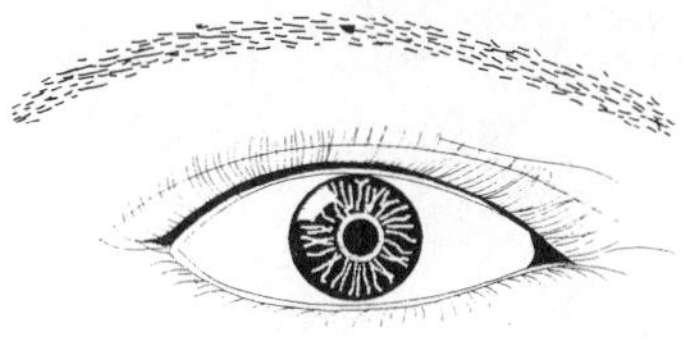

6 A fine tapered line to provide 'natural' enhancement

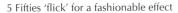

Different eyelining effects: the line produced can be made hard or soft by adjusting the amount of water used.

- Liquid: this type of product is a gum solution containing pigments. It is applied with a brush and gives a heavier effect than cake eyeliner.
- Pencils: eyeliner pencils have a basic formulation of oils and waxes with pigments added. They are produced in a wide range of colours and are usually soft enough to be blended like an eye shadow if a hard line is not required.
- Kohl: this soft black waxy pencil is applied to the inner rim of the lower eyelid to enhance the white of the eye and produce a sophisticated make-up look.

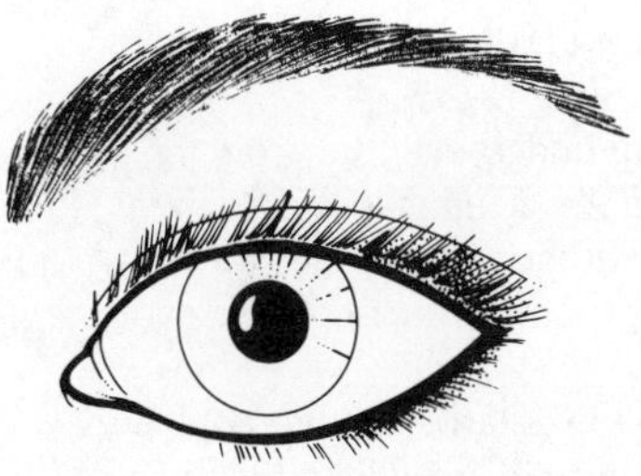

Lining the eyelid inside the lashline makes the eye look smaller. Dark eye shadow and eyeliner are usually applied to the upper and lower lids to compensate for this.

Application

Do	Don't
Use a clean sterilised brush for applying cake or liquid eyeliner.	Press down on the eye when applying eyeliner.
Keep your hand steady when applying eyeliner. If you rest your hand on the client's face, make sure there is a tissue beneath it to protect the make-up.	Apply eyeliner if the eyes are tired, sore or infected.
Lift the eyelid from beneath the brow to ensure the line is drawn right up to the base of the lashes.	
Ask the client to keep her eyes shut when applying eyeliner to the upper lid.	
Soften the eyeline on more mature clients. 'Hard' lines are only suitable for creating fashion effects on younger clients.	

Mascara

Mascara is used to accentuate the eyes by darkening and thickening the lashes. Mascaras are produced in standard colours of black, brown and grey and also in 'special effect' colours such as violet, green, blue and pink.

- Cake: this type of mascara has been available for a long time but became less popular when automatic brush and wand mascaras appeared on the market. Cake mascaras are currently regaining their popularity in salons because they are applied with a brush which is easy to clean and sterilise. The basic formula for a cake mascara combines waxes and pigments in a soap base.
- Liquid: liquid mascaras have been modified to produce a wide range of products with special features, for example waterproof, smudge proof, lash-lengthening, extra-thickening, protein-enriched. Pigments and synthetic resins are contained in a base of water, or alcohol and water, with castor oil added to prevent the film of mascara from becoming brittle. Lash-building ingredients include filaments of rayon or nylon.

> Remember
> If the client's eyes water, sit the client upright. Gently blot moisture from the outer corner of the eye with a soft tissue and allow her to relax for a minute or two. Resume applying the mascara when the eyes have settled down.

Application

Do	Don't
Instruct the client to relax her eyelids while mascara is being applied to the upper lashes.	Apply mascara to the lower lashes if the skin beneath the eyes is loose and crepey.
Lift the skin of the eyelids from underneath the brow to prevent wet mascara touching the face make-up.	Allow mascara to penetrate the eye area.
Apply mascara downwards over the upper lashes then upwards from underneath to give maximum coverage and curl.	Apply mascara if there are signs of infection or if the eyes are feeling sensitive.
Place a tissue underneath the lower lashes before applying mascara to them. Excess mascara will go on the tissue and not on the skin.	Ignore the client if she thinks her eyes are going to water.
Instruct the client to look away from the brush when applying mascara to the lower lashes	
Build up the mascara in fine coats which are allowed to dry between each application. This will help prevent the lashes from clogging together	
Separate the lashes afterwards with an eyelash comb if a more natural effect is required.	

Eyebrow pencil

Eyebrow pencils are used to strengthen the colour of the brows and define their shape. They have a similar formulation to eye liner pencils but have to be harder so that they can be sharpened to a point and applied with very fine feathery strokes. Eyebrow pencils are produced in a limited range of hair colours, for example grey, brown, black.

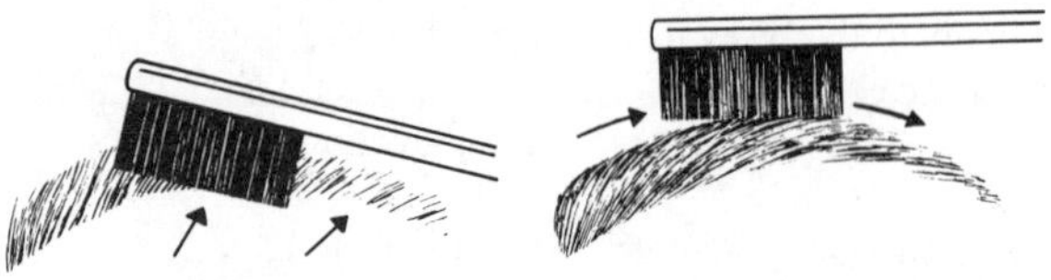

Separate brow hairs   Smooth them into shape

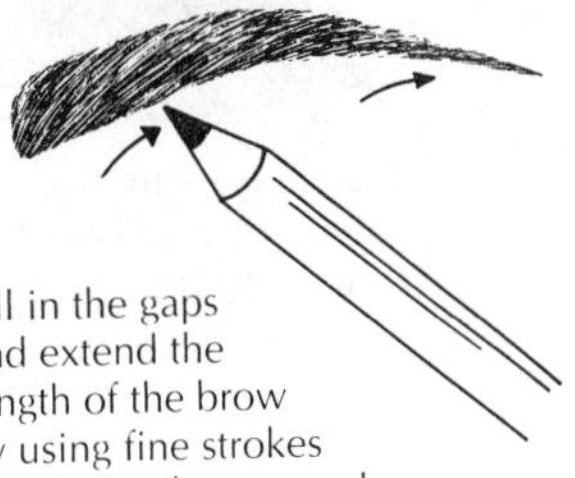

Fill in the gaps and extend the length of the brow by using fine strokes which simulate natural hair growth. Stroke over the line with your finger to produce a fine tapered end

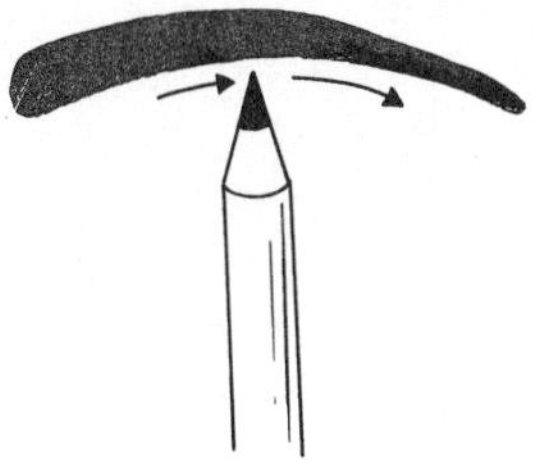

No! ... unless it's for special effects

Application of eyebrow pencil

Application

Do	Don't
Brush the eyebrows into shape before applying the pencil Sharpen the pencil before use. Try to simulate natural hair growth.	Apply the pencil in a heavy unbroken line.

Lip cosmetics

These are available as lipsticks, glosses and pencils and are used to define the mouth by adding colour and enhancing the shapes of the lips. The products share the same basic ingredients of oils, fats and waxes but in different proportions. The vast range of colours of lip cosmetics are derived from lake pigments, which are safe to eat!

- Lipstick: the hardness of lipstick is due to its high wax content. Creamy textured lipsticks contain softening ingredients such as lanolin, mineral oils and petroleum jelly. Mica or bismuth oxychloride is contained for producing a pearlised effect. Lipstick is applied with a brush to outline the mouth and spread the colour evenly over the lips.
- Lip gloss: this has a gel consistency produced by mixing bentonite clay with mineral oils. Lip gloss may be clear or coloured. It gives a temporary 'wet' shine to the lips and can be applied over lipstick or on its own for a more natural look.
- Lip pencil: this may be used to outline the lips before applying lipstick and is a popular retail line. Lip pencils contain a high proportion of hard waxes, which means that they are less likely to smudge than softer lip cosmetics. They are very useful for correcting lip shapes.

Corrective techniques for the lips

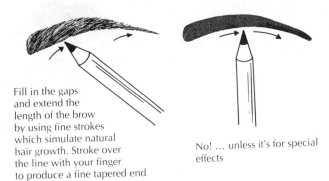

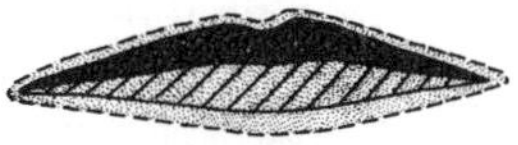

1. Thin lips: draw a lip line slightly outside the natural shape

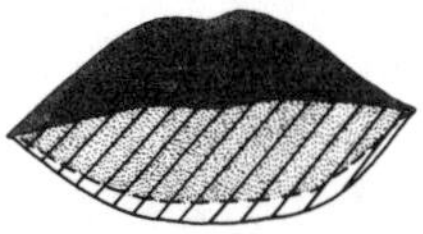

2. Full lips: blot out natural lip line with foundation and powder. Use dark colours to draw just inside the natural shape

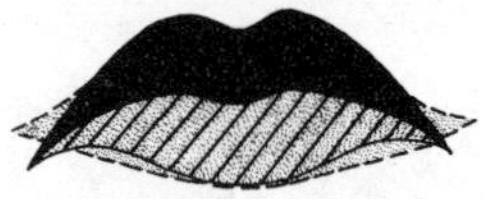

3. Drooping mouth: build up the corners of the upper lip slightly. Join with lower lip line

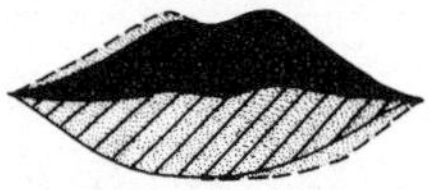

4. Asymmetrical lips: build up lip line where necessary to achieve balance and symmetry

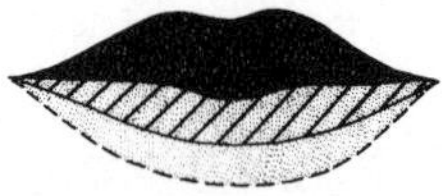

5. Unbalanced lips: draw slightly outside the natural lip line as required

Application

Do	Don't
Use a clean sterilised lip brush Outline the mouth first and then fill in with lip colour. Outline the lips from sides to centre, with the mouth slightly open so that the corners can be reached. Protect the make-up with a tissue when supporting the hand on the client's chin. Blot the first application of lipstick with a tissue. This helps to fix the colour on the lips. Apply a second coat to achieve the final finish.	Apply lip cosmetics if there is an infection present or if the lips are cracked and chapped.

Choosing and using make-up products: Self-checks

1. Why is green moisturiser used?
2. Why is glycerol contained in a foundation?
3. Which ingredient in a foundation is contained for 'good cover'?
4. Why should foundation be blended outwards away from the face?
5. State three reasons for applying face powder.
6. Name one ingredient in a face powder which helps to produce a good finish.
7. Why are pressed powders not suitable for salon use?
8. Give two contra-indications to face powder.
9. Explain the main difference between blushers, highlighters and shaders.
10. Describe how a natural effect is achieved when applying contour cosmetics.
11. State two advantages and two disadvantages of using eye pencils.
12. Give two contra-indications to the use of pearlised eye shadows.
13. Name the main ingredients in a lash-building mascara.
14. Describe how to prevent mascara from smudging when applying it to a client.
15. Give three reasons for applying lipstick with a brush.

Choosing and using make-up products: Activity

1 Think of all the changes which take place during the ageing process and decide how these should affect the choice and application of make-up products. Prepare a talk on this subject which could be given to a local women's group and which would promote the sale of skin-care and make-up products available in your salon.

Hypo-allergenic cosmetics

> Remember
> In the EC and USA the law requires cosmetic companies to conduct very strict safety tests on the materials they use to formulate products. Nevertheless there will always be someone somewhere who is allergic to a substance that most other people tolerate without any problems.

Hypo-allergenic cosmetics are available for people who are irritated by, or are very sensitive to, standard make-up products. They do not contain perfume and, usually, fewer pigments and preservatives are used. The colour range of hypo-allergenic cosmetics is usually more limited than with other make-up products.

Product labelling

By law, ingredients which are known to be irritants or sensitisers must be identified on the product package label, together with any special precautions which must be taken.

Some of the substances which are known to cause adverse reactions in people who are hypersensitive are:

- lanolin: a fatty substance similar to sebum which coats sheep's wool and is used as a softening ingredient in skin creams
- eosin: a red dye contained in some lipsticks
- perfumes: particularly those containing bergamot, lavender and cedarwood
- alcohol: a strong grease solvent and astringent used in cosmetics and skin care products
- cobalt blues: pigments used to produce eye make-up colours
- pearlising agents: ingredients which give make-up products an iridescent (light reflective) effect.
- gums: adhesive and binding ingredients contained in cosmetics.

Eye-irritation

Very strict testing is carried out to ensure that eye make-up products will not irritate the eye or surrounding skin. Only 'safe' pigments are used but, even so, some of them may cause a reaction in people who are hypersensitive.

Hypo-allergenic cosmetics: Self-checks

1 Which types of ingredients in make-up are most likely to cause an allergic reaction?

2 State one advantage and one disadvantage of using hypo-allergenic cosmetics.

Hypo-allergenic cosmetics: Activity

1 Take a sample of make-up products which are used in your salon. Have a look at their labels and see if you can recognise any of the ingredients. Make a note of any references to irritants or sensitisers contained in the products.

Contact lenses

Clients should be offered the choice of either taking out their contact lenses or keeping them in during treatment. Some people find even the slightest pressure on their eyelids when wearing lenses very uncomfortable. They prefer to keep the lenses soaking in a special bath containing soaking solution which they bring with them to the salon. The lenses are replaced at the end of the treatment.

Clients with less sensitive eyes may choose to keep their lenses in place during treatment. This helps to prevent particles entering the eyes and becoming trapped beneath the contact lenses when they are replaced. Whatever the decision of the client, the following precautions should be taken to prevent irritating the eye area:

- be particularly gentle when working on the skin around the eyes
- take care not to touch the eyes with make-up applicators
- avoid using heavy creams around the eyes which could melt and smear the natural lens
- instruct the client to keep the eyes closed when applying powder products
- do not create dust in the atmosphere when transferring powder from the container
- apply powder eye shadows to the eyelids with a slightly damp brush
- use only creamy textured pressed powder eye shadows, not loose, dry ones
- use block or liquid mascara which does not have a high alcohol content
- avoid using a mascara which contains filaments.

Contact lenses: Self-check

1 Explain why particular care must be taken when applying make-up to a client who wears contact lenses.

Make-up for people who wear glasses

The effects of glasses on the appearance of the face depend on the design of the frames and the colour and type of lenses.

Frames

Heavy frames can usually take bolder eye make-up and a strong lipstick colour to provide balance. Lightweight, steel frames look lost in front of a dark, heavy eye make-up. Keep make-up colours soft, but make good use of eyeliner, mascara and eyebrow pencil for defining the eyes and brow shape.

The make-up scheme should complement the colour of the frames. Muted shades of eye shadow are preferable if the frames are a bright colour.

> *Remember*
> People who wear glasses often cannot see well enough to apply their own make-up: recommend eyelash and eyebrow tinting treatments for defining the eyes without make-up, and the use of all-in-one foundations and make-up sticks and pencils. These are easier to use as they do not require detailed brush work.

Lenses

People who are short-sighted wear glasses which enable them to focus at a greater distance: the lenses in their glasses make the eyes look slightly smaller. Long-sighted people wear glasses which help them to focus on closer objects: the lenses in their glasses make their eyes appear bigger. Corrective techniques may be necessary to compensate for the effects of lenses on the appearance of the eyes.

Tinted lenses change the effects of eye make-up colours. Stronger and more contrasting colours may be needed to provide definition.

Make-up for people who wear glasses: Self-check

1 How might a short-sighted client who has been used to wearing glasses look different with contact lenses?

Choosing make-up colours

The colours used to create the make-up should enhance the client's colouring and co-ordinate with the clothes that are being worn. They should also be suitable for achieving the overall effect required by the client.

> *Remember*
> Eye shadow colours, blushers and lipsticks will look stronger and more vibrant against a pale background than a dark one.

Foundation

This is probably the most important colour choice of the whole make-up. Foundation provides the backdrop to the make-up. The depth and tone of the foundation colour influences the effects of all the other products which are applied.

The main considerations when choosing a foundation colour are the natural skin colour and hair colour.

When we are born, the colours of our skin and hair are determined and, because they are natural, they are considered to be the best for us. We are not always satisfied with what we have got, however, and our 'natural' look is the last thing we want!

Ideally, the foundation colour should match the facial skin but this rule does not always work when the hair has been dyed a different colour or when some colour corrective work is necessary to lift the complexion or create a special effect.

Skin colours

Skin can be described as pale, medium or dark with neutral, pink, yellow, red or blue tones. The tones are created by pigment present in the epidermis, blood circulating in the superficial blood vessels and fat contained in the skin.

> Remember
> *Golden, honey* and *tan* shades add warmth; *beige* and *olive* shades neutralise; *rose, golden* and *bronze* shades brighten.

Simple rules can be used to help choose a foundation colour for any shade of skin. Foundation colours should be chosen to:

- match or add warmth to neutral skin tones
- neutralise pink or red skin tones
- brighten yellow' (sallow and olive) or blue skin tones.

> Remember
> A pale, neutral foundation colour would look very drab on a person with light, ash blonde hair. Neutral foundation colours are based on 'green', as are ash-toned hair colours.
>
> A bronze foundation would not be suitable for a client with auburn hair as both colours are based on 'red' which would dominate the make-up.

Hair colours

Hair colours range from the lightest pastel blonde, through brown to darkest blue-black. The tones of hair are usually described as *ash* which is 'cold' and neutral, *golden* which is yellowish and *red* which is warm.

The colour of the foundation should compensate for cold and warm tones in the hair so that there is a contrast which adds interest to the make-up.

Cosmetic manufacturers often create commercially acceptable names to describe make-up colours. The foundation colours recommended in the table are descriptive.

> Remember
> Always patch test the chosen foundation on the client's forehead before applying it to the rest of the face. Check that it does not change colour. Skins which do not normally have a slightly acid surface may turn the foundation orange. A paler, cooler shade is preferable to compensate for this.

Face powder

Translucent powders are the most popular as they are fine and allow the foundation colour to show through. However, there are times when more dense coverage is required, for example when concealing blemishes or applying face powder over a colourless foundation cream. In these cases, a powder should be chosen which matches the shade of foundation.

> Remember
> When making up black skin, it is better to use a golden or bronze powder. Translucent face powder creates a chalky effect on black skin.

Blusher

There is an extensive range of blusher colours which is why this type of product is so versatile. The palest silvery pinks may be used as highlighters, the corals, peaches and reds add warmth and the deep tawny colours and bronzes are often effective as shaders.

When choosing blusher for a natural look, the colour should complement the foundation shade and harmonise with hair colouring and clothing.

The colour of blusher often looks quite different once it has been applied to the face. The effect created depends on the shade of foundation or natural skin colour to which the blusher is applied.

Cool colours

Cool colours have quite a lot of blue pigment in them. They include the purplish and vivid pinks and some reds and bronze shades. Applied to a pale, neutral base, the blue tones in cool colours become emphasised and the overall effect is cold. This may sometimes be the effect required when applying a high fashion or special effect make-up.

Applied to a darker, 'warmer' base, the blue tone of the blusher becomes neutralised by orange tones in the foundation and the effect is no longer cold.

Warm colours

These contain more red and yellow pigments and include the coral pinks, peaches, rusts and orangey-reds.

Choosing foundation colours

	Hair colours						
	Blonde			Brown			Black
Skin colour	**Ash**	**Golden**	**Strawberry**	**Ash**	**Golden**	**Red**	**Blue**
Pale Neutral	Light warm beige Honey beige	Creamy beige Natural beige	Creamy beige Honey beige	Light warm beige Honey beige	Natural beige	Ivory Creamy beige	Ivory Creamy beige
Sallow	Light rose beige Light warm beige	Natural beige	Natural beige Honey	Light rose beige Light warm beige	Natural beige	Natural beige Honey	Light rose beige Light warm beige
Pink	Honey beige	Natural beige	Natural beige	Natural beige	Natural beige	Natural beige	Natural beige
Medium Neutral	Honey Warm beige Rose beige	Natural beige Light tan	Creamy beige Natural beige Honey	Rose beige Warm beige Light golden	Honey beige Light tan Natural beige	Honey beige Light tan	Creamy beige Honey beige
Olive	Warm beige Light tan	Rose beige Light bronze	Natural beige Light tan	Warm beige Rose beige	Rose beige Light bronze	Light tan Warm beige	Rose beige Warm beige
Pink	Honey beige	Natural beige	Natural beige	Warm beige	Olive/beige	Olive/beige	Natural beige
Dark Olive				Bronze beige Golden tan	Bronze beige Medium tan	Warm beige Golden tan	Bronze beige Golden tan
Light brown				Light bronze Clear golden	Light bronze Clear tan	Dark warm beige Clear tan	Bronze beige Clear golden
Dark brown				Golden tan Clear bronze	Clear bronze Dark tan	Dark golden	Dark golden Clear bronze
Ebony/ Blue black				Dark golden Clear bronze	Clear bronze Dark tan	Clear dark tan Dark golden	Bronze Dark golden

> Remember
> Black skins need strong colours of blusher. Blue-toned reds and deep pinks are ideal for applying over golden and bronze foundation shades. Orangey-red blushers are more effective on very dark blue/black skins.

When applied to a pale, neutral base, red and orange tones in the blusher become emphasised and the overall effect is very warm. The effect can look quite natural if the blusher is a pale colour and more dramatic if it is vibrant.

When a very warm blusher colour is applied over a darker warm-toned foundation, the make-up can become too orange or red. The result does not look as natural as when using a 'cooler' shade of blusher.

Contour cosmetics

For highlighters and shaders to be effective, they should be significantly lighter or darker than the base colour without looking theatrical. White, ivory and pale cream highlighters produce more subtle effects on a paler foundation than they do on darker ones.

> Remember
> Very warm brown colours should be avoided for shading: they tend to appear too orange when applied over foundation and act more as a blusher than a shader.

When applying highlighter over a darker foundation, the colour chosen should have the same tone as the base colour, for example very pale peach is effective over warm colours of foundation. Very pale pink looks good over rose-toned shades. Beige is dark enough to be used as a shader over a pale base. A darker foundation colour needs a deeper colour of shader.

The colour density of powder highlighters and shaders makes them more suitable for evening wear, photographic and young, fashion make-ups.

Subtle effects for day wear can be achieved by using different colours of foundation. These should be in the same tone as the base colour. The highlighter should be two shades lighter than the foundation and the shader two shades darker.

Lipstick

A lipstick should be chosen which balances the colour scheme of the make-up with the clothes that are being worn. Strong and vibrant lipstick colours draw attention to the mouth and lower part of the face. They should be avoided if the teeth are discoloured or if the skin around the mouth and chin is blemished. Strong lipstick colours look better balanced with subtle and muted shades of eye make-up.

> Remember
> You should always try and link-sell lipsticks and nail enamels. Most cosmetic ranges offer them in identical colours which is ideal for achieving full colour co-ordination.

A deeper colour of lipstick should be used for outlining the new lip shape if corrective work is being done.

Very pale, pearlised lipsticks help to give fullness to the lips. Pearlised lip gloss has a similar effect.

Deep blue-toned reds, dark purplish-pinks and bronze shades help to reduce the effect of fullness. They are often preferred by people with black skins where large full lips are a racial characteristic.

Eye shadow

Different eye shadow colours achieve different effects, depending on how and where they are applied. The client will often express a preference for a particular eye shadow colour, but different shades and contrasting colours may also be used to create the best effects.

> Remember
> The eyes lose some of their colour with age. Pastel shades of eye shadow compensate for this. They do not drain the eye colour as stronger eye shadow colours would. Pink and lilac eye shadows can make tired eyes look sore. Choose them only when the eyes are clear and bright to tone in with what is being worn.

The eyes and lips are the main focus of colour in the make-up so it is important that the colours chosen harmonise with clothing.

- Dark muted colours, for example charcoal, brown, olive and plum: these are used for defining eye contour and producing a sophisticated look. They are particularly effective on clients who have dark hair colouring and dark eyes. They can be used to produce subtle eyelining effects on people with fairer colouring, particularly more mature clients.
- Pastel colours, for example pale blue, light aqua, pale green and peach: these colours produce very soft effects, particularly when applied to people with blond or grey hair. They emphasise the colour of the eyes when applied in the same tone.
- Very pale colours, for example white, pearl, cream: these have highlighting effects when contrasted with darker eye shadows. They are applied to emphasise the arch of the brow and to help make the eyes appear bigger.
- Soft, muted shades, for example grey, beige, sage and mauve: these produce more subtle effects than the purer eye shadow colours. They are used when a more natural effect is required.
- Bright colours, for example blue, green, yellow, violet and red: great care must be taken when using bright colours of eye shadow. They are fun to use in a fashion or glamour make-up if the client has the confidence to wear them, but they can look very hard and unattractive on more mature or sophisticated clients. Some colours are suitable for use as eyeliner.

> Remember
> Bright blue applied sparingly to the lashline brightens up the whites of the eyes.

Eyeliner

Eyeliner defines the shape of the eye by accentuating the lash line. Colours which blend in with the mascara look most natural. Very dark colours of eyeliner are suitable only for people with dark hair or for achieving dramatic fashion effects. An eyeliner which is in the same tone but darker than the eye shadow will give a softer look.

Mascara

> Remember
> Use a darker mascara if stronger or deeper colours of eye shadow and eyeliner have been applied. The mascara should match the colour of false eyelashes if they are being worn. Fantasy colours, for example blue, green, pink and violet may be used for fun or fashion effects.

The mascara should be the darkest of the eye make-up colours applied. For a natural effect, it should tone in with the hair colour:

Hair colour	Mascara colour
White	Grey
Grey	Grey
Blonde	Brown or Grey
Auburn	Brown
Brownish	Black
Brown	Brown
Black	Black

Eyebrow pencil

> Remember
> Look at the colour tone of the client's hair before choosing the eyebrow colour. A reddish brown pencil would not look right on a client with ash-blond hair.

A colour of pencil should be chosen which looks natural with the hair colour and which complements the rest of the make-up. Care should be taken to avoid applying an eyebrow pencil which is too dark. This would spoil the balance of the make-up.

Choosing make-up colours: Self-checks

> *Remember*
> When designing a special make-up for a client, take time to explain what you would like to do and why you have chosen particular colours. Once the make-up has gained the approval of the client, record details of the colours which were used for future reference.

1. What are the components of skin colour?
2. How does the colour of the hair influence the choice of make-up colours?
3. Why might a foundation change colour on the skin?
4. State three factors which influence the choice of lipstick colour for a client.
5. Why should the mascara be the darkest eye make-up product used in the make-up?
6. State three reasons for giving the client a make-up chart.

Choosing make-up colours: Activity

1. Build up a portfolio of your own make-up work. Photograph those make-up designs which you feel particularly proud of. Include pictures of a wide range of models showing your ability to adapt to any age group, skin colour and occasion. Include in your portfolio details of the make-up products used, particular problems encountered and what you did to resolve them.

   Put a copy of your portfolio in reception to let your clients know what you can do!

Chapter 7

Lash and brow treatments

After working through this chapter you will be able to:

- explain the benefits of treatments for the eyebrows and eyelashes
- apply treatments safely, hygienically and effectively to the lashes and eyebrows
- carry out a skin test for eyelash tint and respond appropriately to the results
- recommend the appropriate eyebrow shape for a client
- advise the client about temporary and semi-permanent false eyelashes
- give appropriate home-care advice.

Eyelash and eyebrow tinting

Well-defined eyebrows and lashes emphasise the eyes and define their shape. They also help to balance the facial features. Tinting the hairs makes them appear darker and thicker. The colour fades gradually with exposure to sunlight and the loss and replacement of tinted hairs.

People with naturally fair eyelashes and eyebrows benefit greatly from having them tinted. They feel more confident in their appearance, particularly when they are not wearing make-up.

The advantages of eyelash and eyebrow tinting treatments are:

- the effect is very natural
- less time is required for applying make-up
- the colour is waterproof and does not smudge or streak
- the facial features appear more balanced, particularly when make-up is not being worn

It is not only fair clients who benefit from eyelash and eyebrow tinting treatments. The colour intensities of the darker tints emphasise the lashes and help to create a more defined eyebrow shape on people with darker hair. Eyelash and eyebrow tinting treatments should be recommended to clients who:

- wear spectacles or contact lenses
- are allergic to or prefer not to wear mascara
- have difficulty in applying eye make-up
- claim not to have time to apply eye make-up
- have had their hair tinted a darker colour
- are due to go on holiday
- participate regularly in active sports
- work or live in a hot environment.

A small amount of eyelash tint is mixed with hydrogen peroxide and the mixture is then applied to the hairs. During the development time, some of the dye penetrates the hairs and becomes oxidised. The dye molecules enlarge and become trapped inside the hairs which then become permanently coloured. The effects of tinting last for between six and eight weeks.

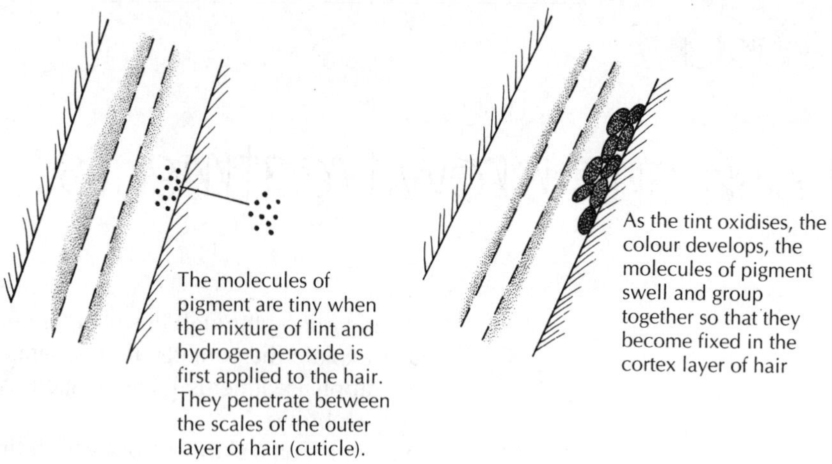

The molecules of pigment are tiny when the mixture of lint and hydrogen peroxide is first applied to the hair. They penetrate between the scales of the outer layer of hair (cuticle).
As the tint oxidises, the colour develops, the molecules of pigment swell and group together so that they become fixed in the cortex layer of hair

Oxidation reaction. For more on hair structure, see Chapter 12, page 264

Choosing a tint

The products used for eyelash and eyebrow tinting are usually available as creams or gels offered in basic colours of black, brown, grey and blue. These colours may be mixed to provide variations in tone. The choice of colour is a matter of personal preference and depends on:

- the client's overall skin and hair colouring
- the type of eye make-up that is normally worn
- the age of the client.

As clients grow more mature, they lose a lot of natural colour from their hair and eyes. Brown or grey tints are preferable to black for producing a softer, more natural effect.

> Remember
>
> Body chemistry can change overnight and allergies develop just as quickly. A client who has been having tinting treatments for years without any trouble must still have a skin test. In this way, both the interests of the client and the salon are safe-guarded.

Suitability for treatment

Eyelash tints contain vegetable dyes and relatively safe chemical dyes such as toluenediamine. When mixed with hydrogen peroxide these ingredients undergo a chemical change which can cause an unpleasant allergic reaction in some people. You must carry out a skin test 24-48 hours before the scheduled tinting appointment to make sure your client is not allergic to the tint.

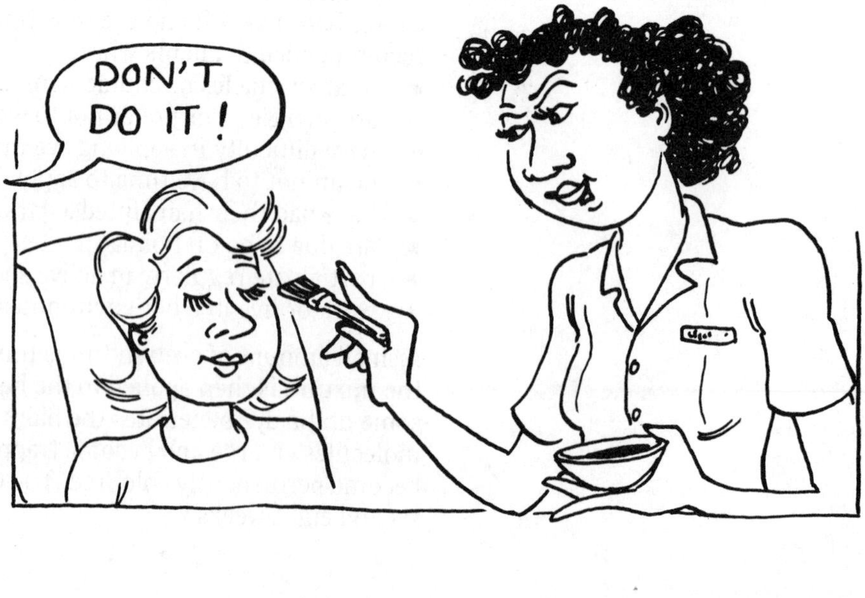

> Remember
>
> You must never use hairdressing products for tinting the eyebrows or lashes. Hair dyes contain strong chemicals such as metaphenylenediamine which are not suitable for using in the sensitive eye area.

> *Remember*
> *Always* read the manufacturer's instructions before mixing eyelash tint. Make sure you use the correct strength of peroxide mixed with the right amount of tint.

Skin test

To do this, you will need:
surgical spirit or mild astringent (to cleanse the skin)
- cotton wool
- applicator (brush or an orange stick tipped with cotton wool)
- a small amount of the desired tint mixed with the correct proportion of hydrogen peroxide.

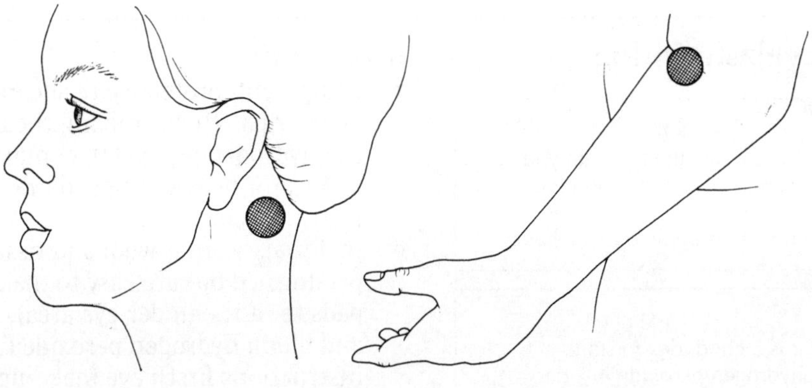

Patch test areas: behind the ear and in the crease of the elbow

The procedure is as follows;

1. Cleanse an area of skin behind the ear or in the crease of an elbow.
2. Apply the prepared tint to the cleansed skin. The test patch should be no larger than a small coin.
3. Leave the tint to develop on the skin for five minutes.
4. Remove excess tint with cotton wool and advise the client about what to do if there is a positive reaction to the test.

Reactions

A positive reaction: inflammation, irritation and swelling of the skin in the test area which may not show up until the next day. In severe cases, the client may feel quite poorly. This client is allergic to the tint and, therefore, not suitable for having eyelash or eyebrow tinting treatments.
- Apply a soothing cream or lotion such as one containing calamine or witch hazel.
- Contact the salon as soon as possible to arrange for the skin to be treated with a special tint remover.

A negative reaction: there is no change in the skin. The client is suitable for treatment. Check that there are no other contra-indications and proceed with treatment.

> *Remember*
> The date of the consultation and skin test and details of the result must be entered on the client's record card.

Contra-indications

Any disorder causing sensitivity of the eyes and surrounding skin is a contra-indication to lash and brow tinting, for example:
- conjunctivitis
- stye

- undiagnosed lumps
- cuts and abrasions
- inflammation and swelling.

If a client were to suffer an adverse reaction to eyelash tinting and claim compensation from the salon, the insurers would require records of the consultation and skin test. These would be considered important evidence to show that *all reasonable care* had been taken when assessing the client's suitability for treatment.

Eyelash tinting

> Remember
> Do not mix the tint until you are ready to use it, or the colour will start developing before the mixture is applied to the hairs.

> Remember
> It is a good idea to store hydrogen peroxide in a dark coloured 'dropper' bottle for use during an eyelash tinting treatment. This helps to prevent the hydrogen peroxide from losing its strength and measures out an accurate amount of peroxide when mixing the tint.

> Remember
> Take care not to irritate the eyes before a tinting treatment, or they may be too sensitive for you to carry on. Use a special eye make-up remover which will dissolve mascara quickly.

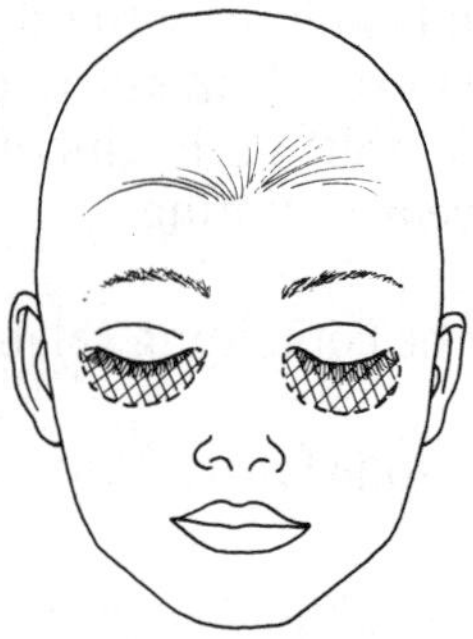

Eyeshields in position

> Remember
> Make sure you do not instruct your client to look up into an overhead light. This could start her eyes watering with disastrous consequences!

You will need:

- equipment: protective headband and towel; small, non-metallic bowl or palette for mixing the tint (a metal one would react with the hydrogen peroxide); container for waste; clean spatula, applicator brush or tipped orange stick; clean eye bath; hand mirror; record card
- materials: cotton wool and tissues; eye shields (these can be bought pre-formed but are easy to make by shaping dampened cotton wool pads to fit the under-eye area); tint (available in black, brown, grey and blue); hydrogen peroxide (usually 10 volume, but check instructions first); eye make-up remover, cleanser, toner, barrier cream or petroleum jelly.

Preparing the client

1. Help the client into a comfortable, semi-reclining position and protect hair and clothing with the headband and towel.
2. Cleanse and tone the eye area. Ensure that all make-up and grease is removed from the lashes .
3. Protect the skin above and underneath the eyes with a barrier cream or petroleum jelly. Take care not to get any of the product on the lashes.

Barrier cream

Barrier cream prevents the tint from staining the skin and spoiling the effect of the treatment. It will also prevent the tint from penetrating the hairs if it touches them.

Use a tipped orange stick or cotton bud to apply barrier cream to the skin above the eyes. When applying barrier cream below the eyes either:

- stroke it directly on to the skin and position the eye shields on top, close to the base of the lashes, or
- coat the underneath surface of the eye shields with barrier cream and slide them in to position.

Applying the tint

Precautions should be taken to ensure that neither the tint nor applicator penetrates the eye. There should not be any problems provided that:

- the tint is applied carefully
- the lashes are not overloaded with tint
- the client's eyes are kept still.

1 Mix the tint (usually 3 or 4 drops of hydrogen peroxide to 1.5 cm of tint) and take up a small amount on the applicator. Ask the client to look upwards, away from the applicator, and cover the lower lashes with tint.

> Remember
> If you prefer to tint the upper and lower lashes together, mix the tint and proceed from point 2, ensuring that you apply enough tint to seep through to the lower lashes without the excess penetrating the eye.

2 Instruct the client to close their eyes and to keep them closed throughout the rest of the treatment. Lift the skin of the eyelids gently from below the brows (this will expose the base of the lashes) and apply the tint. Take up more tint on the applicator as required. Ensure even coverage of the lashes from base to tip, making sure that you do not miss the shorter hairs which grow near the inside corners of the eyes.

3 Cover the eyes with slightly dampened cotton wool pads. This will help to keep the client's eyes closed and trap in warmth which aids the development of the tint. A client who prefers not to wear eye pads will need leaving a little longer for the tint to develop.

4 Note the time and allow between 10 and 15 minutes for the tint to process, according to the manufacturer's instructions. The colour should be checked at intervals and tint re-applied if necessary.

If the client complains of uncomfortable prickling or the eyes begin to water, remove the tint immediately using damp cotton wool pads and rinse the eyes with clean, warm water contained in an eye bath.

Apply damp cotton wool pads soaked in witch hazel to cool and soothe the eye area. Do not proceed with tinting until the eyes have calmed down and, only then if you are sure that the client is suitable for treatment.

Possible causes of eye irritation are:

- very sensitive skin
- too much or incorrect strength of hydrogen peroxide used
- something in the eye, for example excess cleanser, eye make-up, cotton-wool fibre, eyelash tint
- inadvertently poking the eye with the applicator.

5 Hold the eye shields and cotton wool pads together at their outer edges and remove them in one swift action, enclosing any excess tint. Remove any remaining tint with clean, damp, cotton wool pads.

> Remember
> Contact lenses must not be worn when tinting the eyelashes. Advise the client beforehand to bring in some soaking solution and a container for the lenses so that they can be kept safely on the trolley during treatment.

6 Finally, wipe over the area with skin tonic to remove all traces of barrier cream.

7 Offer the client a hand mirror and seek approval of the final result.

8 Enter details of the treatment on the client's record card.

Tinting the eyebrows

1 Prepare the skin and brows in the same way as for treating the lashes. Apply barrier cream or petroleum jelly around the eyebrows and lift hairs from the skin using an orange stick. Apply the tint with a fine brush or orange stick tipped with cotton wool, working gradually from the outer and underneath hairs towards the centre.

> Remember
> The development time for tinting the brows is much shorter than for the lashes, usually between one and three minutes.
>
> Care must be taken to prevent the brows from becoming too dark as this can create an unattractive 'hard' effect.

2 After one minute, remove a little tint from the inner corners of the eyebrows and check how the colour is developing. Apply more tint and repeat colour checks at one minute intervals until the desired effect has been achieved.

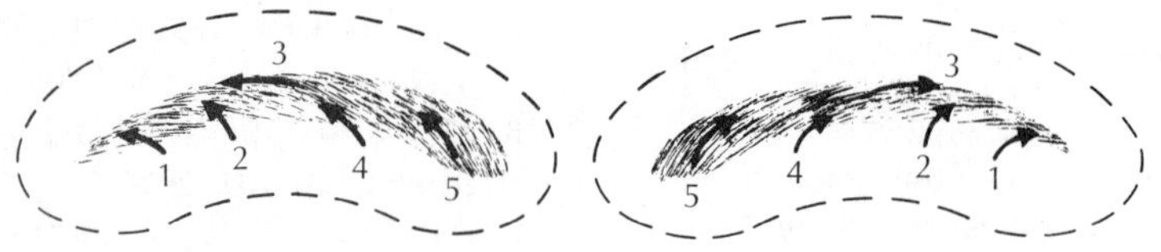

Applying tint to eyebrows

3 Remove tint with clean, damp cotton wool pads.

4 Wipe over the area with skin tonic to remove all traces of barrier cream.

Assessing results

A successful tinting treatment produces the required colour changes to the lashes or brows without staining the skin.

Even the shortest eyelashes should be coloured evenly from their base. Blond roots after an eyelash tinting treatment show that not enough care was taken. The skin fold of the eyelid was probably not lifted away from the base of the hairs when applying the tint.

> Remember
> If you wish to colour and shape the brows in the same treatment, tint the hairs first and then use the tweezers. This prevents over-stimulating the skin before applying tint.

The tint will not have coloured the lashes or brows successfully if:
- there was grease or make-up left on the hairs
- old tint was used
- the hydrogen peroxide had lost its strength
- the tint and peroxide were mixed incorrectly
- the tint was removed too early.

Do not shape the eyebrows if there is any skin or eye irritation following the tinting treatment.

Eyelash and eyebrow tinting: Self-checks

1 When would be particularly good times of the year to promote eyelash and eyebrow tinting treatments?

2 State three specific benefits of eyelash tinting for a client who wears contact lenses.

3 Explain briefly how the hairs become coloured by eyelash tint.

4 Why do the effects of eyelash tinting last for only six to eight weeks?

5 State two reasons for giving a client a skin test.

6 Why should details of the skin test be written on the client's record card?

7 Describe a positive reaction to a skin test.

8 List the contra-indications to eyelash and eyebrow tinting.

9 Give three possible causes of a client's eyes watering during an eyelash tinting treatment.

10 State two advantages of applying cotton wool pads over the eyes after tint has been applied.

Eyelash and eyebrow tinting: Activity

1 Visit your wholesaler and have a look through suppliers' catalogues to find out the range of tinting products available. Compare their prices, ingredients, colour ranges and instructions for use. Try to work out which product represents the best value for money.

Eyebrow shaping

Shaping the brows emphasises the eyes and helps give character to the face. The most popular method of shaping is by plucking with tweezers. Automatic tweezers are used to remove the bulk of excess hairs growing beneath the eyebrows. Manual tweezers create the final shape.

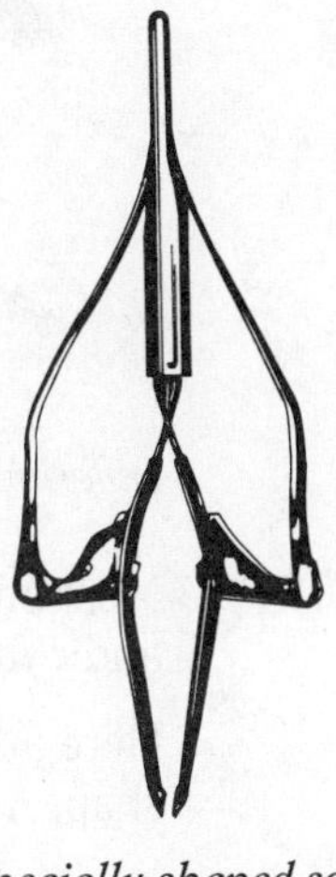

The sides of the tweezers are specially shaped so that they can be held comfortably and squeezed together quickly to operate the automatic plucking mechanism.

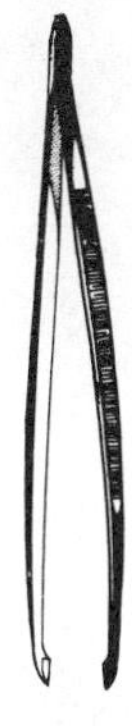

The more familiar traditional type of tweezer which requires the operator to perform the gripping and plucking action.

The eyebrow hairs grow in skin which lies over the base of the frontal bone at the upper part of the eye socket. The thicker hairs which make up the general shape of the brows protect the bony prominence.

Finer hairs grow further down towards the eye socket. These finer hairs are more obvious in darker people. They tend to give a heavy appearance to the brows which dominates the upper eye area. In fair people, these hairs are less conspicuous but they spoil the effect of eye make-up.

> Remember
> A regular fortnightly eyebrow trim is usually all that is required once the client's desired eyebrow shape has been achieved.

By removing excess hair, the skin becomes smoother and more suitable for make-up. Eye shadows can be blended more evenly producing a softer and more professional finish.

Choosing an eyebrow shape

Eyebrow shapes come in and out of fashion as often as make-up looks change. For younger clients, fashion may be the only influence on their choice of eyebrow shape.

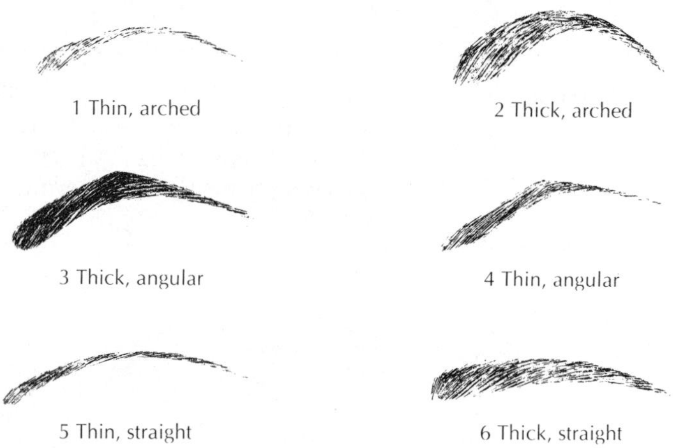

Different fashions in eyebrow shapes

Most clients prefer a shape which suits their face, emphasises their eyes and complements or corrects their natural eyebrow shape.

Here are some guidelines to help you measure up for an eyebrow shape.

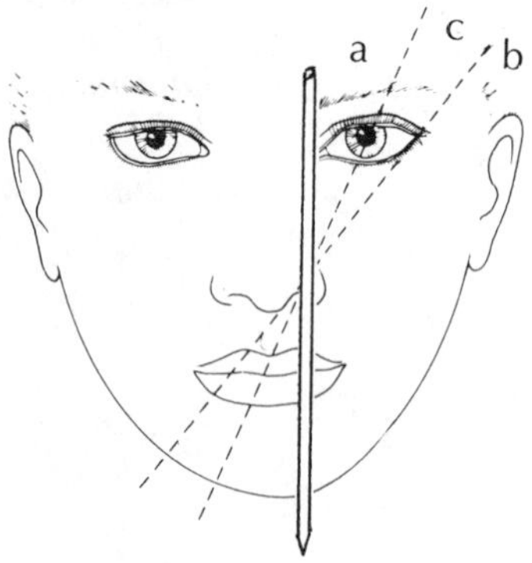

1 Position a clean orange stick vertically at the sides of the nose so that it crosses the brow. You will need to remove any hairs growing in area (a).

2 Swivel the orange stick round so that it crosses the brow on line with the outer corner of the eye. Eyebrow hairs growing in area (b) will have to be removed.

3 Re-position the orange stick so that it crosses the brow on a line which passes through the centre of the eye. The hairs in area (c) should be removed to produce the highest point of the eyebrow arch.

With experience, you will develop a trained eye which will help you to make quick, reliable assessments without going through this procedure.

Creating effects

The natural shape, thickness and spacing of the eyebrows determine what can be achieved by plucking. The basic guidelines may need adapting for dealing with particular problems. Sometimes, a little eyebrow pencil is needed afterwards to achieve the final effect.

Close-set eyes

Eyes which are less than one eye's width apart need the illusion of extra space created between them. This can be helped by increasing, slightly, the distance between the eyebrows and extending the length of the brows beyond the normal guideline.

Eyes too wide apart

Eyes which are more than one eye's width apart need to look closer together. This can be achieved by reducing the distance between the brows and finishing the shape slightly inside the normal guide-line.

Brows which meet

- Eyebrows which meet in the middle produce a frowning effect. Clear hairs from above the bridge of the nose to draw the brows apart.

'Droopy' eyebrows

- Eyebrows growing too far down at the sides make the eyes look sad or tired. Shorten the brows so that they do not extend beyond the outer corners of the eyes.

Thick untidy eyebrows

- The brows look heavy and the eyes lack definition. Clear excess hair from above the socket and create an arch. This emphasises the eye shape and surrounding bone structure.

Excessive eyebrow hairs on very mature skin

- Excess hairs emphasise the effects of loose skin and slack muscle tone in the eye area. Clear the excess hairs and create an arch at the outer edges of the brows to give a more youthful lift to the eye area. Do not make the brows too thin. Thicker eyebrows are more sophisticated than thin ones and produce a softer, more natural shape.

The shape and thickness of the eyebrows can be adapted to help balance the facial features.

Face shapes

Long

The brows should be of medium thickness and taper off slightly. They should be kept almost straight to divide the length of the face and draw attention across its width.

Square

A smooth tapering arch is best to soften the effects of an angular face shape. Do not make the brows too thin or they will be lost on a face with heavy bone structure.

Heart

An arched brow which is not too thin will help to balance the deeper and wider upper part of the face without drawing attention to the highest points of the forehead.

Pear

Angular brows with a fairly high arch at the outer corners help to widen the forehead and balance it with the heavier bone structure of the lower part of the face.

Diamond

A well-defined angular arch helps to square off the forehead and balance it with the widest part of the face.

Round

Eyebrows which are quite thick at the inner edge and taper off into a high angular arch draw attention away from the fullness of the face and help create an illusion of extra length.

Preparing for eyebrow shaping

> Remember
> Tweezers which have been cleaned and then stored in a jar of sterilising fluid are ready for use at a moment's notice.

You will need:

- headband and towel
- jar of sterilising fluid containing automatic and manual tweezers and scissors
- clean eyebrow brush
- container of cotton-wool pads, tissues and a bowl for waste
- eye make-up remover, cleansing lotion, toner, surgical spirit, witch hazel, soothing antiseptic cream
- eyebrow pencil
- hand mirror and record card.

Make sure that you will be working in good light when giving an eyebrow shaping treatment. This will help you to produce good results and will reduce the risk of nipping the skin with tweezers. Ideally, a magnifying lamp should be used which will show up even the finest hairs.

> *Remember*
> A client who is anticipating pain will definitely feel pain! Help your client to relax by ensuring that she is warm enough and seated or lying in a comfortable, semi-reclining position.

> *Remember*
> If the tweezers pick up grease they will not be able to grip the hairs well. The treatment will take longer, the skin will become more sensitive and the results will probably not be effective.

> *Remember*
> If eyebrow shaping is being combined with a tinting treatment, tint the brows first and then pluck them.

> *Remember*
> It is important to discuss your intentions with the client , particularly if there is going to be a significant change in appearance.
>
> Offer the client a hand mirror so that you can show her what you have planned. Explain what the benefits are going to be.
>
> Seek approval before you go ahead: once the hairs have been plucked out, they cannot be put back!

> *Remember*
> If the eyebrow hairs are very long, they should be trimmed first with scissors to make plucking more comfortable.

> *Remember*
> Be careful when using the tweezers. Examine the area you are working on closely. If you are over zealous when plucking, you may remove hairs which were effectively concealing a scar.

Preparing the client

Many clients come to the salon for eyebrow shaping treatments because they find the treatment too uncomfortable to do for themselves. A thick growth of dark, strong eyebrow hairs can be particularly painful to remove if the skin and hairs are not prepared properly.

1. Use the headband to keep the client's hair off the face and cover upper clothing with a towel.
2. Remove make-up from the eyebrow area and cleanse the skin and hairs.
3. Wipe over with a toner to remove any traces of grease
4. Check the area for contra-indications:
   - diseases or disorders of the skin
   - cuts and abrasions
   - lumps and swellings
   - recent scar tissue
   - hypersensitive skin
   - sensitive or infected eyes.
5. If it is safe to proceed with treatment, brush the eyebrows upwards to separate the hairs and then brush them into their natural shape.
6. Assess the client's preferences relative to the natural growth and shape of the brows and give appropriate advice.
7. Warm the brow area by using a facial steamer or by applying cotton-wool pads dampened with hot water. The walls of the hair follicles normally have a tight grip of the hairs contained in them. Warming the area helps to relax the follicles so that they loosen their grip and the hairs comes out more easily and with less discomfort.

Shaping the brows

Plucking begins above the bridge of the nose where the skin is less sensitive. The eyebrows are then worked on alternately, removing a few hairs at a time until the bulk of excess hairs has been removed. Automatic tweezers make plucking much more comfortable because they can be used very quickly and can clear a lot of hair before the client has time to think painful thoughts! (Many clients are reassured by the rhythmic clicking of automatic tweezers and find the sound relaxing.) Manual tweezers achieve the final eyebrow shape.

Use the following techniques to ensure a comfortable, safe and effective eyebrow shaping treatment:

- keep the skin taut: this helps to deaden the pain nerve endings. It also makes the hairs stand on end so that they are easier to grip. There is less chance of nipping the skin [
- pluck hairs out in direction of growth: hairs will be removed cleanly from the follicle. They will not break off at the surface of the skin
- re-apply warm pads: particularly when plucking coarse hairs, keeping the area warm makes the treatment more comfortable
- work as quickly as safety allows: it does not matter if the automatic tweezers do not pluck out hairs every time so long as the whole area is cleared within a reasonable time

- monitor the skin: check for signs of skin sensitivity and do not continue if there is an extreme reaction to the treatment
- brush brows into shape regularly: keep an eye on how treatment is progressing, particularly when doing detailed work with the manual tweezers. Make sure the eyebrows are shaped evenly and at the same level.
- remove plucked hairs: do not leave loose hairs on the skin. Transfer them to a clean tissue or cotton-wool pad
- keep tweezers clean: during the treatment, wipe over the ends of the tweezers regularly with surgical spirit. This removes any adhering hairs and skin cells and keeps the tweezers disinfected.

> *Remember*
> Good hygiene is essential when shaping the brows. Empty hair follicles provide a route for bacteria to enter the skin.

Completing the treatment

The treatment is not finished until you know the client is pleased with the results: wipe over the brows with witch hazel to soothe the skin and reduce redness. Brush the eyebrows into shape and offer the client a hand mirror to examine the brows. Finally you should seek the approval of the client.

If any adjustment is needed, the brow area will have to be warmed again before using the tweezers. If the client is satisfied with the treatment, apply some soothing antiseptic cream to prevent the skin from becoming infected.

Advice for home care

If adequate precautions have been taken, any slight pinkness will disappear quickly after eyebrow shaping and the skin will soon return to normal. A more sensitive reaction to the treatment may take longer to calm down. The client should be advised to apply soothing antiseptic cream regularly and to refrain from applying make-up to the skin while it is still pink.

Details of the treatment and any retail sales should be entered on the client's record card before she is escorted away from the treatment area.

Cleaning up

It is important to clear up immediately after treatment so that the next client can be attended to promptly.

- Dispose of waste immediately after treatment and return soiled linen to the laundry.
- Wash the tweezers and eyebrow brush in detergent and rinse thoroughly under clean running water.
- Immerse the brush in a suitable disinfectant and then place it in an ultra-violet cabinet.
- Return the tweezers to soak in sterilising fluid or wipe them over with surgical spirit and place them in the ultra-violet cabinet. Look after your tweezers: if they become damaged, they are of no use to you. Always release the hinges on automatic tweezers when storing them and oil the joints regularly to ensure a smooth action. Keep the tips protected and do not use them for any other purpose: if they become scratched, they will collect germs.

> *Remember*
> The tweezers will need turning halfway through the sterilising period to make sure that all sides are treated with the UV rays.

Eyebrow shaping: Self-checks

1 Why are automatic tweezers preferable to manual for removing the bulk of eyebrow hairs?

2 What hygiene precautions should be taken before and during an eyebrow-shaping treatment?

3 What steps should be taken to ensure the comfort of the client during eyebrow shaping?

4 Why is the treated area wiped over with witch hazel after eyebrow shaping?

5 State three factors which influence the choice of eyebrow shape for a client.

6 How often should a client return to the salon for an eyebrow shaping treatment?

False eyelashes

False eyelashes are used extensively when applying make-up for fashion photography and cat-walk modelling. They are also popular for achieving glamour effects when the client's natural lashes need more enhancement than can be achieved with mascara or eyelash tinting. False lashes are fun to wear and are particularly popular during the party season at festive times of the year. They are available in black and brown and are made from natural hair or nylon. There are two types:

- temporary: supplied as pre-shaped strips which are attached with a special adhesive to the edge of the eyelid
- semi-permanent: available as individual lashes or in small clusters of two or three which are attached to the base of the natural eyelashes with a special adhesive.

> Remember
> You must never use any other type of adhesive for attaching false eyelashes.

False eyelashes must not be applied if:

- the client has very sensitive eyes
- the eye or surrounding skin is infected
- the eyelid is swollen or inflamed
- the client has previously experienced an allergic reaction to eyelash adhesive. Although false eyelash adhesives are relatively safe, it is wise to test the client's skin sensitivity to them before treatment. This is done in the same way as you would for an eyelash tint.

Choosing false eyelashes

The client must have the confidence to wear false eyelashes so it is important to consult with her first and give appropriate advice. You will need to consider:

- reasons for use: there is no point in going through the comparatively lengthy procedure of applying individual lashes if they are intended to be worn only for a single event
- facial characteristics: the length and thickness of the lashes must suit the size and shape of the eyes and balance with the face shape. Strip lashes should be the same colour as the mascara. The colour of semi-permanent lashes should match the natural ones
- client's personality: although most clients prefer their false eye lashes to look natural, more extrovert ones may want a more obviously glamorous effect

> Remember
> If the client wears glasses, make sure you choose lashes which will not touch the lenses and cause irritation when moving the eyes.

- personal preference: strip lashes are very effective but they usually look heavier than individual ones. They are quick to apply and can be removed easily by the client.

Semi-permanent lashes look and feel more natural and are particularly effective when applied to fair lashes which have been tinted. They do, however, need looking after carefully. Some lashes may become detached and need replacing.

Temporary (strip) lashes

Strip lashes are worn to make the natural lashes look thicker and longer. They are usually applied to the eyelids as complete strips, but the base can be cut down into shorter sections, depending on the client's requirements. Lashes on a fine base look more natural than ones on a thicker, heavier base.

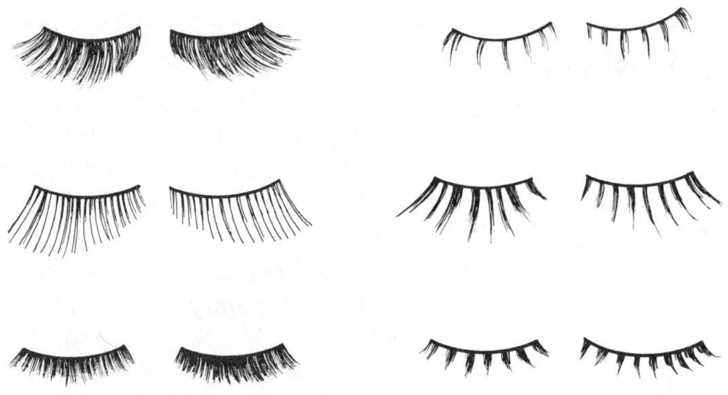

Strip lashes come in various thicknesses, lengths and shapes for achieving different effects.

Applying temporary (strip) false eyelashes

Strip lashes are applied at the end of the make-up procedure. This way, they do not need washing as often and they last longer. Applying an eyeline first helps to conceal the base of the strip so that the lashes look more natural.

Preparation

You will need:
- the chosen set of false eyelashes
- tube of adhesive
- pair of clean manual tweezers
- clean mascara brush
- eyebath (in case of an accident)
- tissues
- hand mirror.

If the lashes are new, measure the strip against the edge of the eyelid. If necessary, shorten the strip from the outside edge to avoid removing the shorter lashes, which are shaped specially to fit comfortably near the nose.

A new strip is easier to apply if it is made more pliable. This is done by moulding the strip in to a half-moon shape to fit the eyelid.

Place the false eyelashes on a clean tissue with the lashes facing away from you.

Applying the lashes

False eyelashes can be applied from in front of or behind the client, depending on which position she is in. Working from behind will give you a better view and the client is less likely to be distracted. The client's eyes should be kept closed when applying the lashes.

1. Apply a small amount of adhesive to the knuckle of one hand.
2. Using the tweezers, pick up an eyelash strip in the centre on the lash side.
3. Stroke the base of the strip through the adhesive so that there is a fine line evenly distributed along its length. Do not get adhesive on the lashes.

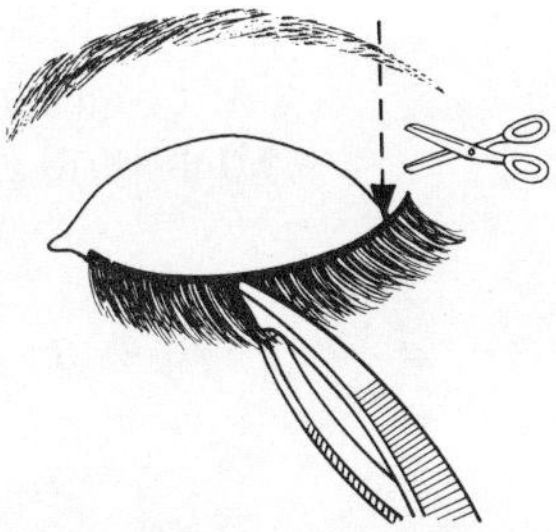

Measuring up for eyelash application

4. Using your free hand over a tissue, lift the brow area slightly to ensure a good fit close to the base of the natural lashes.
5. Line up the tweezers with the centre of the eyelid and press the strip gently in to place, making sure the lashes follow the direction of natural hair growth.

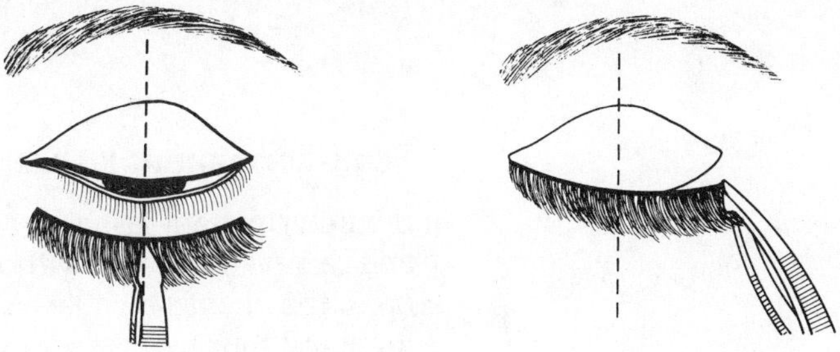

Attaching the lashes

6. Secure the inner and outer corners of the strip. Do not get adhesive on the tweezers or natural lashes.
7. Apply the remaining strip in the same way.
8. When the lashes are quite secure (after approximately 2 minutes), ask the client to open her eyes and gently press the false eyelashes and the natural ones together with clean tweezers.
9. Use a clean mascara brush to blend the false eyelashes with the natural ones.
10. Offer the client a mirror and ensure that she is satisfied with the result.

> Remember
>
> When applying strip lashes to the lower eyelid, ask the client to look upwards and secure the lashes in the same way, but underneath the lower lashes.

Removing and cleaning the lashes

Hold the eyelid taut and pull the strip away from the outer edge towards the inner corner of the eyelid. The adhesive can be removed from the strip quite easily and the lashes replaced in their box until required.

Over a period of time, the lashes will collect dust and traces of mascara. To clean them, wipe over with eye make-up remover and then wash the lashes in warm soapy water and rinse well.

To curl the lashes:

1. Wrap a tissue once around an even-barrelled pencil
2. Place the clean false eyelashes on the pencil, over the tissue, with the inner edges of the strips together. Make sure the lashes are evenly dispersed along the pencil.
3. Roll the pencil along the rest of the tissue, enclosing the lashes. Secure the tissue tightly at both ends with rubber bands.

Alternatively, eyelash curlers may be used. These press the strip into shape and can also be used for curling the natural eyelashes.

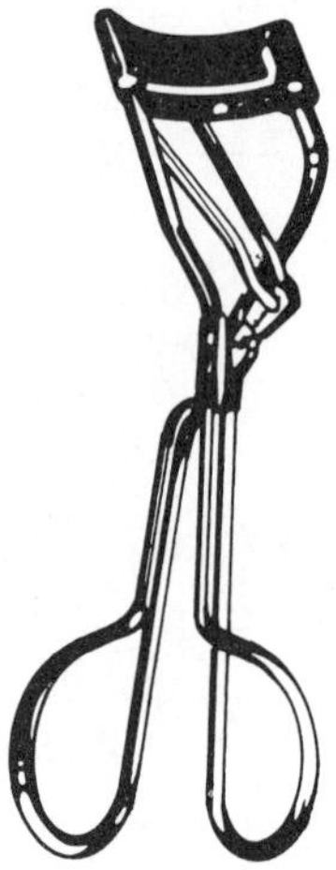

Semi-permanent lashes

Semi-permanent lashes produce a more natural effect than strip lashes and can even be worn without eye make-up. They are applied directly on to the client's own lashes and, if treated carefully, will stay in place for about four weeks so long as the supporting eyelash is secure.

Applying semi-permanent false eyelashes

These lashes are attached individually to the client's natural eyelashes, so take much longer to apply than the strip type. Great care is needed to prevent adhesive or lashes penetrating the eyes.

The client should be in a semi-reclining position with you working from behind. Good lighting is essential. You will need:

- a selection of false eyelashes
- adhesive (transparent or black, depending on the colour of lashes)
- a piece of foil
- special eyelash adhesive solvent
- clean tweezers

- a clean eyebath (in case of accidents)
- a clean headband
- tissues
- a hand mirror.

Semi-permanent lashes are usually supplied in three lengths: short, medium and long. The number and type of lashes you will need depends on the length of the client's own lashes and the effect she requires.

1 Secure the client's hair off the face with the headband.

2 Ensure that the natural lashes are scrupulously clean and dry.

3 Using the tweezers, remove the lashes individually from the pack and arrange them on a tissue in the order that they will appear after attachment. The lashes should be facing away from you.

4 Shape the foil into a small cupped shape and squeeze into it a small amount of adhesive. The foil helps to keep the adhesive the correct consistency and saves you the job of cleaning up hardened adhesive afterwards.

5 Raise the client's head slightly to reduce the risk of adhesive running into the eye.

6 Select the cluster of lashes which is due to be placed centrally and pick it up with the tweezers so that the knotted base is exposed.

7 Dip the knot into the adhesive, making sure that none gets on the tweezers.

8 Ask the client to look downwards, but not to close her eyes.

9 Using your free hand over a tissue, lift the brow area to release the fold of skin from the base of the natural lashes.

10 Carefully locate the false eyelash over a centrally placed natural one. Stroke the knot slightly along its base to distribute the adhesive and then ease it back up the natural lash so that it settles on top. Hold the lash in place for a few seconds.

11 Apply the corresponding lash to the other eye and continue in the same way, working alternately between the eyes to achieve a balanced effect.

12 When all the upper lashes have been applied and the adhesive has dried, ask the client to open her eyes gently and allow a few seconds for her to get used to them. Check that they are comfortable and apply lower lashes if they are required.

13 Offer the client a mirror and ensure that she is satisfied with the result.

14 Enter details of the treatment on the client's record card.

> Remember
>
> Keep checking the eyes to ensure that the different lengths of lashes have been applied in the right place and that the eyes match.

> Remember
>
> When applying lower lashes, ask the client to look upwards and secure the lashes in the same way but underneath the natural eyelashes.

Removing individual false lashes

The client should be advised never to pull off the false lashes: the underlying natural ones will also be lost. If many hairs were removed in this way, the eyelids would be left bald. Besides spoiling the appearance of the eyes, this would remove the protection given to them by the lashes.

The procedure for removing the lashes is as follows:

1 Secure pre-shaped, dampened cotton wool pads beneath the eyes, close to the base of the lashes.

2 Tip one end of an orange stick with cotton wool and soak it in the special solvent.

3 Ask the client to close her eyes and apply the solvent to the base of the lashes.

4 Allow the solvent to penetrate the adhesive for about 10 seconds and then ease the false lashes away with a gentle rolling action of the orange stick.

5 Finally, wipe over the eyelids and lashes with a mild skin freshener.

There are always risks involved when working so closely around the eyes, particularly when applying chemical adhesive and extensions to the natural eyelashes. You must work with a very steady hand to avoid the following problems:

- adhesive entering the eye: do not use an excessive amount of adhesive. Only the knotted base of the false lash should be covered.
- false lash entering the eye: the client's eyes must be kept still and remain relaxed. The false lashes should follow, exactly, the direction of the natural eyelashes and should never be placed at an angle to them.
- eyes watering: this may be a reaction to penetrating the eye, but can also occur if the client is nervous about you working so close to her eyes. It is up to you to put the client at ease: reassure her and build up her confidence beforehand. If the client's eyes start watering during the treatment, sit her up and ask her to keep her eyes closed. Offer her a tissue to dry the eyes.

Mild watering without an obvious cause will usually settle down quite quickly and you may proceed so long as the eyes have not become too sensitive.

Heavy watering accompanied by intense irritation suggests that the eye has been penetrated, probably by adhesive. You must immediately fill an eyebath with clean warm water and help the client to flush out the irritant.

It is not safe to continue the treatment if the eyes remain sore or sensitive.

- top and bottom lashes sticking together: make sure the client does not close her eyes during the procedure and keep the skin above the eye lifted until the adhesive has set.
- irritation or sensitivity to the adhesive: a patch test beforehand should establish the client's sensitivity to the adhesive. If irritation occurs during the treatment, you must not continue. Remove any lashes which have been applied and help your client with an eyebath.

> Remember
> Eyelashes keep growing for approximately four months. They then enter a resting phase and eventually fall out to make way for a replacement hair. The lashes do not all fall out at the same time, but one or two may due to be replaced when you attach false lashes to them.

Explain this to your client. If some lashes are lost during the week following application, it is good policy to replace them at no extra cost to the client.

Home care

The client should be particularly careful when removing eye make-up and cleansing her face. Although the adhesive is strong, it does not embed the false lash into the skin. Any rough treatment which dislodges the false lash will also affect the eyelash to which it is fixed.

Mascara may be applied to the lashes but it is best to keep this to a minimum to avoid attracting dust particles which may accumulate in the longer lashes and cause irritation.

Eye make-up remover pads may be recommended for cleaning the lashes.

False eyelashes: Self-checks

1 List the contra-indications to applying false eyelashes.

2 State four factors which influence the choice of false eyelashes for a client.

3 How should a new pair of strip false eyelashes be prepared for application?

4 How is a natural effect achieved when applying strip lashes?

5 What advice should be given to a client following application of strip false lashes?

6 How can you ensure that the effects on the eyes match each other when applying individual false lashes?

7 When are individual false lashes preferable to strip ones?

8 State the possible causes of discomfort around the eyes following application of individual false lashes.

9 What advice should be given to a client following application of individual false lashes?

10 State one retail product which could be sold to a client who has had individual false eyelashes applied.

False eyelashes: Activity

1 Practise achieving different effects with false eyelashes and photograph the results. You could either:
a) incorporate this activity into your make-up portfolio, or
b) use the same model each time so that the effects of different lengths, colours and thicknesses of lashes upon the eyes is more obvious. Adapt the eye make-up according to the effect you are trying to achieve.

Chapter 8

Examining the hand and nails

After working through this chapter you will be able to:

- ▶ carry out an examination of the hands and nails
- ▶ understand the structure and growth of nails
- ▶ recognise and respond to a full range of nail diseases and disorders
- ▶ recognise and respond to skin disorders affecting the hands
- ▶ give advice on specific hand and nail problems.

Assessing the hands and nails

It is important that the hands and nails are clean so that an accurate assessment can be made of their condition. Examination should take place in good light, preferably under a magnifying lamp. The client's hand jewellery should be removed.

1 Examine the palms and backs of both hands: note the colour and texture of the skin. Is it soft and smooth or dry and rough? Look for any cracks or breaks in the skin. Are there any signs of infection?

2 Look at the skin between the fingers: are there any signs of dryness and flakiness? Is there any skin irritation where rings are usually worn?

3 Inspect the cuticles: notice if they are dry and hard or soft and pliable. Are there are any splits or hangnails? Are any of the cuticles excessively thick?

4 Examine the skin around the nails: is the skin intact and are there any signs of infection?

5 Study each of the nails: are they smooth, flexible and slightly pink? Do they look and feel strong or are they all different shapes and sizes? Are there any splits or breaks?

You will need a very good background knowledge of normal and abnormal nail growth.

Structure and growth of nails

The parts of the nails that we can see are dead. They have no blood supply, no nerves and no means of taking in nourishment from the outside. This can cause confusion when products and treatments claim to 'nourish' or 'feed' the nails. The true source of food for the nails is the blood which supplies the 'living' matrix cells, just behind the nail fold where the eye cannot see.

Strong nails depend on a supply of blood which carries, to the matrix, the breakdown products of a healthy, balanced diet, rich in protein and calcium. Meat, cheese, milk and eggs are particularly good sources of nourishment for the nails.

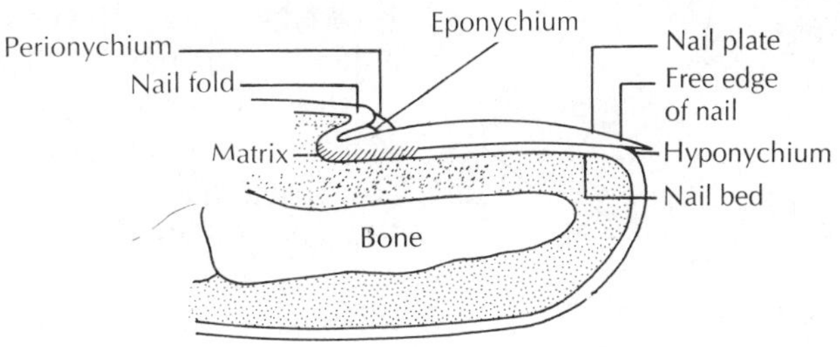

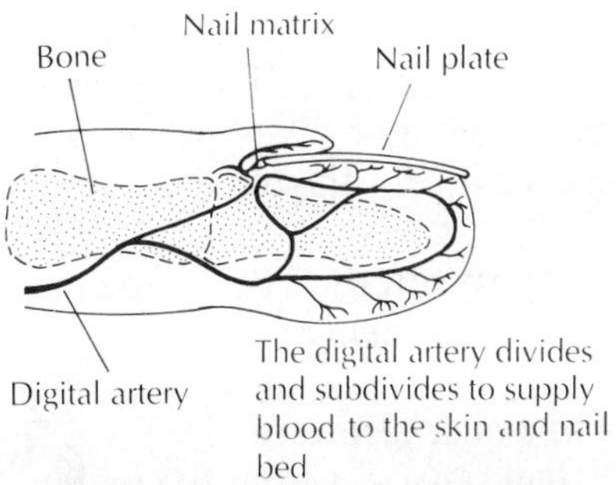

Blood supply to the nail and nail bed

The matrix is the site of nail formation. Some of the protein keratin is deposited here, which is then carried in the cells as they travel along the nail bed. Keratin makes the nails hard and gives them strength. The journey from the matrix to the end of the fingertip takes approximately six months and, during that time, changes take place which convert the soft living cells into compacted layers of dead cells, held together with a little moisture and fat.

As the cells move along the nail bed, more keratin becomes deposited in them so that, by the time a free-edge has developed, the nails are perfectly structured to perform their important protective function.

Without nails, the delicate nerve endings and blood vessels in the ends of the fingers would soon become damaged. The nails give support from above which enable the fingers to perform many important functions. They also concentrate the sense of touch.

Parts of the nail

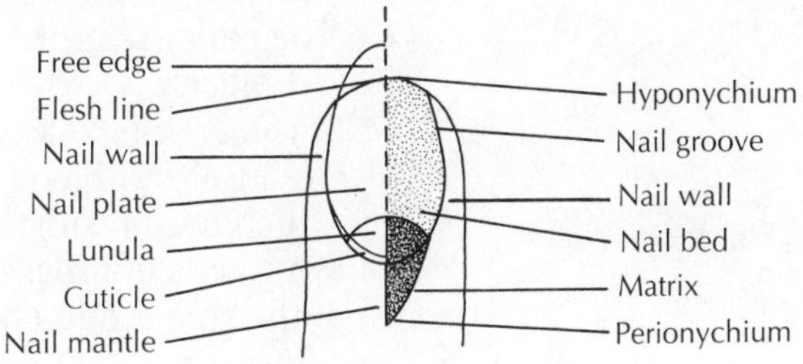

- Cuticle: this is divided in to two parts. The main, outer portion surrounding the nail is the *perionychium*, which develops from the stratum corneum of the epidermis. It covers about a fifth of the developing nail. Beneath this lies the less significant *eponychium*, a thin layer which adheres to the nail plate. The function of the cuticle is to protect the matrix by forming a barrier.
- Lunula: commonly known as the half moon, the lunula is situated on all the nails, but is generally only visible on the thumbs. The pale colour is due to the relative looseness of the nail plate over an area of very dense fibrous tissue. The cells in the lunula are only partially keratinised.
- Nail walls: these pads of skin which surround the nail on three sides help to cushion the nail from external damage and to hold the nail in place.
- Nail plate: this is the main body of the nail, made up of specialised cells of the stratum lucidum layer of the epidermis. Ridges on the under surface fit firmly into ones on the underlying nail bed. The cells of the plate have an overlapping, stacking arrangement which, together with keratin, make the nails hard and strong.

- Free edge: this is the extension of the nail plate which does not adhere to the nail bed, hence its white colour. The free edge is the hardest part of the nail.
- Matrix: this is the only living part of the nail. The cells are contained in an area of dense fibrous tissue in the dermis called the mantle. The reproductive processes of the nail take place at the matrix and a vast network of blood and lymphatic vessels maintains the healthy functioning of the cells.
- Nail bed: this is composed mainly of dermal tissue containing blood vessels and nerve endings. A thin layer of the stratum germinatum connects the nail bed to the nail plate. If a nail is removed, this layer of epidermis remains in contact with the nail. Ridges in the nail bed connect with the plate above, keeping the nail firmly in place as it grows. The nail bed is responsible for the pinkish colour of the nail.
- Nail grooves: these are deep ridges underneath the sides of the nail along which the nail moves as it grows. They help to direct the nail along the nail bed.
- Hyponychium: this is the area of skin which rests directly underneath the free edge where the nail separates from the nail bed.

Nail growth

Here are some facts about nail growth.

- The average rate of nail growth is between 0.5 and 1.2 mm. per week. Toe nails grow much more slowly than finger nails and take between 12 and 18 months to replace themselves entirely.
- The nails are growing all the time but the rate slows down as you get older.
- If you are ill, your nails suffer just like your skin and hair. This is because your blood supply concentrates on those parts of your body which need restoring to good health. As you get better the state of your nails improves.
- If the skin around or underneath a nail becomes inflamed, the rate of growth of that nail speeds up.
- The nails of the long fingers grow faster than those of the thumbs and little fingers.

Nail disorders

Nail disorders do not create a problem for the therapist. The basic manicure procedures can be adapted for a variety of conditions and supported with appropriate home-care advice.

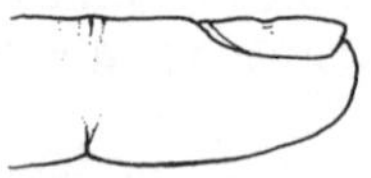

If the matrix is damaged through injury or impaired blood supply, the resulting nail is always malformed. Common illnesses such as flu temporarily affect the supply of blood to the matrix and, consequently, the nail-forming cells suffer. *Horizontal ridges* appear across every nail as the affected cells emerge from under the nail fold. Of course these cannot be seen until two or three weeks after the illness. As the general state of health improves, so does the health of the matrix and new normal cells replace the damaged ones, which eventually grow out. Clumsy manicure practices can also cause ridging of the nails when too much pressure is applied during the cuticle work.

Severe damage to the matrix is more serious. For example, trapping the finger in a car door, besides being extremely painful, can interfere with the arrangement of cells at the matrix. The injury can cause bleeding under the nail, which eventually turns black. If the bleeding is extensive, the nail may fall off or become permanently distorted.

A *blue-black* nail indicates bruising of the nail bed as a result of injury. Occasionally this can happen before losing the nail entirely.

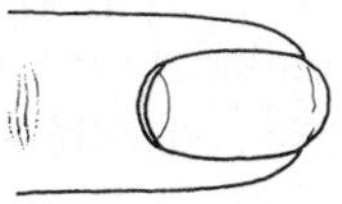

Fat and moisture keep the nails flexible and the layers of cells compacted into a smooth plate. They can be removed easily if the hands are not properly cared for, causing *dry, flaking nails (onychorrhexis)*. Detergents are designed to dissolve grease and they are just as effective on skin and nails as they are on dirty dishes and laundry! Dry, flaking nails and chapped skin are common complaints which particularly affect the busy housewife who does not make the time to protect and moisturise the hands between chores. Normally, the nails contain 18% of water. If this amount is increased greatly, for example after soaking, the nails become very soft. If the amount is considerably reduced, the nails become brittle.

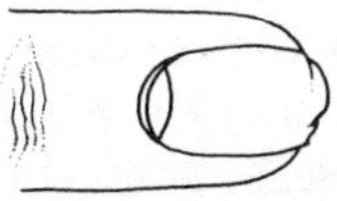

Splitting nails can be due to the repeated increase and decrease of water content, so that the nails change from soft to brittle frequently during the course of the day. Other external causes include injury, excessive use of solvents and detergents or careless filing of the nails. If the condition is accompanied by dry hair and skin, there may be a glandular disorder present. Ill health often causes the nails to become brittle. Dry cuticles lead to hangnails, where hardened pieces of skin split away from the sides of the nail and cuticle.

A few isolated *pits* or *dimples* in the nail are common and do not usually indicate a serious disorder. Deep pitting of the nails may be caused by psoriasis, in which case there is usually an accompanying skin condition.

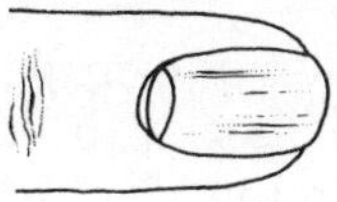

Vertical furrows or *grooves* may appear on the nail as the result of minor external injury. The furrows may split, allowing dirt to enter. As the new nail grows, healthy cells replace the damaged ones and the problem disappears.

The excessive use of nail hardeners containing formaldehyde can cause the nail plate to separate from the nail bed. Loose nails (*onycholysis*) can also accompany skin diseases such as psoriasis and eczema.

Some deeply pigmented nail varnishes produce yellow stains on the nails, particularly when worn without a base-coat. The stains are unsightly but harmless. Brown staining of the nails and surrounding skin is usually evident in heavy smokers.

White spots (*leuconychia*) occur, usually, as a result of minor injury which causes air to become trapped between the layers of cells. They are harmless and grow out eventually. White spots present on every nail can indicate a calcium deficiency, but this is very rare and not likely to be met in the beauty salon.

Spoon-shaped nails (koilonychia) are due to an accumulation of cells under the free edge. Some people are born with the condition but, for others, it can be a symptom of anaemia and when this is treated the nail condition disappears. Koilonychia sometimes occurs in people who have an over-active thyroid gland.

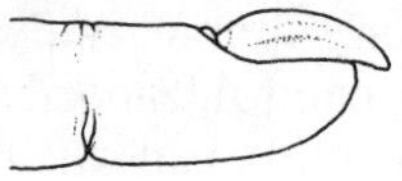

Very thick nails (onychauxis) usually accompany the ageing process, but they can be caused by an internal disorder.

Blue nails are associated with poor blood circulation. The fingers have a bluish tinge and the hands feel very cold. The nails do not actually turn blue, but they lack the healthy pink colour that would normally show through the nail plate.

Eggshell nails are thin, white and much more flexible than normal nails. In this condition, the nail plate separates easily from the nail bed and curves up at the free edge. Eggshell nails can be caused by chronic illness or nervous disorders.

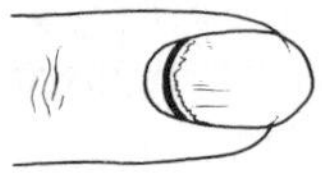

Pterygium is a condition where there is an excessive amount of cuticle growing over the nail plate. In extreme cases the nail plate is virtually covered in cuticle skin and has to be treated medically.

Nail diseases

> Remember
> The general signs of disease are inflammation, swelling and pus around and sometimes underneath the nail plate. Some conditions show a green, yellow or black discoloration of the nail, depending on the nature of the infection.

Nail diseases are conditions of the nail and surrounding skin which result from bacterial, fungal and viral infections. Nail diseases contra-indicate manicure. This means that a manicure must *not* be given. Besides the high risks of spreading the diseases by using tools and materials which have been in contact with them, the condition could be worsened by disturbing the infected area. The manicurist is also at risk through personal contact. A client with a diseased nail should be referred to a doctor for medical treatment.

It is unlikely that a client with a severe nail disease would keep an appointment for a manicure treatment, particularly where the symptoms are accompanied by pain. However, a therapist might recognise the initial signs of disease and advice resulting in prompt medical attention could save the client a lot of discomfort and inconvenience.

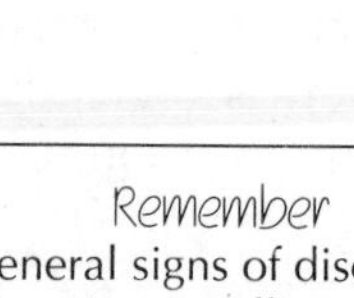

The main route for infection is through broken skin or damaged cuticle. *Paronychia*, the most common of all nail diseases, usually starts off as hangnail or following loss of cuticle from part or whole of the nail. Bacteria enter the 'live' tissue behind the nail fold and a swollen throbbing condition results with the formation of pus around the nail border. Housewives, cleaners, bar workers, chefs and hairdressers are particularly at risk, as their jobs require them to have their hands continuously in and out of water. These occupations have the highest incidence of *chronic* paronychia, an advanced form of the condition which involves infection by a fungus (vegetable parasite) as well as bacteria. The nail becomes discoloured as the fungus becomes embodied in the nail. The doctor will usually prescribe an anti-fungal ointment and antibiotics to clear the infection. The best way of preventing paronychia is to keep the hands dry and the cuticles soft and pliable.

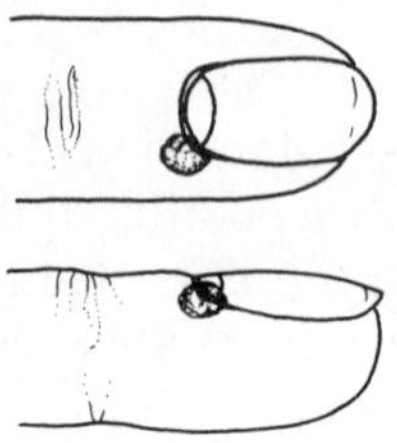

Ringworm of the nail (onychomycosis or tinea unguium) is another infection caused by a fungus. The most common form consists of whitish patches which can be scraped off the nail surface. Alternatively, yellow streaks appear in the nail substance. The disease invades the free edge and spreads down to the nail root. The nail plate becomes spongy and furrowed and is sometimes completely detached. Often, after medical treatment, the nail remains malformed.

Nail biting

Bitten nails are unsightly and, in extreme cases, can lead to permanent deformities. Unfortunately, people who bite their nails are usually so embarrassed about their habit they are reluctant to consider manicure treatments. They feel happier hiding their hands than seeking expert advice! In fact, there is much that can be done by a professional manicurist to improve the appearance of bitten nails and a client who can be persuaded to have regular manicure treatments will be far more encouraged to break the habit.

The main problems associated with nail biting result from chewing the cuticles and skin around the nails once the free edge has been destroyed. Recurrent attacks of bacterial infection around the nail are not uncommon, due to exposing the live skin of the nail walls and transferring bacteria from the teeth.

Three stages can be seen in the process:

- stage 1: finger tips appear bulbous due to the lack of a free edge. Soreness is probably present due to biting the nail plate away from the nail bed. The border of nail is rough as layers separate. 'Spicules' are created which tempt the next chewing session!
- stage 2: the cuticles have become involved. Constant friction has caused them to thicken and grow over what is left of the nail plate. Invariably, damage to the cuticle results in hangnails and paronychia.
- stage 3: warts are a frequent complication of nail biting. They are due to a virus and are, therefore, infectious. There are various forms of medical treatment depending on the severity of the condition. Very often it is the treatment of the warts which finally puts an end to the nail-biting habit.

Disturbance of the matrix cells over a prolonged period of nail biting can affect the formation of the replacement nail.

How manicures can help

Having bitten nails does not mean no nails. So long as there is some remnant of nail available, the therapist has a job to do! Professional manicures encourage the client by improving the appearance of the nails and by making them less easy to chew. This is achieved by:

- filing the nails into a regular shape and bevelling the split layers so that the edges become smoother
- softening, lifting and removing excess cuticle from the nail plate. (A warm oil treatment is particularly useful before doing this)
- buffing the nails which helps them to grow and gives them a healthy glow.

Many traditional home-care treatments for bitten nails involve some sort of punishment! These include:

- wearing brightly coloured enamel which looks ghastly once it has been bitten
- painting foul-tasting products on the nails which leave a strong, bitter taste in the mouth if the nails are chewed
- wearing cotton gloves, sitting on the hands or finding some absorbing manual activity to do at recognised peak chewing periods, for example when watching television.

Whatever your feelings about the reliability and practicality of these recommendations, there is no doubt that professional manicures produce immediate improvements which help to give hope to a client with a nail-biting problem.

You will have to be patient, and accept that it is going to take more than one treatment to convert your client. Educate, encourage and persevere!

Skin disorders affecting the hands

Many skin diseases involve the hands but some are more likely to appear there than on other parts of the body. This is mainly due to them being exposed and in contact with potentially harmful substances or other sources of infection through touch.

> Remember
> It is not just the nails which are examined before a manicure. The condition of the skin of the hands also influences the manicure procedure and the advice for home care.

> Remember
> An allergy to nail enamel affects the skin of the face. Advise against nail enamel if the client suffers from eczema of the face.

Eczema and dermatitis

Eczema and dermatitis are often referred to separately but have the same symptoms: both conditions start off with redness or duskiness of the skin. Small lumps appear which blister and form scales. There is usually intense itching.

Eczema (from a Greek word which means *to boil over* - you should already have a fairly good idea of what this disorder looks like!) is usually caused by factors inside the body or by an inherited or acquired instability of the skin. People suffering from eczema often suffer from asthma or hay fever as well. Dermatitis (also from a Greek word, and meaning inflammation (*-itis*) of the skin (*derma*) results from factors outside the body, for example contact allergies. An allergic dermatitis reaction usually shows up within 24 hours of contact with the offending substance.

Nail enamel is a common cause of allergic contact dermatitis, as are metals, cosmetics, hair dyes, deodorants, drugs and household materials.

Both these conditions should be treated by a doctor. The skin of the hands should be excluded from the manicure. Basic nail shaping, cuticle work and buffing is permissible. Nail enamel is not contra-indicated but it will draw attention to the hands. This is not always advisable for a client with eczema or dermatitis.

Warts

Warts occur commonly on the fingers, and less frequently on the palm of the hand. They are usually skin-coloured or a greyish brown, raised and with a rough surface which tends to itch. The centre of the wart is often depressed with a dark centre.

Warts are due to a virus and contra-indicate manicure treatment because they are contagious. Substances can be bought from the chemist which help to destroy the wart chemically. There are medical treatments for warts, but most of them tend to disappear spontaneously.

Whitlow

A whitlow is a bacterial infection of the soft pad at the tip of a finger or thumb. It is often confused with paronychia, which affects the skin around the base of the nail. There is a build up of pus which can not escape due to the thickness of the skin. As a result, intense pain occurs which reaches a peak after two or three days.

Manicure is contra-indicated due to the infection present. Treatment is medical and usually involves lancing the swelling and prescribing a course of antibiotics.

Rheumatism and arthritis

Rheumatism is a general term for pain, with or without stiffness, which affects the muscles and joints. It describes a symptom of a disorder rather than being a disorder itself. Rheumatism covers many conditions including arthritis.

Arthritis is a general term for inflammation of a joint. The condition can follow injury or bacterial infection but, more commonly, it results from the wear and tear of ageing. The joint swells, stiffens and becomes painful. The overlying skin takes on a red, shiny appearance. In severe cases, the whole hand appears deformed.

Great care is required when massaging the hands of a client with arthritis. Joints which are inflamed must not be over-stimulated.

Examining the hands and nails: Multiple choice quiz

1 Nails receive nourishment from the:
a) matrix
b) blood supply
c) keratin
d) nail bed.

2 The cuticle must be kept pliable so that it does not:
a) bleed
b) grow too thick
c) split
d) look untidy.

3 Keratin is a:
a) mineral
b) blood vessel
c) disorder
d) protein.

4 Keratin makes the nails
a) hard
b) soft
c) flexible
d) pink.

5 Permanent damage may result from injury to the:
a) free edge
b) nail fold
c) cuticle
d) matrix.

6 The cuticle protects the:
a) nail
b) hyponychium
c) matrix
d) lunula.

7 The free edge is a different colour from the rest of the nail because it:
a) contains more keratin
b) does not lie over blood vessels
c) gets damaged more easily
d) does not lie over the matrix.

8 The function of nail grooves is to:
a) guide the nail
b) strengthen the nail
c) protect the nail
d) straighten the nail.

Examining the hands and nails: Self-checks

1 Can you explain why:
a) An illness like 'flu can cause ridges in the nails?
b) Detergents cause the nails to flake?
c) The nails might be discoloured?
d) A whitlow is painful?
e) White spots in the nail usually disappear?
f) Diseases should not be treated in the salon?
g) Manicures are good for bitten nails?
h) A doctor may prescribe antibiotics for treating a disease of the skin or nails?
i) Special care is required when giving a manicure to a client with arthritis in the hands?
j) Warts on the fingers spread easily?

2 Answer *true* or *false* to each of the following statements:
a) The nails get thicker with the ageing process.
b) Toe nails grow faster than finger nails.
c) A young person's nails grow faster than an elderly person's.
d) Nail disorders can be treated by a beauty therapist.
e) Horizontal ridges in the nail usually grow out.
f) If swelling is present, a manicure may be given, but great care must be taken.
g) Ringworm of the nail is caused by a fungus.
h) People with asthma often suffer from eczema as well.

Examining the hands and nails: Activities

1 Role play: with a partner acting as a client, make an examination of the hands and nails. Make sure that they are clean and that you are working in good light.

Comment on the general condition of the skin and nails and then on specific disorders which may be present. Identify the conditions by name, explain the cause and describe the symptoms.

Write down your findings and then ask a supervisor to confirm that you are right.

Provide advice on home care, explaining the specific benefits to the client

2 Study the diagrams of the nail. Learn the functions of the various parts.
a) Without cheating, see if you can draw identical, accurately labelled diagrams. The larger your diagrams, the neater they will be. Check your diagrams against the originals.

b) Ask a partner to test your knowledge of the structures of the nail. They should ask you about their locations and functions.

3 Make out a revision chart to help you learn the diseases and disorders of the nails and hands.

List the conditions down one side and make columns for:

- appearance
- cause/s
- manicure indicated/contra-indicated
- salon treatment
- special care.

Pick out the key points from the information that has been provided. Remember, the chart is for quick reference.

Design your chart so that there is enough space to fit all the information. Study the chapter closely before deciding on the exact layout of the chart.

Chapter 9

Manicure and hand treatments

After working through this chapter you will be able to:

- prepare the equipment and materials for a manicure
- state the purpose of each item of equipment
- maintain equipment safely and hygienically
- describe the contents of manicure preparations and their uses
- provide a manicure treatment
- understand hand and arm massage techniques
- provide special treatments for the hands and nails
- explain the effects of treatments for the hands and nails
- give advice on home care.

Preparing for manicure

The preparation of tools and equipment does not begin minutes before the manicure is due to start. The cleaning and tidying procedures which conclude one treatment actually help towards preparing the next.

Tools which have been cleaned, sterilised and stored hygienically can be used safely, even at a moment's notice, to treat an unexpected client.

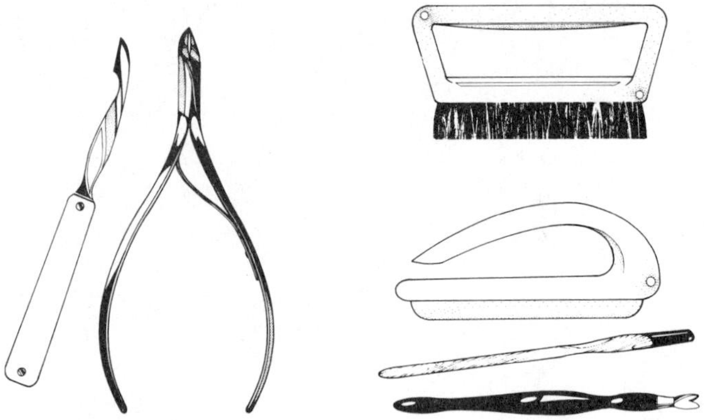

Tools and equipment

You will need the following:

- nail scissors: the lightweight, curved blades adapt to the convex shape of the nails. They cut the nails without weakening them. Nail scissors are used for removing excessive length before the nails are shaped with an emery board
- emery boards: professional emery boards are long, strong and flexible with a coarse side for reducing the length of strong nails and a fine side used for achieving the final shape and smoothing the free edge

> Remember
>
> Emery boards and orange sticks are made of fibrous materials which are absorbent. There is no effective way of cleaning and sterilising them. It is best to offer these items to the client for home use after the treatment.

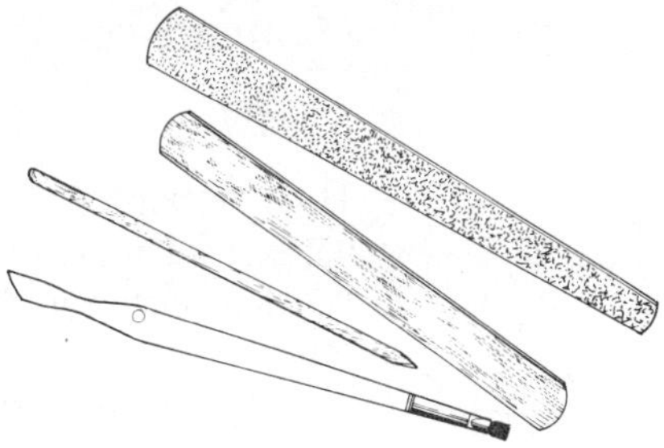

- orange sticks: the bevelled end is used for pushing back pre-softened cuticles and, also, for transferring small amounts of cream from pots. The pointed end is always used tipped with cotton wool for cleaning around the nail border, the cuticles and under the free edge
- cuticle knife: the straight cutting edge of the knife is sharp and must be used with great care when scraping away eponychium from the surface of the nail plate
- cuticle nippers: the small pointed blades are used to trim away excessive cuticle in one continuous piece. The nippers are also used to remove hangnails
- nail brush: this is used to remove all traces of treatment preparations from the nails and cuticles after soaking
- spatula: used for transferring hand cream from the jar for massage
- buffer: covered with chamois leather, it spreads paste polish over the nails and buffs them up to create a sheen.

> *Remember*
> It is not enough to clean and sterilise tools after use. They must be stored hygienically to avoid contamination.

Good quality tools will last a long time if you look after them properly:

- use the tools only for their professional purpose
- apply lubricating oil regularly to the screws and hinges of cutting tools
- store cuticle nippers with the spring released
- regularly check the blades of cutting tools and have them sharpened professionally
- store cutting tools in an ultra-violet cabinet or in a clean case wrapped in tissue with the blades well protected.

> *Remember*
> Scratched or damaged blades can not be cleaned and sterilised effectively. Do not risk spreading germs by using tools in poor condition.
> Stiff or broken hinged tools do not have a smooth action. They are more difficult to control and are likely to cause damage.

Other general items which you will need for manicures and hand treatments are:

- disinfectant: kept in a small jar for soaking the cutting edge of metal tools during the treatment procedure
- tissues: tools which are not kept in disinfectant are wrapped in or laid on clean tissue until required
- cotton wool: used for tipping orange sticks and applying liquid preparations to the hands and nails
- towels: for protecting the immediate treatment area and drying the hands
- three bowls: one lined with a tissue for the client's jewellery, one for waste and one for the soaking water. The bowl of soaking water is the last item to be prepared before the manicure: a small amount of liquid soap is added to very hot water, so that by the time it is needed the solution has cooled to a comfortable temperature for the client
- manicure cushion: to support the client's hands between the various stages off treatment. Alternatively, a towel can be folded in to a roll for the same purpose
- surgical spirit: for cleansing the hands and cleaning equipment.

> *Remember*
> For hygiene reasons you must give each client a clean towel. Do not dry your own hands on the client's towel.

Manicure products

Nail enamel remover

This contains a solvent which dissolves the enamel so that it may be wiped off the nail plate. Acetone is the most frequently used solvent but it has a very drying effect which can cause the layers of the nail to separate. For this reason, a small amount of oil or glycerol is usually included in the formulation. Acetone-free removers, which are less harsh on the nails, have become popular. They contain solvents such as ethyl, amyl and butyl acetates and toluene.

> Remember
> Why nail enamel thickens: some evaporation of solvent takes place every time the top is removed from the nail enamel bottle. The same processes which cause the enamel to thicken and dry on the nails also occur in the bottle if the top is left off or not tightened sufficiently after use. If enamel is allowed to build up around the neck of the bottle this prevents a good seal with the top and thickening occurs. Nail enamel also thickens if it is stored in a warm room or in direct sunlight.

Nail enamel thinners

Ethyl acetate is one example of a solvent used to thin down nail enamel which has thickened. A few drops of thinners is added to the enamel at least twenty minutes before the manicure to ensure that it dissolves evenly in time for application. Nail enamel removers are not suitable as thinning agents as their oil content causes the enamel to separate and discolour.

Cuticle cream

Cuticle cream is used to make the cuticle pliable so that it can be pushed back and lifted without causing damage or discomfort. White soft paraffin, lanolin and mineral oil are examples of emollients contained in cuticle cream to soften the skin. Dry, flaking nails also benefit from the softening and lubricating effects of cuticle cream.

Cuticle remover

Potassium hydroxide is alkaline and caustic (burning). In cuticle remover it is combined with water to produce a milky consistency, and glycerol, which is a humectant. Cuticle remover works by breaking down the eponychium so that it can be scraped away gently from the nail plate with a cuticle knife. It can also be used as a nail bleach. Cuticle remover makes the skin dry, sore and irritated if left in contact for too long. Make sure the skin and nails are rinsed well after it has been used.

Buffing paste

Buffing paste is used to smooth out ridges on the nail plate and helps to remove surface stains. Buffing the nails with paste creates a natural looking polished effect which is sometimes preferred to coloured nail enamel. An abrasive ingredient such as stannic oxide is included in the formulation. Other abrasive ingredients which are sometimes used are talc, silica, kaolin and chalk.

Nail enamels: base-coats, top-coats and coloured enamels

These products share the same basic formula: a *film-forming plastic* such as nitrocellulose, a plastic resin such as aryl sulphonamide, formaldehyde to give gloss, a *plasticiser*, usually castor oil, to give flexibility to the plastic film and help prevent the enamel from cracking and a mixture of *solvents* which dissolves all the other ingredients and evaporates so that the enamel dries on the nail. The most commonly used solvents are ethyl acetate, butyl acetate, amyl acetate, toluene and alcohol. Pigments provide colour and a pearlised effect is achieved by the addition of an ingredient such as guanine or bismuth oxychloride.

Base-coat is applied before coloured nail enamel to prevent staining of the nail plate and, also, to provide a smooth adherent surface for the nail enamel. Special ridge-filler base coats are available.

Top-coat seals and protects the coloured nail enamel. It helps to harden the surface of cream textured nail enamels so that they are more resilient to knocks. The extra ingredient contained in pearlised enamels has a similar effect so a top-coat is not required.

Hand cream

As well as making the skin feel soft and smell nice, hand cream provides slip for the massage: this means that the therapist's hands glide smoothly over the skin without causing friction and discomfort. A typical formulation combines an emollient such as lanolin or glycerol with water, emulsifiers, colour and perfume.

Hand lotion

Hand lotion contains the same basic ingredients as hand cream but with a higher percentage of water. Pump dispensers are available which prevent contamination of the lotion and minimise wastage during use. Hand lotion spreads easily and does not leave a sticky film on the skin as some creams do.

The following items are extras which may be required for individual clients.

Nail bleach

Buffing paste and cuticle remover have mild bleaching effects but it is useful to have a small supply of 20 volume hydrogen peroxide available to work on more stubborn stains, for example those caused by nicotine.

Nail hardener

This can be used on fragile nails which have a tendency to split It is painted on and allowed to soak into the nail. The active ingredient is usually aluminium potassium sulphate (alum) or zirconium chloride.

Nail strengthener

Powder acrylic nail hardeners are mixed to a paste with liquid plastic to produce a coating which sets and reinforces the nail.

Nail white pencil

This special pencil contains titanium dioxide to help whiten a free edge which has become discoloured. It is moistened before applying to the under side of the nail tip.

Nail repair kit

This consists of fibrous tissue and a special adhesive which are used to bond and strengthen a split in the nail. Acrylic strengtheners are also available which are applied directly to the split and harden when in contact with air.

Quick dry spray

This solvent based preparation is used to speed up the rate at which the enamel dries on the nail. It is much better for nail enamel to be allowed to dry naturally but, in emergencies, it is useful to have this product available.

> Remember
> Keep your tools, equipment and materials in good order so that you do not have to hunt for them during the treatment.

Some salons have portable manicure trolleys or baskets which contain all the necessary products and equipment. These help to save time when setting up a treatment and take up very little storage space, but because they have shared use, assumptions can be made that they are adequately stocked and equipped and that they have been left clean and tidy. You are advised never to assume! Always make time before the treatment to make sure that everything is prepared so that no time is wasted once the client arrives.

Preparing for manicure: Multiple choice quiz

1 Nail scissors have curved blades so that:
- a) the nails can be shaped to an oval
- b) there is less risk of cutting the skin
- c) the nails can be shaped before filing
- d) the nails are not weakened when cutting them.

2 A cuticle knife is used for:
- a) cutting off excess cuticle
- b) scraping away eponychium
- c) preventing the build up of perionychium
- d) preventing the formation of eponychium.

3 The manicure equipment should be kept tidy to:
- a) impress the client
- b) prevent the spread of infection
- c) prevent wasting time
- d) avoid losing equipment.

4 Oil is contained in nail enamel remover to:
- a) counteract the drying effect of the solvent
- b) dissolve the nail enamel
- c) improve the texture of the nail enamel remover
- d) soften the nails.

5 Emery boards should not be used for more than one client because they:
- a) wear out quickly
- b) spread disease
- c) cannot be kept hygienically
- d) are discarded after use.

6 The main purpose of a base coat is to:
- a) prevent the nail enamel from peeling
- b) prevent the enamel from staining the nails
- c) keep moisture in the nails
- d) strengthen the nails.

7 Plasticiser affects the texture of nail enamel by giving it:
- a) flexibility
- b) a high gloss effect
- c) a pearlised effect
- d) strength.

8 The caustic ingredient of cuticle remover is:
- a) acetone
- b) bismuth oxychloride
- c) glycerol
- d) potassium hydroxide.

9 The effect of an emollient is:
a) drying
b) softening
c) soothing
d) cleansing.

10 One example of an emollient contained in manicure preparations is:
a) kaolin
b) lanolin
c) nitrocellulose
d) acetone.

Preparing for manicure: Self-checks

1 Which items of manicure equipment are suitable for sterilisation in an autoclave?

2 How should orange sticks and emery boards be stored before use?

3 What special care is required to keep cutting tools in good working order?

4 Why is disinfectant required for the manicure?

5 How can the thickening of nail enamel be prevented during storage?

Preparing for manicure: Activities

1 Visit a wholesaler and study the full range of manicure products and equipment available. Find out if any new products have come on the market. Try to compare the quality of different ranges of tools. See if you can tell the difference between cheaper and more expensive ones.

Take away product information leaflets and price lists to keep safely in a file for future reference.

2 Check the nail enamels in your salon: test the texture of the enamel enamels which have been opened. Thin them down with solvent if necessary.

Check that the necks of the bottles are clean before replacing the caps. The cotton wool should be saturated with solvent before use so that dry fibres do not get into the enamel. Wear rubber gloves for doing this job.

Manicure procedure

'Are you sitting comfortably?' This is probably the first question you will ask your client at the beginning of the manicure and it is just as important that you can answer 'yes' as well. The effects of bad posture get worse over the course of a working day, causing premature fatigue and aches and pains. Slouching strains the back, neck and shoulders and restricts proper breathing, reducing the oxygen supply to the body. The following checklist will ensure comfort for both you and your client:

- the client and the therapist should be positioned close enough to avoid stretching and straining the arms during the manicure.
- sit upright with back straight and shoulders relaxed
- your seating should be firm and at the correct height
- sit with your legs together and not crossed
- make sure you work in good light to avoid 'peering' over the client's hands.

> *Remember*
> Place jewellery in a bowl where it can be seen to be safe by the client.

1 Ensure that the client's hands and arms are free from clothing and jewellery.

2 Wash and dry your own hands, preferably where the client can see you. Evidence of good hygiene practice is always reassuring for a client and shows that you are working to professional standards.

3 Examine the hands and nails. If nail enamel is being worn it will have to be removed before you can make an accurate assessment. While you are checking that there are no contra-indications, note any conditions which may need special attention during the manicure. If there are signs of neglect they will need discussing with the client and advice given regarding their home care.

> *Remember*
> It takes at least twenty minutes for nail enamel thinners to be effective. If the enamel is too thick, add two or three drops of thinners, secure the cap and roll the bottle between your hands. Do not shake the bottle as this fills the cap with enamel and floods the cuticles during application.

4 Explain the purposes of the manicure relative to the condition of the client's hands and nails. If the client wishes to wear enamel, establish which one she requires and check that the texture is suitable for application.

5 Wipe over both sides of the hands with surgical spirit on a cotton wool pad. This cleans the hands without softening the nails before filing. Surgical spirit, unlike many other liquid antiseptics, is an antiseptic that is tolerated by most skins.

6 Establish whether the client is left- or right-handed: proceed on the opposite hand. This ensures that the hand which suffers the most wear and tear has a longer soaking period which benefits the nails, skin and cuticles.

> *Remember*
> Do not rub the nail with the cotton wool pad and remover, or the nail enamel colour may spread over the surrounding skin. This will need treating with more nail enamel remover, which is bad for the skin and takes up time during the manicure.

7 Apply nail enamel remover with a cotton wool pad held between your index finger and middle finger. Press the pad firmly onto the nail for a couple of seconds then slide it off the nail, squeezing gently against the nail plate to remove all traces of dissolved enamel.

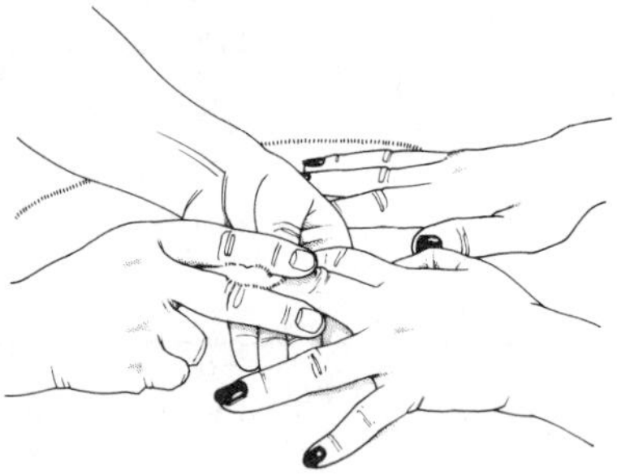

> *Remember*
> Do not cut down the sides of the nails as this will weaken the bridge and the nail may snap off or split.

8 Pull back the nail walls gently from the sides of the nail plate to expose any enamel which might otherwise be hidden. Use a tipped orange stick and nail enamel remover around the nail border so that the nails are left absolutely clean.

> *Remember*
> There is no point in buffing at this stage of the manicure if buffing with paste is required as an alternative to nail enamel later. Make sure you know exactly what the client wants before you start the treatment.

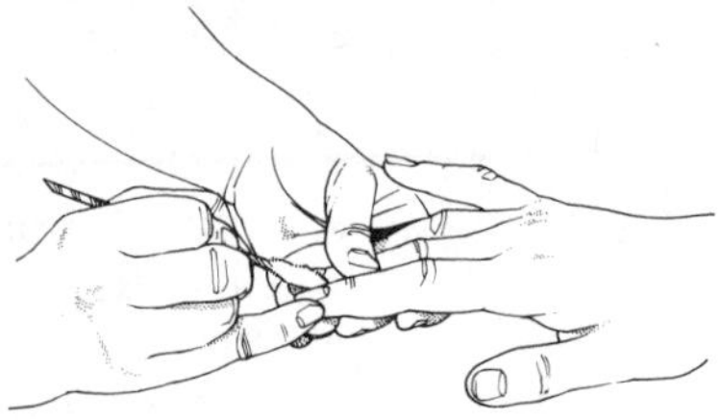

9 Nails which are excessively long may need cutting before filing. Apply a little pressure from above with your thumb when using the scissors. This helps to give support and minimises disturbance at the base of the nail. Cut across the free edge of the nail, leaving the nail slightly longer than the desired length.

10 Working on the first hand, file the nails from sides to centre towards the nail tip. Hold the emery board as near to the end as possible. This produces long flowing strokes and gives the nails a smooth edge. Never use a two-way sawing action with the emery board. This creates heat which dries out some of the moisture within the nail and causes the layers to separate.

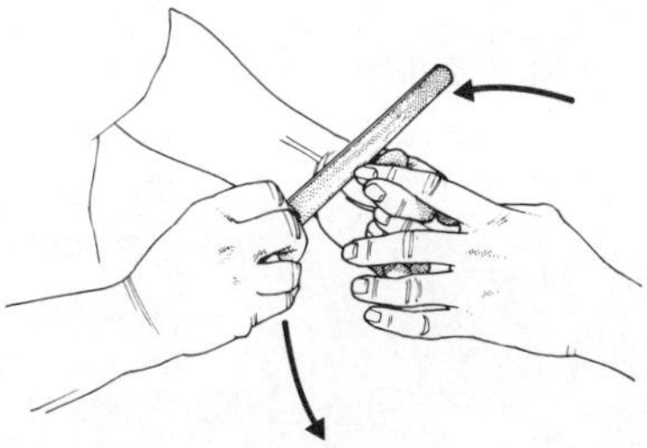

11 Buffing can be done after filing, without paste polish to stimulate the blood supply to the nail bed, or with paste polish to help smoothen the nail for a later application of nail enamel. Use the buffer briskly but lightly, applying approximately 15-20 strokes per nail in one direction only, towards the free edge.

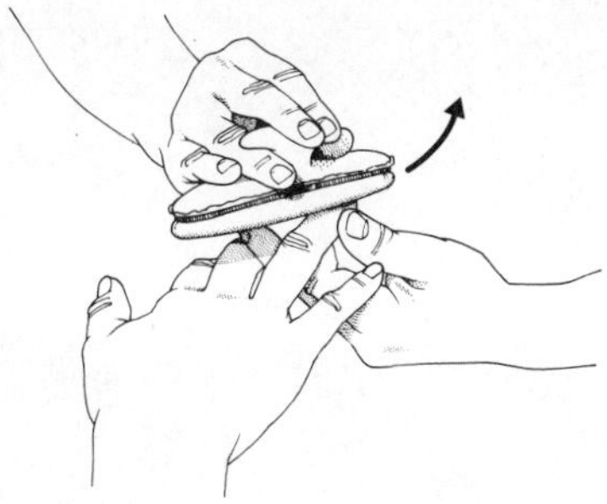

12 Use the blunt end of an orange stick to transfer a little cuticle cream to the client's nails. Massage the cream well into the cuticles.

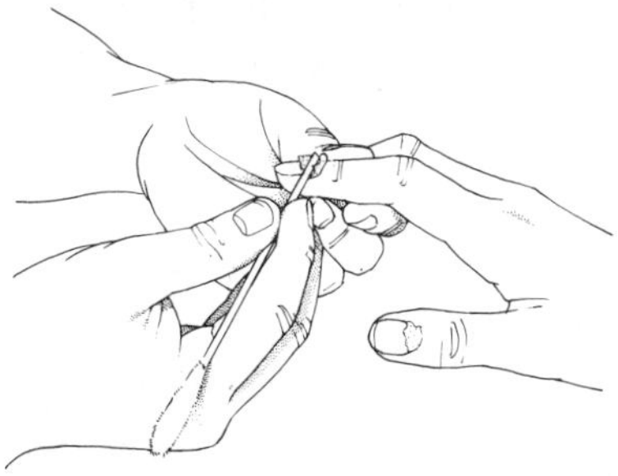

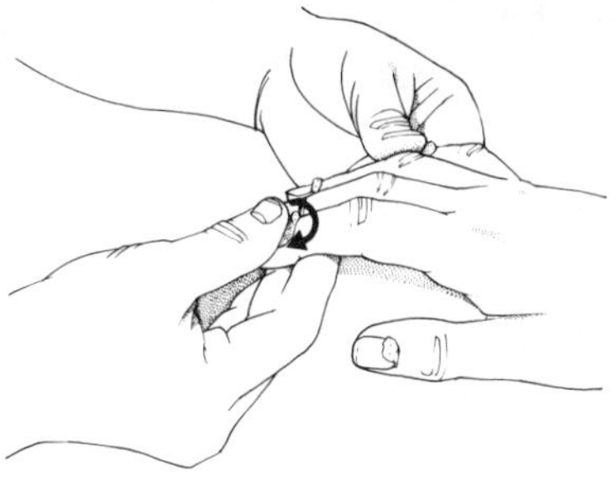

Remember
If you apply too much pressure when working on the cuticles at the base of the nail, you may disturb activity at the matrix. This shows up as ridges in the nail as the damaged cells grow along the nail bed.

> Remember
> Cuticle remover has a bleaching effect which helps to whiten the free edge.

13 Soak the fingers in the prepared soapy water and repeat the filing and cuticle massage on the second hand. Dry the first hand thoroughly and put the second hand in to soak.

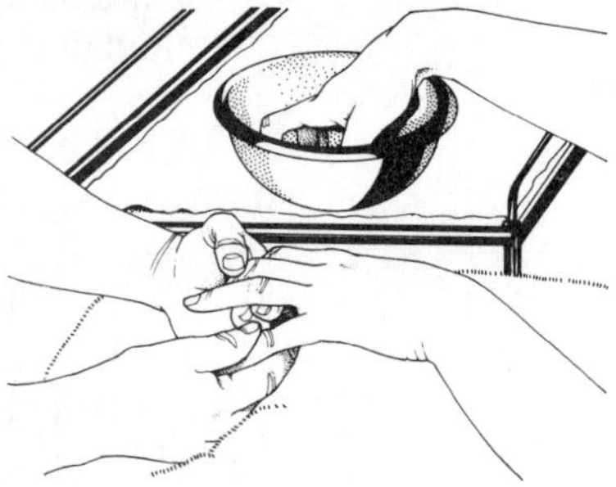

> Remember
> Never angle the knife so that the cutting edge is vertical. The blade may not look sharp; but it can penetrate the nail if not used carefully.

14 Apply cuticle remover with the pointed end of an orange stick tipped with cotton wool. With the flat side of the stick resting on the nail plate, gently push back the cuticles, working around the nail border with small, circular movements.

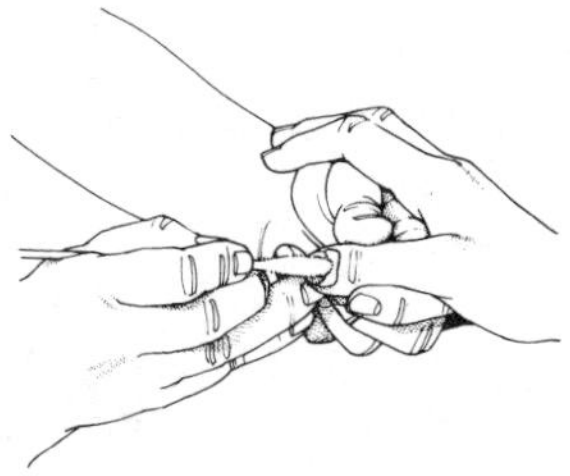

15 Gently lift and clean under the cuticles with the tipped end of the orange stick and cuticle remover. Use the same stick to clean under the free edge.

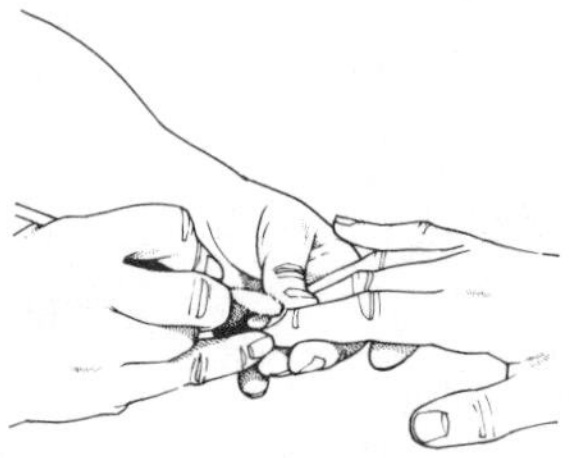

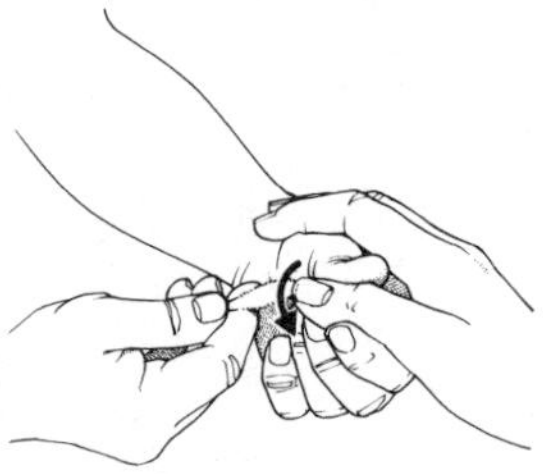

16 Use the cuticle knife gently to loosen eponychium from the nail plate. The blade should be used wet and kept as flat to the nail surface as possible to avoid scratching it. Work round the nail border with small circular movements, keeping the cutting edge facing towards the main body of the nail.

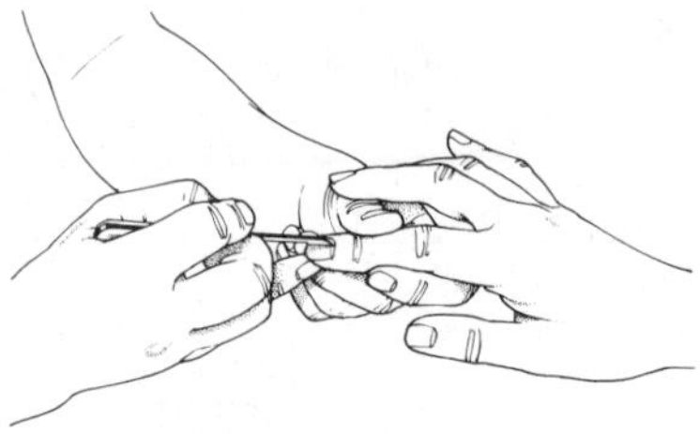

17 Take the other hand out of soak and dry it thoroughly. Rinse the nails of the first hand and scrub them to remove all traces of debris and cuticle remover. Dry the nails, pushing the cuticles back gently with the towel. Repeat steps 14-17 on the second hand.

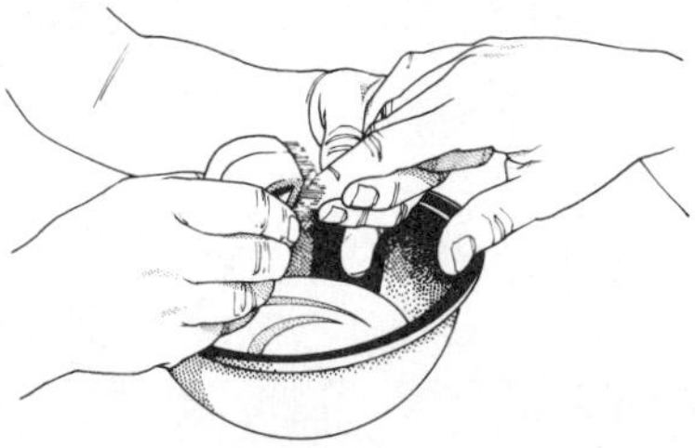

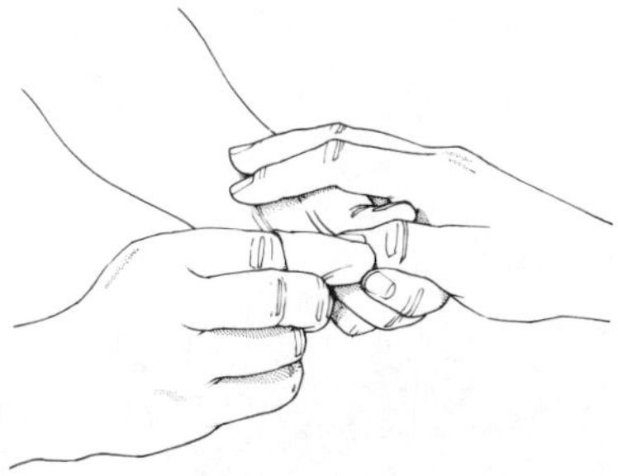

18 Use the cuticle nippers to remove any excessive or damaged cuticle. Place the pointed end of the nippers slightly under the lifted cuticle. Squeeze the blades together to ensure a clean cut is made before releasing the blades and moving further along the cuticle. Do not pull the nippers away without releasing the blades or the cuticle will tear back to the live skin and bleed. Apart from being painful, this would provide a route for infection.

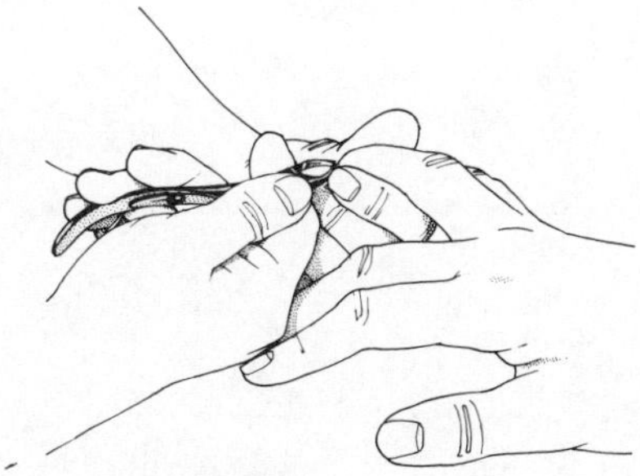

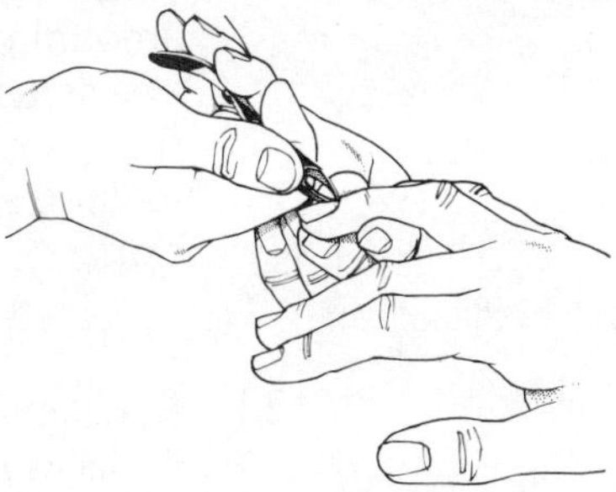

19 Use the smooth side of the emery board to remove any roughness which may have developed around the free edges of the nails.

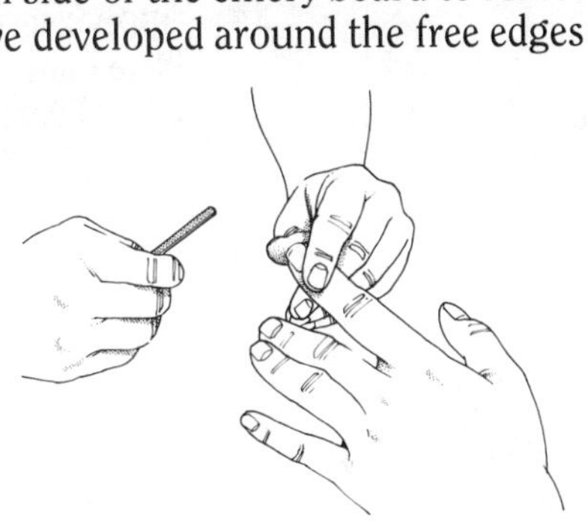

20 Apply either hand cream or lotion to the hand and forearm and proceed with the massage. Re-apply lotion or cream as necessary during the massage to prevent friction. See page 00 for the massage sequence.

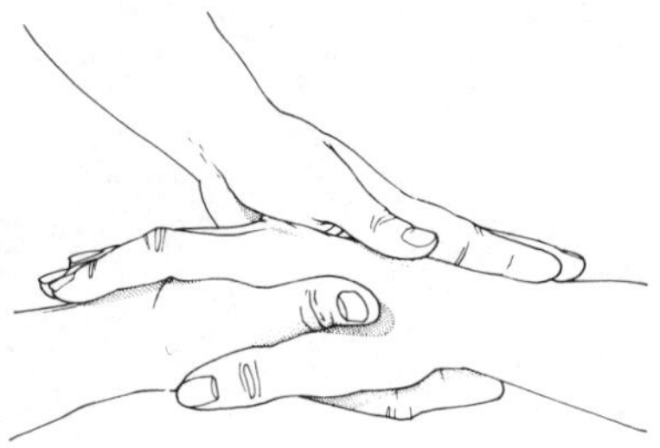

21 The massage leaves a film of grease on the nails which must be removed before the next stage of the manicure. Wipe over the nails with nail enamel remover on a cotton wool pad. Nail enamel will not adhere to the nails if grease is present.

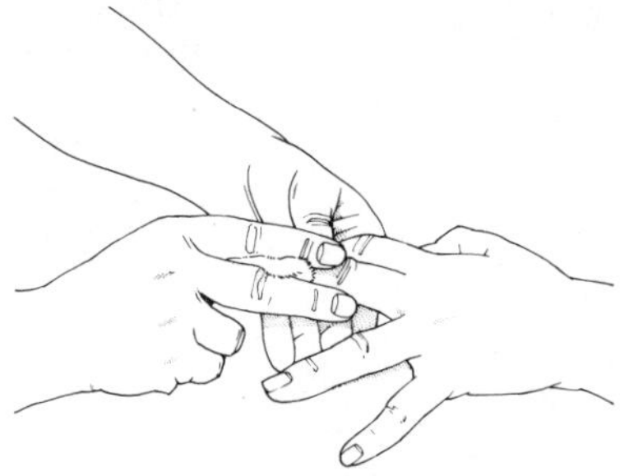

22 If buffing is required as an alternative to nail enamel, apply a tiny amount of paste to the centre of each nail with an orange stick and smooth it towards the free edge with the pad of the ring finger or thumb. Buff the nails until you have created a healthy looking shine. Take care not to spread paste over the surrounding skin.

23 If nail enamel is going to be applied, make sure that the client replaces jewellery beforehand to prevent smudging.

24 Applying nail enamel is very skilled and needs practice. Apply a base coat, then two coats of a coloured enamel and then a top coat. Pearlised enamels do not require a top coat.

> Remember
> You must be able to produce a smooth even finish to the enamel which covers the nail plate without touching the cuticle.

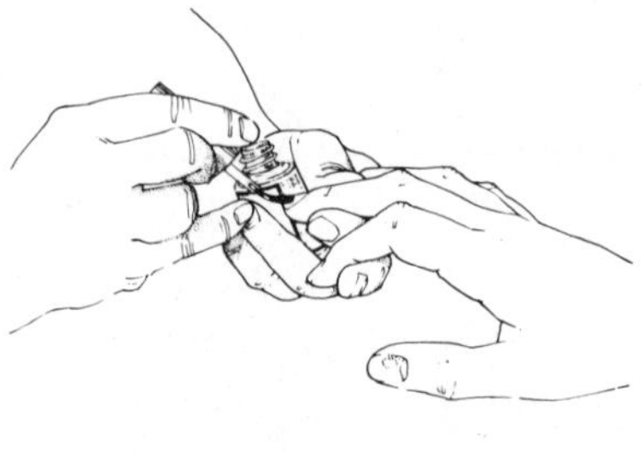

> Remember
>
> Method 1 ensures a smooth edge up to the cuticle. Method 2 is more suitable for narrow nails.

> Remember
>
> The nails are curved so it may be necessary to turn the fingers slightly in either direction to ensure full coverage by the enamel.

Practise using no more than four strokes for each nail to avoid 'over working' the enamel and causing streaks where wet enamel is applied over enamel that has started to dry.

Method 1 *Method 2*

25 Following the application of each coat, lightly touch the tip of the thumb nail to test whether the enamel has dried. It is important to allow each coat to dry before applying another, otherwise the enamel smudges easily and the effect of the treatment is spoiled.

26 While the nails are drying, advise the client about products which may be purchased from the salon for home use.

Record details of the client's treatment and purchases and escort them away from the area.

Manicure procedure: Self-checks

1. State three ways of avoiding backache when giving a manicure treatment.
2. Give three reasons for examining the client's hands before a manicure.
3. Why should the nail enamel colour be chosen at the beginning of the manicure?
4. Why is the orange stick used tipped with cotton wool?
5. How does buffing the nails *without* past polish benefit the nails?
6. Why is cuticle cream used *before* cuticle remover in the massage sequence?
7. State two precautions which should be taken to avoid scratching the nail plate with the cuticle knife.
8. Give three examples of damage which can occur by using incorrect manicure techniques.
9. How should the nails be prepared for nail enamel after the hand massage?
10. Why is it important to apply nail enamel with the minimum number of strokes?

Manicure procedure: Activities

1. Work on building up your speed, using the emery board in the correct way.

   Find as many volunteers as you can to let you practise. Keep a check on the nail shapes and ask for your 'client's' comments regarding the final result.

2 Practise buffing the nails quickly without 'bashing' the nail plate. Lightweight strokes are required which will not hurt the client or damage the nail bed.

3 Male manicures: in a small group or with a partner, consider how the basic manicure techniques should be adapted for treating a man.

Discuss the reasons for the differences and then - find a man to practise on!

Structure of the hand

The hand has a very intricate structure which influences the way the massage is performed. The basic movements are adapted according to the size, shape and position of the underlying tissues. This ensures that maximum benefits are achieved from the massage.

A closer look at the structure of the hand helps us to understand the effects of the massage. Starting from the top, the skin is made up of three main layers:

- the epidermis: the outer, protective covering of the body. The cells at the base of this layer are living. They gradually move up to the surface and die
- the dermis: a deeper, fibrous, supportive layer. Made up of different types of protein fibres, this layer contains blood vessels, nerves, hair follicles, sebaceous glands and sweat glands.
- beneath the dermis is a subcutaneous (adipose) layer which stores fat (see page 67).

The uppermost layer of the epidermis is called the *stratum corneum*. It is made up of dead cells containing the protein *keratin*. The role of the stratum corneum is to protect the deeper living layers of the skin. It is thickest on the palms of the hands and the soles of the feet where extra protection is required against friction.

Some jobs, such as gardening, cause dirt to become ingrained deep into the stratum corneum. Even after scrubbing, the evidence remains trapped between the cells for several days until they are finally shed.

It is important to keep the epidermis soft and flexible so that it does not crack and allow germs to enter. Sebum and sweat combine on the surface to lubricate the skin and make it supple. They also help to keep the skin in a slightly acid state which prevents harmful bacteria from penetrating the skin.

The deeper layers of the epidermis contain the skin's natural moisture which bathes the living cells and helps to keep the skin soft. Sebum provides an almost waterproof coating which helps to stop natural moisture from escaping.

The skin of the palm of the hand is thick, ridged, and has no hair or sebaceous glands. It does, however, have more sweat glands than many other areas of the body.

Supply of blood to the hand and forearm

> Remember
> Muscles and bones also need a good supply of blood to remain healthy.

The arteries carry blood, which contains oxygen bound to a chemical called *haemoglobin*. Living cells need oxygen. Blood containing oxygen is bright red: when the skin is given a stimulating massage, the walls of the arteries expand and become nearer the surface of the skin, so that it appears pink.

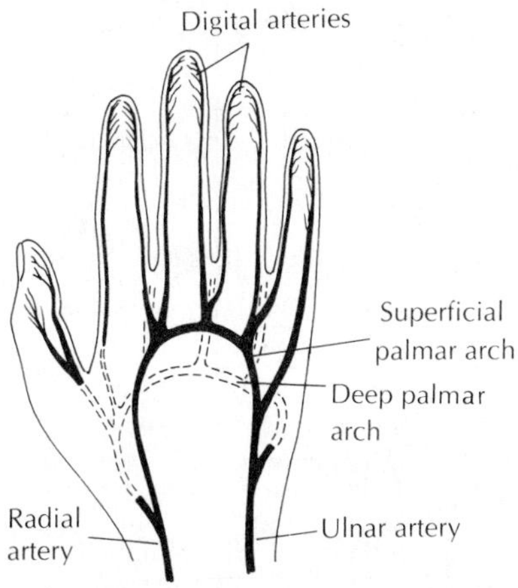

Blood supply to the hand

Blood which has had its oxygen removed by cells is bluish in colour and is returned into the system by veins. (Sometimes main veins can be seen quite prominently on the backs of hands of people with pale skin.) Blood also carries the breakdown products of digestion. The food we eat is converted into nutrients which living cells use to keep them healthy.

When the cells have taken up oxygen from the blood and used the nutrients they need, they create waste products which are taken away in the veins with carbon dioxide. Carbon dioxide is later converted into oxygen. Picture

Capillaries form a branched network of tiny thin-walled vessels which link the arteries, tissues and veins and circulate blood around the body.

Muscles

The power behind joint movements is supplied by the muscles. Muscles are most powerful at the point of their insertion, i.e. where they are attached to bones. Movements occur as a result of a muscle contracting. Muscles which bend the parts they are attached to are called *flexors*; muscles which straighten the parts they are attached to are called *extensors*. *Abductor* muscles pull parts away from the centre of the body; *adductor* muscles pull parts towards the centre of the body.

Muscles work in pairs to produce movements at joints. The following diagram identifies the muscles by their actions. Muscles are made up of fibres and always pull in the direction of the muscle fibres.

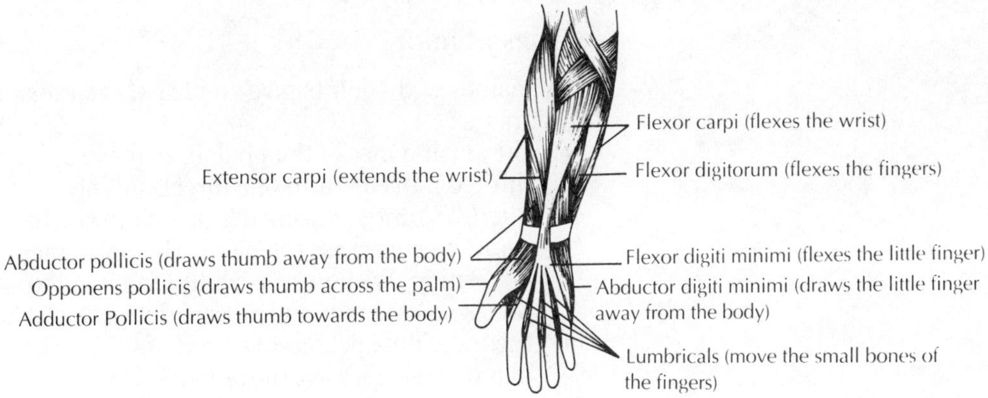

Muscles of the hand

Bones

The *radius* and *ulna* are the long bones of the forearm. The ulna is situated on the little finger side of the arm. There are eight *carpal* bones in the wrist arranged in two rows. The five long bones in the hand are the *metacarpals*. They are different lengths and each one moves with one of the five *digits* (fingers and thumbs). The thumb is the most specialised digit and contributes most to the hand's dexterity.

Fourteen small bones make up the digits. There are three in each finger and two in each thumb. These bones are called *phalanxes*.

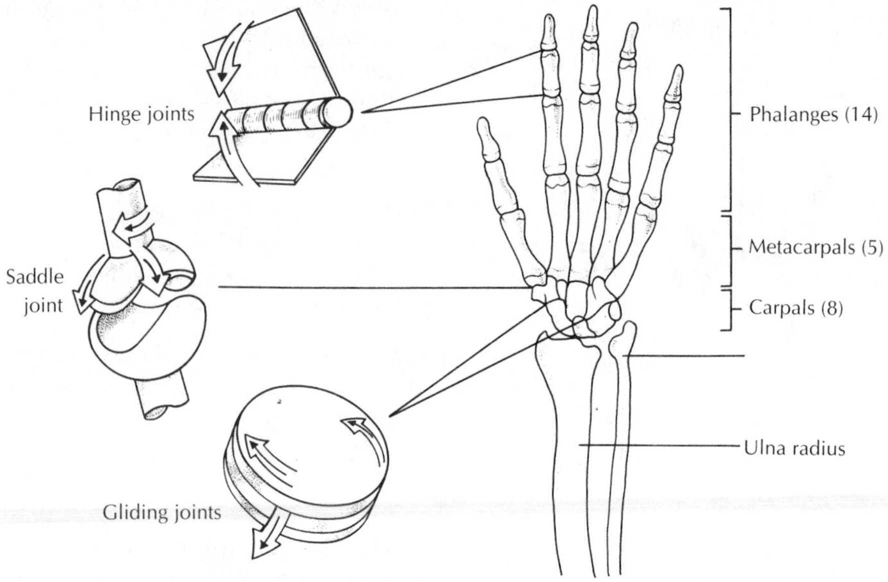

Bones of the hand

Wherever two bones come into contact there is movement between them at *joints*. Bones are bound by *ligaments*, which limit their movement and prevent dislocation.

Joints

Joints make up the main 'engineering' of the hand. Muscles and bones work together to produce a variety of movements which make everyday activities possible.

Types of joint

The names of the joints give an idea of the range of movement which occurs there:

- the small bones of the phalanxes move at *hinge* joints. There is limited movement in one direction only.
- a *saddle* joint connects the thumb to the hand and allows it to rotate freely across the palm. This movement is known as opposition. Without this ability the hand would be just a claw. Its precise movement and powerful grip would be severely limited.
- the individual pebble-like bones of the wrist *glide* over one another in a mainly sideways movement.

Structure of the hand: Multiple choice quiz

1 The function of the epidermis is to:
a) water proof
b) support
c) protect
d) cover.

2 Dry chapped skin is lacking:
a) sweat
b) moisture
c) sebum
d) blood.

3 Muscles pull in the direction of the:
a) fibres
b) bones
c) hand
d) joints.

4 The saddle joint at the base of the thumb helps the hand to:
a) move towards the body
b) move away from the body
c) grip
d) turn.

Structure of the hand: Self-checks

1 a) What is the function of muscles at joints?
b) Why do muscles work in pairs?
c) Name the main vessels which supply blood to the hand.
d) Why does the blood in veins have a bluish colour?

2 a) Where are the carpal bones situated?
b) Name the bones which connect with the carpal bones.

Structure of the hand: Activity

1 Draw life-size diagrams. Draw around your hand with fingers apart and then fill in the shape. Use your own hand and the diagrams in this chapter as a guide.

Using this method, draw different diagrams to show each of the following:
a) bones of the hand and wrist
b) muscles of the hand
c) blood supply to the hand

Label your diagrams fully.

Hand massage

Massage is not just rubbing in hand cream. If that was the case, the client might just as well be handed the bottle and be told to get on with it! Skilfully applied massage movements help to relax the client, make the joints more supple and leave the skin feeling smooth and refreshed. Besides helping the skin to absorb the hand cream or lotion, the massage increases the flow of blood to the area, providing essential nutrients for the muscles, bones, skin and nails. The removal of waste products from the area is also speeded up. Exercises are included in the sequence which help to ease stiffness and improve the mobility of the joints. The basic massage procedure is made up of *effleurage* movements, which are relaxing, and *petrissage* movements which are stimulating:

- effleurage: long, flowing, stroking movements performed with the fingers and palms of the hand. Very little pressure is used. Every massage sequence begins and ends with effleurage. Effleurage soothes the nerve endings and helps to remove loose surface skin cells
- petrissage: deeper, rhythmic, localised circular kneading or friction-type movements which have stimulating effects. Petrissage increases the rate at which blood flows through the skin and underlying muscles, and removes loose surface skin cells and waste matter.

The joints of the fingers and wrists are put through their full range of movements, sometimes against a resistance. This stimulates the circulation of blood through the joints and helps to increase their suppleness and flexibility.

Hand massage sequence

1a

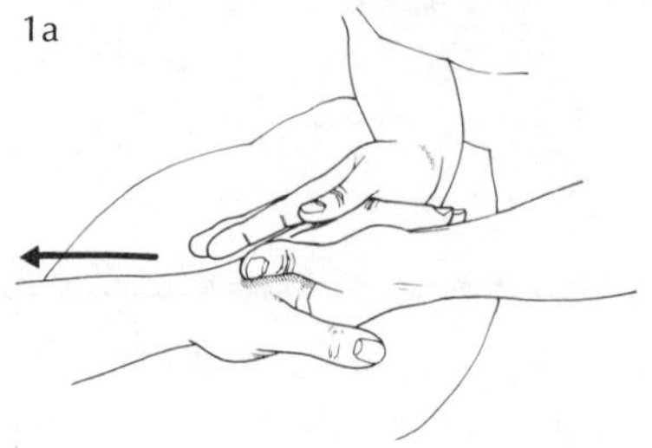

1b

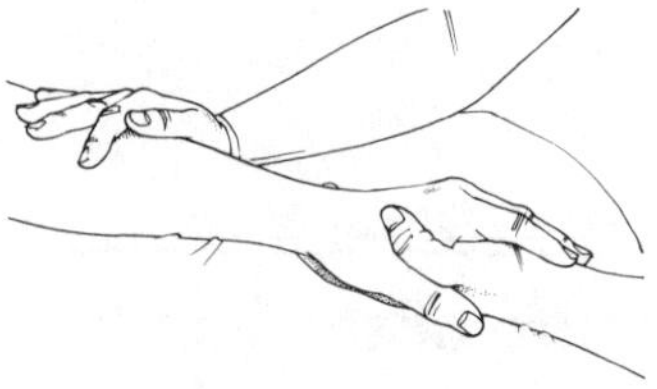

1a, b Stroking (effleurage) from fingers to elbow, six times with each hand

2

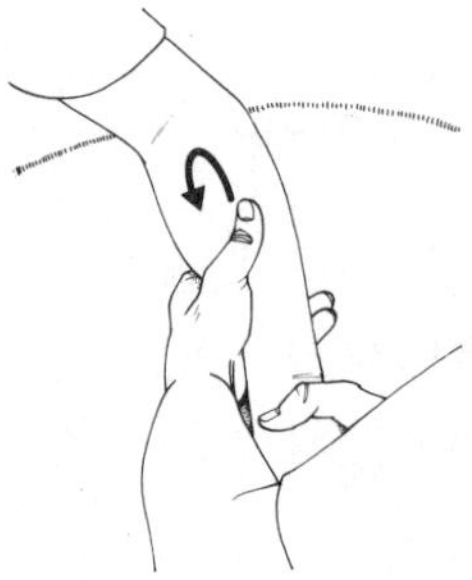

3a

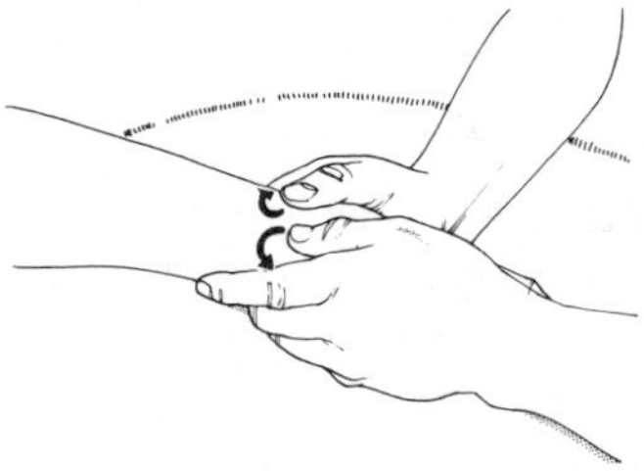

2 Thumb kneading (petrissage) on forearm

3a, b Thumb kneading (petrissage) to wrist and back of hand

3b

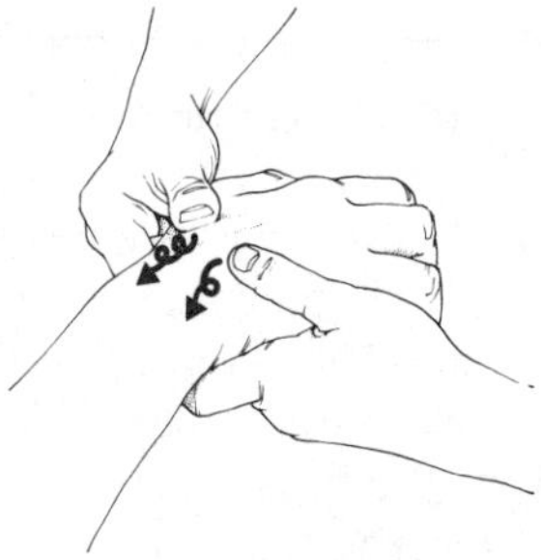

4

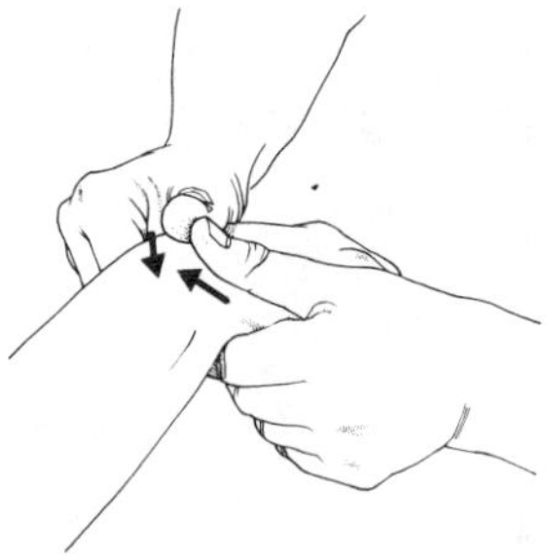

4 Cross thumb frictions (petrissage) to back of hand

5a

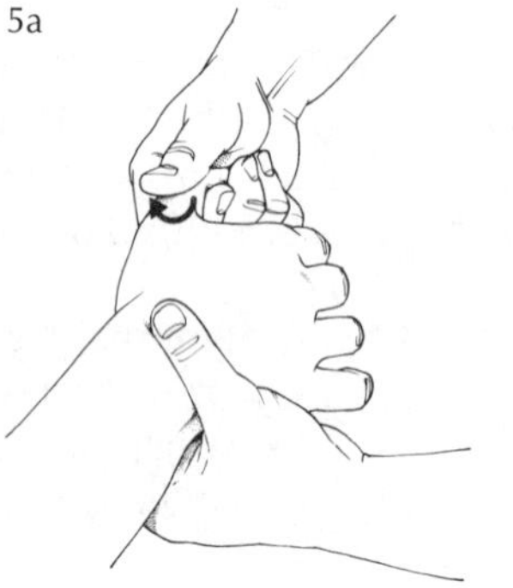

5b

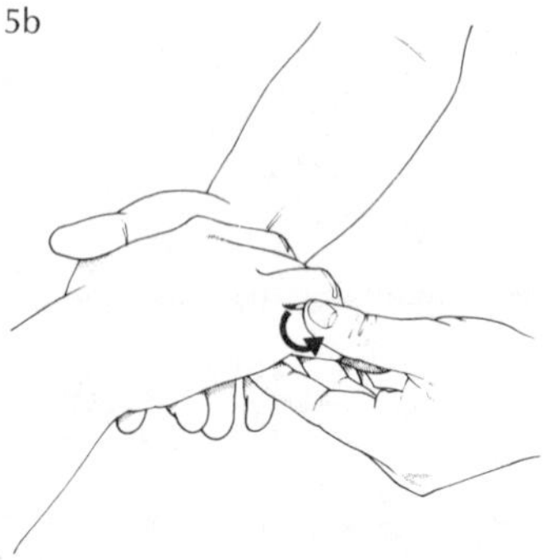

5a, b Thumb kneading (petrissage) to joints of fingers and thumbs

6 Pushing against a resistance (exercise) six times with each finger and thumb

6

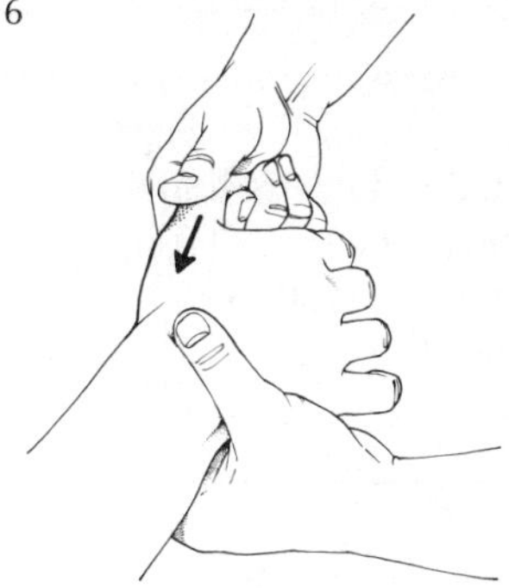

7 Turning the hand over

7

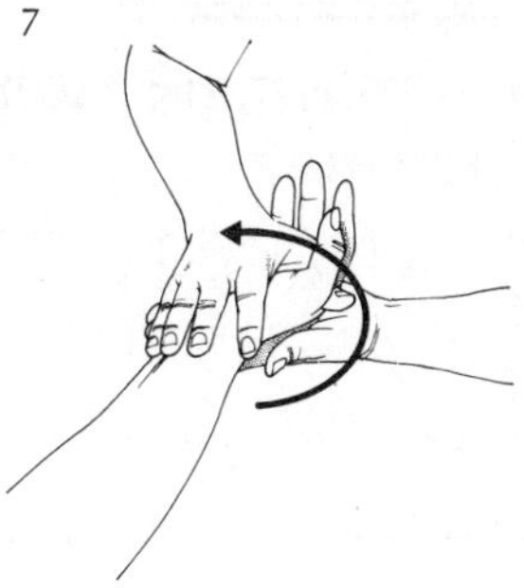

8 Stroking (effleurage) from fingers to elbow, six times with each hand

8

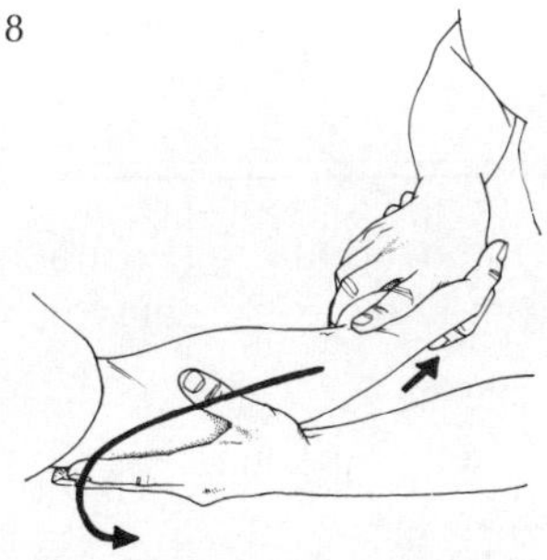

9 Thumb kneading (petrissage) from elbow to palm

9

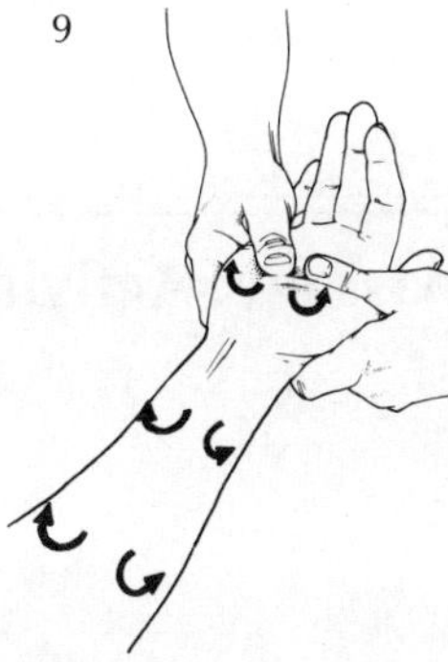

10 Finger rotation (exercise) six times with each finger and thumb

10

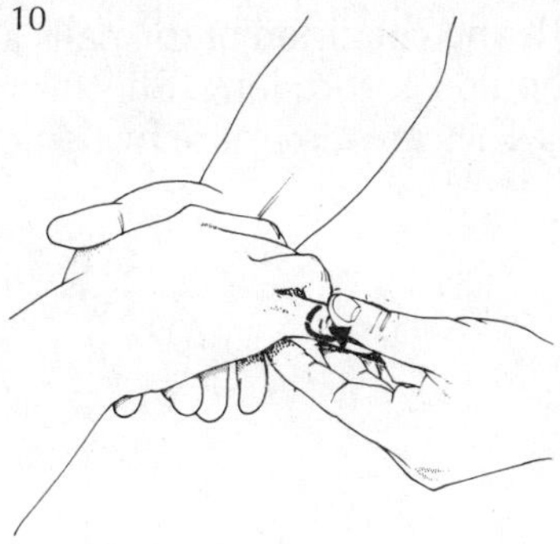

11 Wrist rotation (exercise) six times in each direction

11

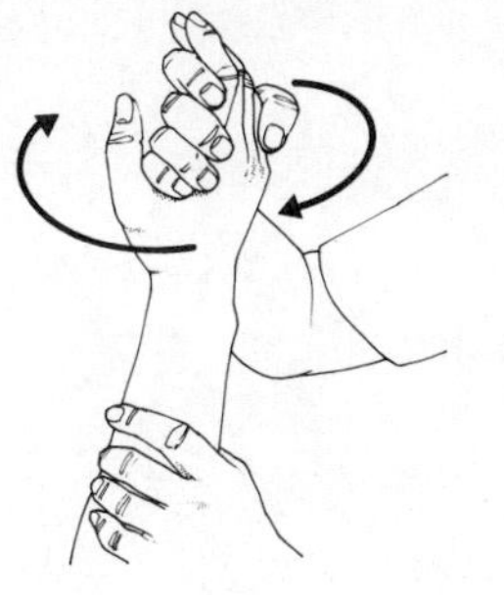

12

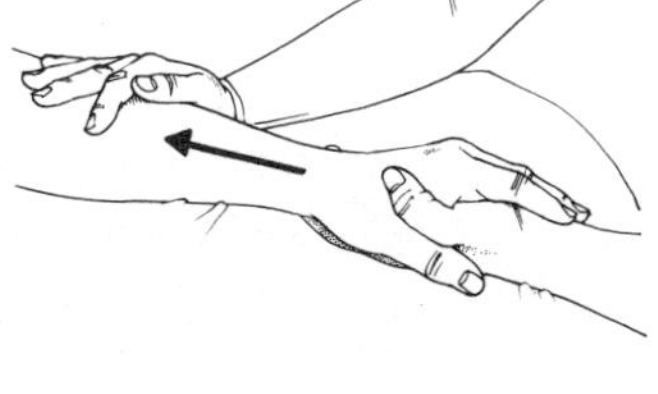

12 Stroking (effleurage) from fingers to elbow

Hand massage: Multiple choice quiz

1 The main reason for using hand cream in the massage is to:
a) make the skin smell nice
b) prevent friction and discomfort
c) encourage retail sales
d) cleanse the skin.

Hand massage: Self-checks

1 a) State two differences between effleurage and petrissage massage movements.
b) Describe the effects of petrissage on the epidermis.

2 a) What are the benefits of stimulating the blood supply during a massage?
b) Describe one massage movement which stimulates the supply of blood to the muscles in the palm.

Hand massage: Activity

1 Practise the hand massage using cream on one hand and lotion on the other. Compare the rates at which the products are absorbed by the skin.

Decide whether the massage feels different to give using the different products.

Examine the skin after the massage and note any differences. Ask your model which product they prefer.

Choosing a nail shape

The length and shape of the nails nail should enhance the overall size and shape of the hands and be practical for the client's occupation. The strength and condition of the nails are also important. Only very strong nails should be worn long. Shorter nails are much less likely to break or split. They are also more hygienic.

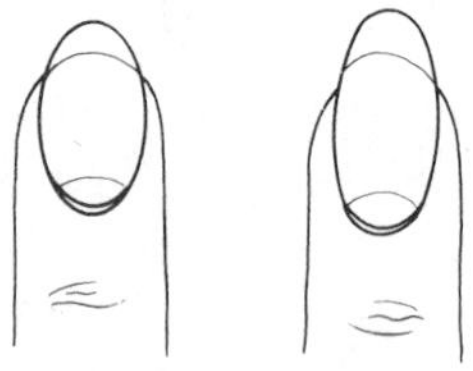

Oval nail: generally considered to be the most attractive shape, oval nails give the effect of length without producing a fragile point.

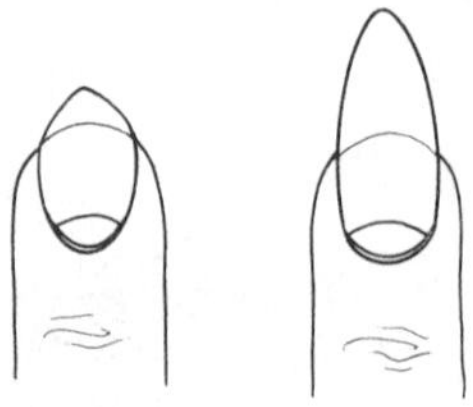

Pointed nail: clients who are impatient for their nails to grow sometimes shape them into a point so that they look longer. This is the worst thing they could do: a pointed nail will soon snap off.

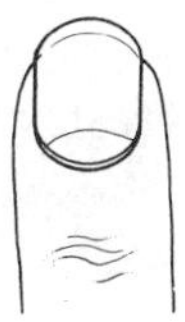

Square nail: short square nails are often preferred for their work by clients such as food handlers and beauty therapists.

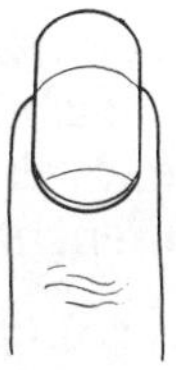

Long square nails flatter long, tapering fingers but the corners should be rounded off to reduce the risk of them breaking.

Choosing a nail shape: Multiple choice quiz

1 Long pointed nails are:
- a) recommended for clients with strong nails
- b) recommended for clients with long, slender hands
- c) not recommended at all
- d) only recommended when they are practical.

2 The width of the nails depends on:
- a) the structure of the hands
- b) the length of the nails
- c) the effects of the nail enamel colour
- d) the client's occupation.

3 The condition of the nails influences their length and shape because:
- a) strong nails need the corners squared off
- b) weak nails should be an oval shape
- c) strong nails can be any shape
- d) weak nails should be kept short.

Choosing a nail enamel

The nail enamel colour should match the client's lipstick and co-ordinate with the clothes that are being worn. This creates a total effect which looks good and makes the client feel confident about her overall appearance.

There may be times when what seems the perfect nail enamel is not the best choice:
- Very bright nail enamel colours draw attention to the hands and are not suitable if the client suffers from arthritis or has an obvious problem skin or nail condition.
- Dark enamels make small nails look even smaller.
- Orange, peach or beige-toned enamels emphasise the bluish tinge of skin with poor blood circulation.
- Pearlised enamels have a reflective quality which draws attention to any imperfections of the nail.

The next best nail enamel is the one which tones in with the overall colour effect without emphasising the client's less attractive features.

Creating effects

Leaving a narrow strip free from enamel at either side of the nail creates an illusion of extra length and gives a more slimline effect.

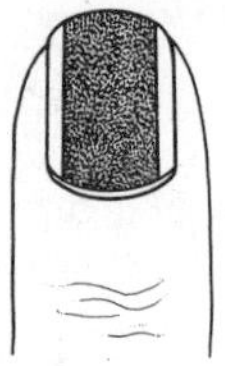

New make up looks are designed to complement the seasonal changes in fashion. Nail cosmetics help to achieve the total effect. The trend towards good skin care and more natural looking make-up has made French manicures very popular.

A high gloss, clean and natural effect is created by using either white pencil, enamel or tape to brighten the free edge followed by a very pale tinted translucent nail enamel.

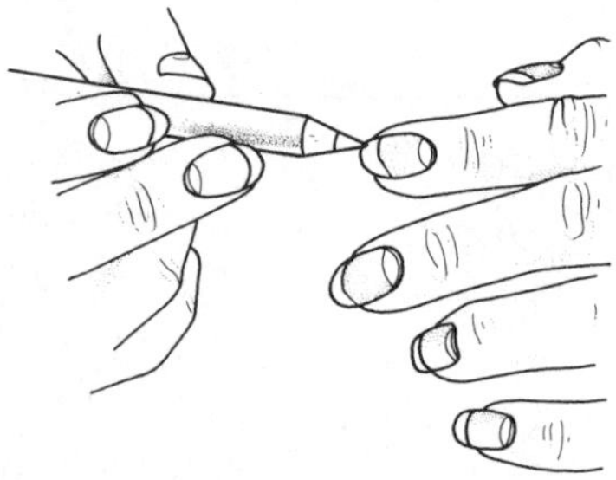

Using a white pencil to create a high gloss effect

Nail art

Nail art provides something a little bit different for the more extrovert client wanting to express their individuality.

Fine sable brushes or an airbrush are used to produce personalised designs on the nails. Coloured enamels or gels are used, some of which are 'cured' with an ultra-violet light to harden them and preserve the design. Very intricate patterns require a lot of skill and they are usually applied to false nails so that they can be kept for longer.

> Remember
> A salon with a serious commitment to specialised nail treatments can develop very good retail sales by providing hand jewellery and nail accessories.

Nail art accessories include gem stones, pearls, chains, lace, glitter, fine tape and transfers. For the therapist with a lot of artistic talent and the patience to practise, there is no limit to the range of creative possibilities with nail art.

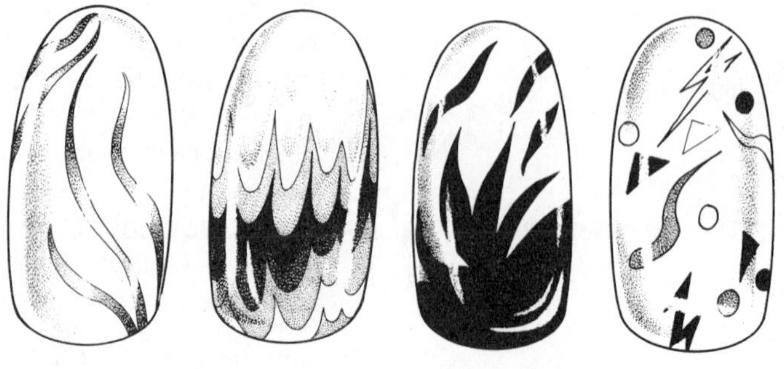

Examples of nail art

Choosing a nail enamel: Multiple choice quiz

1 The best choice of nail enamel for a client with pale hands and narrow nails is:
a) a bright, pearlised enamel
b) a pale, plain enamel
c) a dark, pearlised enamel
d) a pale, pearlised enamel.

2 A client with arthritis who wants to wear nail enamel should be advised to:
a) have a French manicure
b) have a pale plain nail enamel
c) have a dark plain enamel
d) have a pale pearlised enamel.

3 Personalised nail art designs give the client:
a) individuality
b) fashion effects
c) colour co-ordination
d) a total look.

Choosing a nail enamel: Activities

1 Choose five contrasting nail enamels and apply one to each of your nails on one hand.

Note how different enamel colours look next to your skin colour and, also, their effects on the nails themselves.

Ask a few friends if they will let you do the same to them.

2 The next time you are at a beauty exhibition, find the stands where professional nail artists are demonstrating their talents and see how they achieve their effects.

Have a look at the range of accessories which are available.

Allergy to nail enamel

Some people are particularly sensitive to substances which are tolerated without any problem by the rest of us. Contact with the substance, even for a very short time, can cause a severe allergic skin reaction. In some cases, other organs of the body also become involved.

The nail plates are dead, so although they can be affected by nail cosmetics, they cannot become allergic to them. An allergy to nail enamel is much more likely to appear on the face or neck as a result of touching the skin and bringing it into contact with the offending ingredient of the nail enamel.

> *Remember*
> Itchiness invariably leads to scratching, which breaks the skin. This allows bacteria to enter and cause disease.

A typical allergic reaction to nail enamel consists of itchiness, inflammation, swelling and blistering at the site of contact, followed by weeping, drying and flaking of the skin. The most commonly affected sites are the eyelids, around the mouth, the sides of the neck and the upper chest.

Formaldehyde resin is thought to be the ingredient of nail enamel most likely to cause an allergic reaction. Products are now available which do not contain formaldehyde.

There have been rare cases reported of allergic reactions to nail enamel which have affected the nail bed. The cause of these has been deep pigments in poor quality enamels which have penetrated the nail plate and reacted with the living skin tissue beneath.

Allergy to nail enamel: Self-checks

1 Describe a typical allergic reaction to nail enamel.

2 a) Why is it unusual for an allergy to nail enamel to affect the nail bed?
b) How can an allergic reaction which affects the nail bed be prevented?

3 Fill in the missing words:

The ingredient of a nail enamel most likely to cause an allergy is.________ . This is contained in the enamel to give it.__________ The allergic reaction appears where the product has been in.___________.with the skin. The areas of the body most commonly affected are the.__________, around the.___________, the sides of the.___________ and the upper.__________. The name given to this reaction is.__________ __________. There is a risk of infection caused by.____________.the skin.

Allergy to nail enamel: Activity

1 When you visit the wholesaler, have a look at the labels on the nail enamels and see if there are any advertised as 'formaldehyde-free'. Make a note of their name.

Also, write down the names of 'acetone-free' nail enamel removers.

Minor nail repairs

Unlike a cut in the skin, there is no way of healing a broken nail. The edges of a split can, however, be bonded together quite successfully with an instant acrylic nail strengthener. This type of product contains ingredients such as rayon fibres, which reinforce the weak area of the split. Alternatively, an acrylic nail hardener can be applied.

Some clients prefer to disguise a split by having a false nail applied. This has an immediate cosmetic effect but can sometimes worsen the split when the false nail is removed.

Before the arrival of acrylic nail products, the traditional type of nail repair involved the use of fibrous tissue and a liquid fixative or glue to patch the damage.

The kits are still available and the method continues to be used by therapists who are sufficiently skilled to be able to apply a strong and resilient smooth repair that is suitable as a base for nail enamel.

> *Remember*
> Do not cut the tissue as this will produce a demarcation line which will show through the enamel. Tearing the tissue also produces a stronger repair.

1 Make sure the nail is clean and then measure the tissues against the damaged area.

2 Choose one which is a suitable width and then tear it to shape so that the final patch is slightly larger than the area needing repair.

3 Saturate the tissue patch with mending fixative and use the bevelled end of an orange stick to transfer it to the area for repair.

4 Working from the inside of the patch outwards, smooth over the tissue with the flat side of an orange stick. This disperses air from underneath the patch which could cause it to bubble. It also blends

the fibres of the tissue on to the surface of the nail, providing a smooth finish.

5 When the patch has dried, apply a coat of nail fixative over the entire nail surface and allow it to dry.

6 If the nail is being capped, apply fixative to the tissue extension and underneath the free edge. Use the orange stick to fix the extension in place.

7 A final smoothing of the patch and nail border can be achieved with a little nail enamel remover applied on the pad of the thumb.

Minor nail repairs: Multiple choice quiz

1 Mending tissue should be torn to size in order to:
a) prevent wastage
b) provide a smooth finish
c) absorb the mending fixative
d) make the patch last longer.

2 The tissue patch is sealed on to the nail with:
a) mending fixative
b) solvent
c) base coat
d) nail enamel.

3 The size of the tissue patch should be:
a) slightly smaller than the damaged area
b) slightly larger than the damaged area
c) the same size as the damaged area
d) the same size as the nail.

4 The repair may be finally smoothed over with:
a) the flat end of an orange stick
b) mending fixative
c) nail enamel remover
d) base coat.

Minor nail repairs: Activity

1 Practise applying tissue repairs until you can manage to produce one which does not show through the nail enamel application.

When you have reached this stage, try to work out what you are doing differently from when you first started to practise!

Special treatments for hands and nails

With a little imagination, the therapist can design a variety of special luxury treatments for the hands and nails. Many beauty therapy treatments designed for other areas of the body can be adapted quite easily, for example face masks and vibro massage, which could encourage a manicure client to try a facial or body treatment for the first time.

It is important to keep up with new product developments so that regular clients do not have long to wait to try something new, and special promotions can help to attract new clients.

Here are some well established special treatments for the hands and nails.

Warm oil treatment

This is given immediately before the hand massage and involves soaking the hands and nails in a good quality vegetable oil which has been warmed up in a hot water bath. Almond oil is ideal but it is expensive. Olive oil is also good but its distinctive smell is retained by the skin after the treatment. Arachis (peanut) oil is a very acceptable, cheaper alternative.

Warm oil treatments are particularly beneficial for clients with dry skin and cuticles and flaking, fragile nails. Sometimes the nails alone are treated.

1 Before beginning the manicure, pour enough oil in to a small bowl to cover the nails up to the first joint of the fingers and thumbs. Cover the bowl and place it in a slightly larger container to one side of the manicure table.

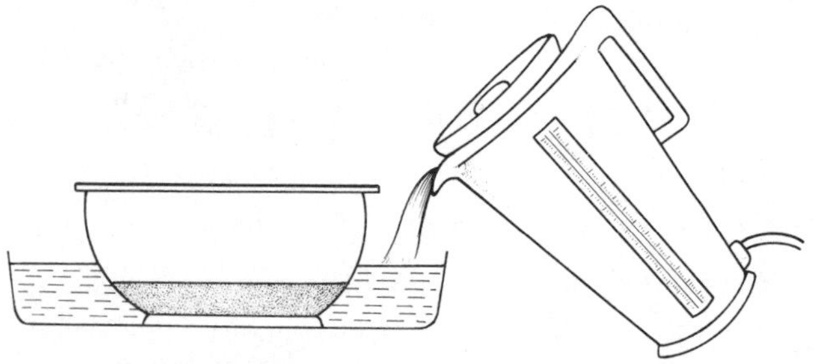

2 As the second hand goes into soak, pour boiling water into the outer container. The heat will gradually transfer to the oil, ensuring that it does not get too hot.

3 When cuticle work is complete and the free edge has had a final smoothing, remove the inner bowl from the water and position the client's fingers and thumbs so that they are covered with warm oil.

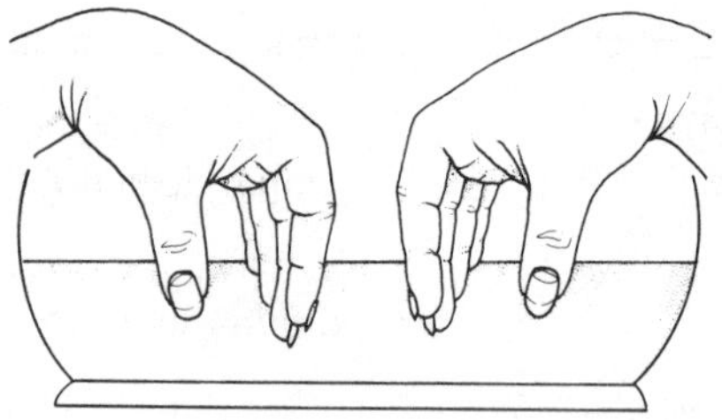

4 Leave the nails in soak until the oil has cooled down, usually about 10-15 minutes. One at a time, lift the hands out of the bowl and proceed to massage the oil well in to the cuticles and over the rest of the fingers and hand.

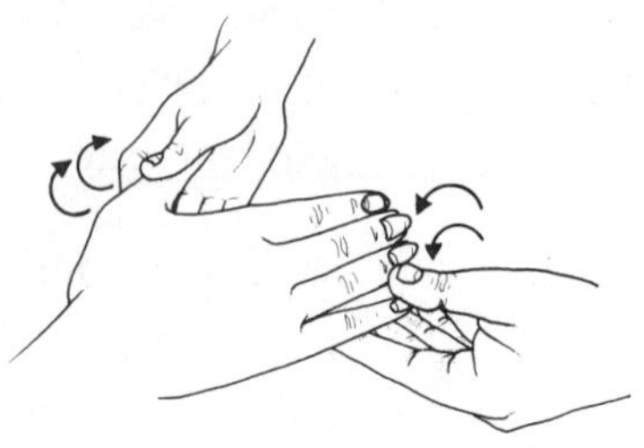

Ideally, the remaining fine film of oil should be left to soak into the nails and skin, and nail enamel should not be applied. The palms of the hands can be de-greased by wiping over with witch hazel. In some manicure procedures, a warm oil treatment substitutes soaking the nails in soapy water. This means that the cuticles have the advantage of being softened by the oil before being lifted and pushed back.

Paraffin wax treatment

In this treatment, layers of melted paraffin wax are built up to form a glove which covers the hand and wrist. The wax glove is then either wrapped in foil or sealed with plastic and wrapped in a towel to retain the heat.

Over the next few minutes the temperature of the skin rises enough to stimulate the sweat glands and sebaceous glands. As a result, the skin is deep cleansed and softened. The heat which is produced stimulates the flow of blood which benefits the skin and muscles.

Clients who suffer from rheumatism may benefit from the heating effects of the treatment.

Paraffin wax can be applied immediately before the hand massage, or afterwards to increase the absorption of hand cream.

Paraffin wax is usually purchased in 1 kilo blocks which melt at around 43 °C (110 °F). The temperature of the wax is raised to approx. 49 °C (120 °F) before being applied to the skin with a brush or by immersion in a special paraffin wax bath.

1 A wax bath is thermostatically controlled. Switch it on at least 30 minutes before you will need it.

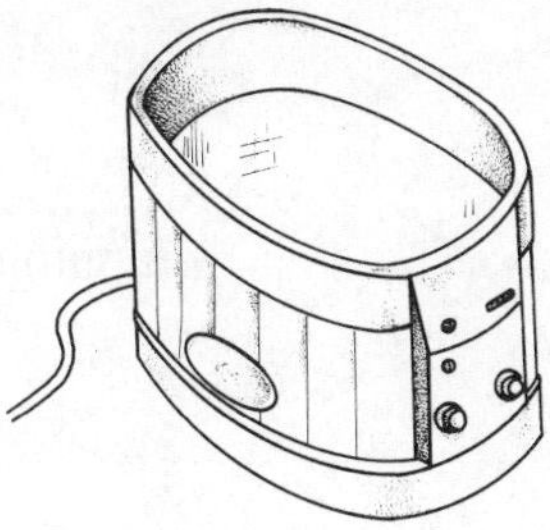

2 Test the temperature of the wax on the inside of your wrist before applying it to the client.

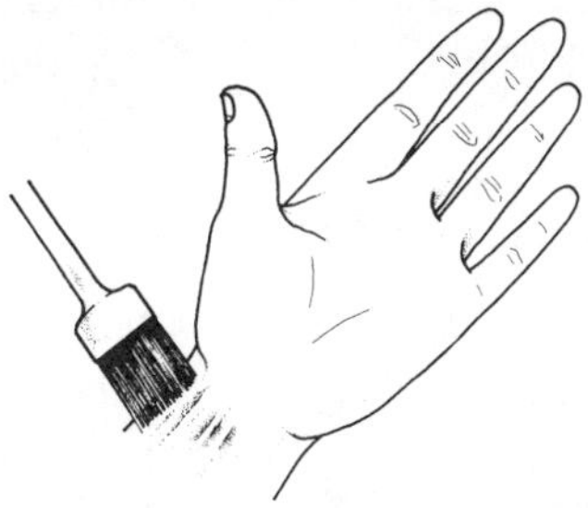

3 Immerse the client's hand in the wax to just above the wrist. As you lift the hand out of the bath, a layer of wax sets on the skin.

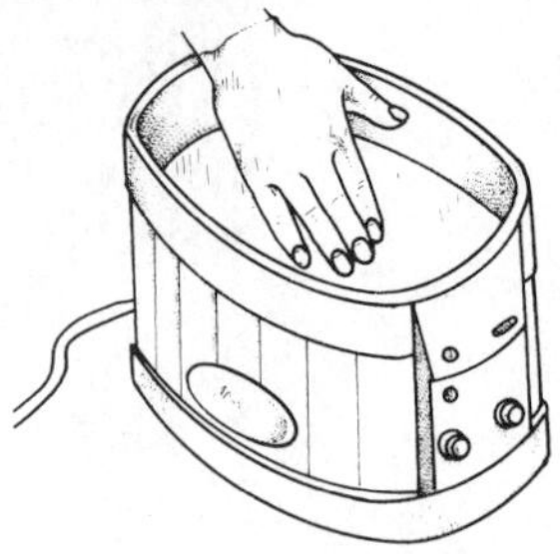

4 Repeat five or six times until a white wax 'glove' has formed.

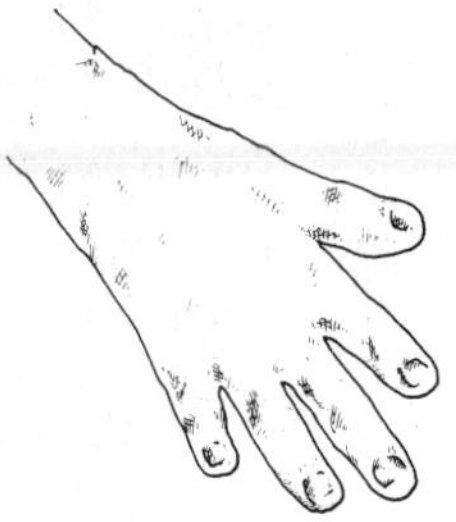

5 Seal the wax-coated hand in a polythene bag or wrap in foil and keep covered with a towel to keep in the heat.

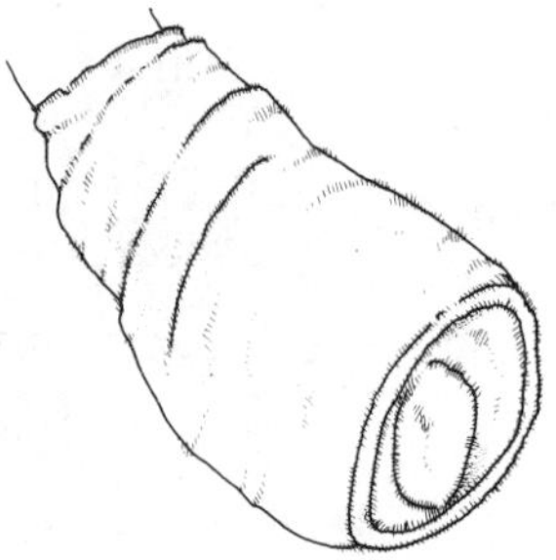

6 After twenty minutes, remove the towel and then the wax film and wrapping in one firm sliding movement.

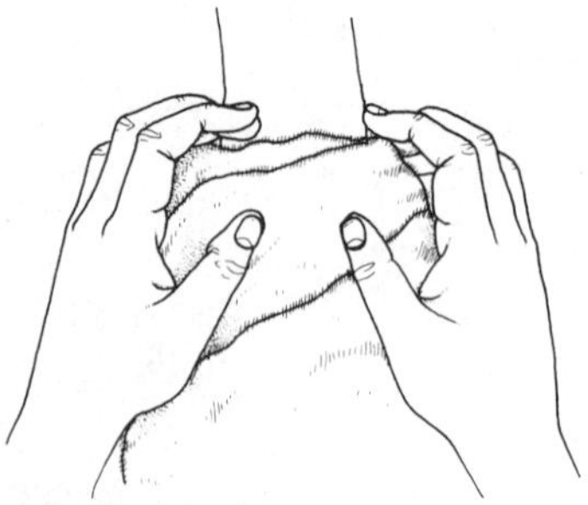

> Remember
> The fine waxy film left on the nails will have to be removed with nail enamel remover if nail enamel is going to be worn.

Safety points

1 Some baths have an outer water vessel which heats up like a kettle. The heat is then transferred to an enclosed metal sided wax container. Always make sure that the water level has been topped up so that the heating element does not burn out.

> Remember
> If you do spill paraffin wax on clothing or bed linen, peel off the wax and then cover the stain with brown wrapping paper. Use a hot iron over the top to melt the wax. Once the excess has become absorbed into the paper, the item can be washed as normal.

2 Make sure that the client's skin does not touch the metal sides of the bath. A paper towel placed over the rim of the bath helps to avoid painful contact between the skin and hot metal.

3 Protect the surrounding area with old towels or plastic sheets. Although the wax sets quickly once it is exposed to air, there is a slight risk of spilling or dripping the wax.

4 Used wax and wrappings should be disposed of immediately after use in a sealed container.

Hand rub

An abrasive rub is particularly good for lifting out dirt or stains which have become ingrained in the skin. (Gardeners, fruit pickers and DIY enthusiasts will understand!) Products are available which combine a granular material such as oatmeal, ground fruit stones, poly chips or plastic granules with a conventional cleansing cream.

- Lanolin and coconut oil are often added to soften the skin and prevent the hands from chapping.
- Glycerine may be contained to help restore the skin's natural moisture balance.
- Clay is sometimes added which sets on the skin and is then gently massaged off, loosening surface skin cells and trapped dirt.
- One of the oldest hand rub treatments uses salt and a little water mixed together to form a paste. This is massaged all over the hands until the skin goes pink. The salt is then rinsed off with clean, warm water.

A salt rub leaves the hands feeling very clean and smooth but be careful to inspect the hands first for cuts or breaks in the skin. If you rub salt into these, it will be painful.

Special treatments for hands and nails: Multiple choice quiz

1 The beneficial effects of a paraffin wax treatment are achieved mainly by:
   a) heating the skin
   b) cleansing the skin
   c) softening the skin
   d) soothing the skin.

2 The correct working temperature for paraffin wax is approximately:
   a) 42 °C
   b) 52 °C
   c) 39 °C
   d) 49 °C.

3 The temperature of the wax should be tested on:
   a) the back of the therapist's hand
   b) the back of the client's hand
   c) the inside of the client's wrist
   d) the inside of the therapist's wrist.

4 The hand is wrapped up after wax has been applied in order to:
   a) protect the client's clothes
   b) keep wax off the towels
   c) retain heat in the wax
   d) stimulate the sweat glands.

5 Wax which has been used should be:
a) melted and recycled
b) disposed of immediately in a waste bin
c) disposed of in a sealed container
d) boiled up and filtered.

Special treatments for hands and nails: Self-checks

1 a) Give three characteristics of an oil which make it suitable for a warm oil treatment for the hands and nails.
b) Name one oil which has these characteristics.

2 a) Why is oil heated for giving a hand treatment?
b) How is the oil prevented from getting too hot?

3 a) Why should the hands and nails be massaged after they have been soaked in the oil?
b) State the general contra-indications to warm oil treatments.

4 List the safety precautions which should be taken when preparing and applying a paraffin wax treatment.

5 Explain how the abrasive effects of a hand rub benefit the hands.

6 Name three granular materials which may be contained in an abrasive hand cleanser.

7 Why would you recommend a hand rub treatment to a client?

Special treatments for hands and nails: Activity

1 Consider the full range of treatments and products available in your salon. Suggest which ones would be suitable as a special treatment for the hands.

Try some of them out, but bear in mind the cost of giving the treatment if you are using large quantities of products.

Home care

Giving advice on home care is an important part of the professional service and should include selling the client good quality hand and nail care products from the salon's retail range.

Clients have confidence in purchases which are backed up with a trusted professional's recommendation. It is also easier to monitor a client's progress with a home-care routine if you are familiar with the products that are being used.

Having convinced your client about the benefits of regular professional manicures, you need to give advice on how the hands and nails can be maintained in good condition between treatments.

You should check how well the hands are usually protected from everyday activities and if there are any aspects of the client's job which might affect the condition and appearance of the hands and nails.

Here is some general advice for hand and nail care.

Washing

- Use mild soaps or hand cleansers which are not too drying.
- Remove rings before washing the hands so that soap does not build up behind them and irritate the skin.
- Rinse the hands thoroughly with lukewarm water and dry them properly with a soft towel: skin creases which are left soggy crack and become sore.
- Always use hand cream or lotion after washing to lubricate and soften the skin.

Protecting

- Wear household gloves for wet jobs and any activities involving the use of chemicals. When this is not practical, apply barrier cream beforehand. If working with the hands submerged in hot water, rubber gloves should not be worn for longer that fifteen minutes at a time as sweat builds up on the hands which irritates the skin.

> Remember
> Wearing a barrier cream for doing dirty jobs makes cleaning the hands afterwards very much easier.

If water or detergent gets inside the gloves while they are being worn, they should be removed immediately and allowed to dry thoroughly before being worn again. Sprinkling talc inside the gloves helps to keep them dry.

- Wear a barrier cream and gloves when going out into a cold climate. Use a richer hand cream during the winter months.
- Keep a supply of hand cream close to the kitchen sink and in the bathroom, which can be used each time the hands are washed or rinsed.
- Massage the hands with cream each evening just before going to bed.
- Rub cuticle cream into the nails and cuticles at bed time to keep them soft and pliable.
- Always apply a base coat under nail enamel to protect the nails and prevent them from becoming stained.
- Avoid using nail enamel remover too often. Acetone-free removers are less harsh on the nails.

Strengthening

> Remember
> Nibble cheese, celery and carrots when you're feeling peckish. They are much better for you than sweets and crisps!

- The health and strength of the nails depends on a good supply of protein and, also, iron, calcium, potassium, Vitamin B and iodine.
- Eat a balanced diet which contains all the nutrients essential for good health/-/they are good for your skin and nails too.
- Apply strengtheners to reinforce weak nails and make them less likely to break or split.
- Use an emery board to neaten a rough free edge or split nails. Metal files should be avoided as they create heat in the nails which dries out the natural moisture and weakens them.
- Buff the nails to a healthy pink shine before going to bed. This stimulates the supply of blood to the nails.

Exercising at home

The exercises described in the massage procedure require the therapist to 'lead' the movements and support the joints being exercised. The following hand exercises can be practised at home to improve the circulation, increase the strength of the hands and make the fingers and wrists more flexible. They are particularly beneficial for people who suffer from arthritis or rheumatism. Just a few minutes are needed regularly when the hands are not busy. After a shower or bath is a good time when the muscles are warm and relaxed. (Why not try them yourself now while you are reading?!)

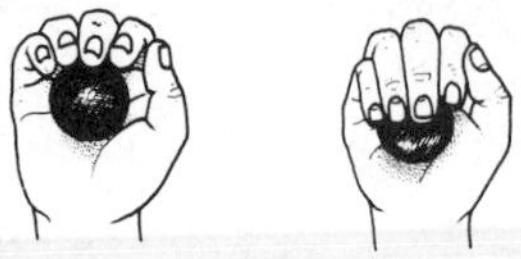

The tight squeeze

Grasp a squash ball in the palm of the hand and squeeze it tightly. Repeat until you can feel the strain. Relax your grip and repeat with the other hand.

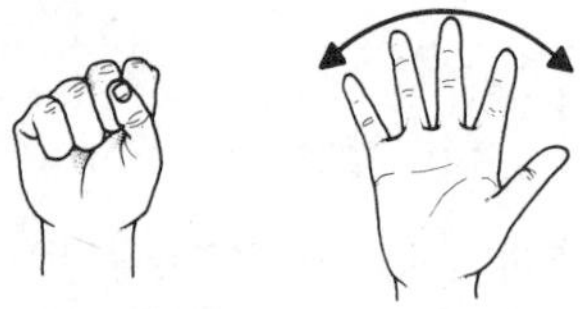

Fist and flare

Clench both fists very tightly. Hold a second, then flare the fingers out in front of you as wide apart and as stretched as possible. Repeat six times.

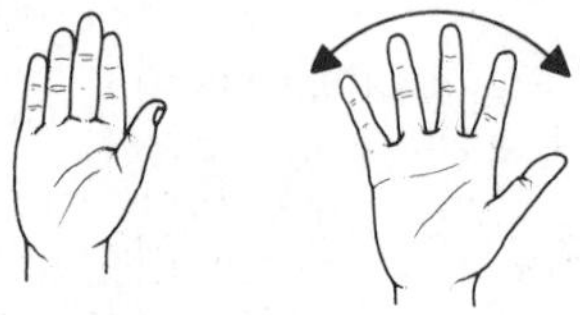

Finger spread

Hold arms straight out in front of you with hands forward, palms down and fingers straight and pressed tightly against each other. Thrust the fingers apart, spreading them as much as possible. Repeat six times.

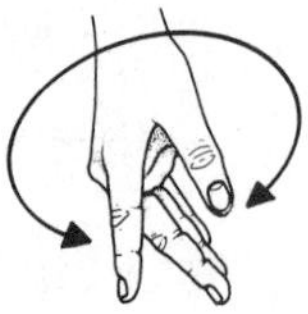

Wrist circles

Let the hands droop, then rotate them from the wrist making as full circles as possible, ten times in one direction then times in the other.

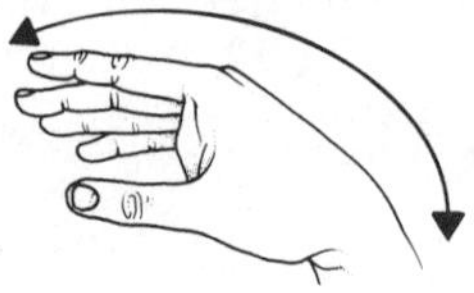

Royal waves

Keep the hands relaxed, palms facing downwards and then move them gracefully up and down, waving slowly from the wrists. Repeat ten times.

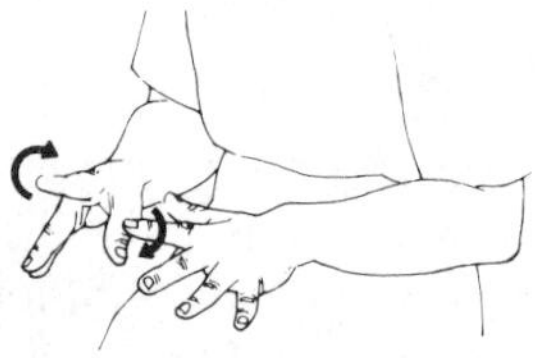

Piano playing

If you are not an accomplished piano player, use the table top instead to rap out the William Tell Overture! All the joints in the fingers and thumbs should get exercised, particularly if you play at double speed!

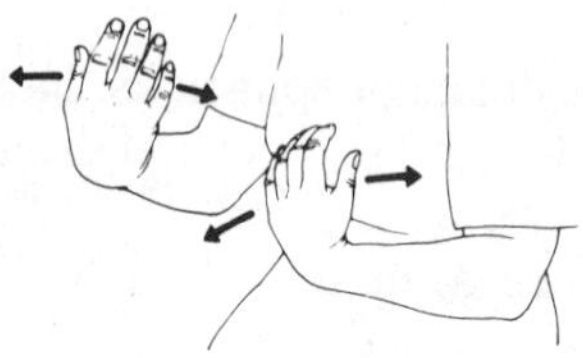

Shake and rest

Finally, with hands and wrists relaxed, shake them both vigorously at the same time for about twenty seconds.

Following the exercises, sit comfortably with your hands completely relaxed on your knees for two minutes.

Chapter 10

Nail technology

After working through this chapter you will be able to:

- appreciate the range of nail technology services
- advise on the suitability of different nail systems
- prepare the nails for treatment
- provide a range of false nail treatments
- provide advice on after care.

Artificial nail systems

The work of a nail technician is concerned mainly with creating natural looking false nails from materials such as acrylic, porcelain, fibreglass and gel. The false nail is produced either as a coating for a poor quality natural nail to give it strength as it grows, or as an extension to the natural nail to create extra length. Whatever method is used, nail treatments are very profitable and there is considerable scope for associated retail sales.

There are many different artificial nail systems and technology is advancing at such a rate that new improved methods seem to be appearing all the time. Fortunately, the companies who distribute nail systems in the UK provide very good training which ensures that technicians keep updated. The main focus of research and development work in nail technology is producing a nail which not only looks natural but feels and reacts like a strong, healthy natural nail: it is comfortable, lightweight, flexible, resilient and not prone to cracking or splitting.

> Remember
>
> Do not soak the hands in water immediately before applying or building up false nails. Moisture which remains on the nail or in the nail substance could become trapped under the artificial structure and cause a fungus to grow.
>
> A fungicide is usually applied during the treatment procedure as further precaution against infection.

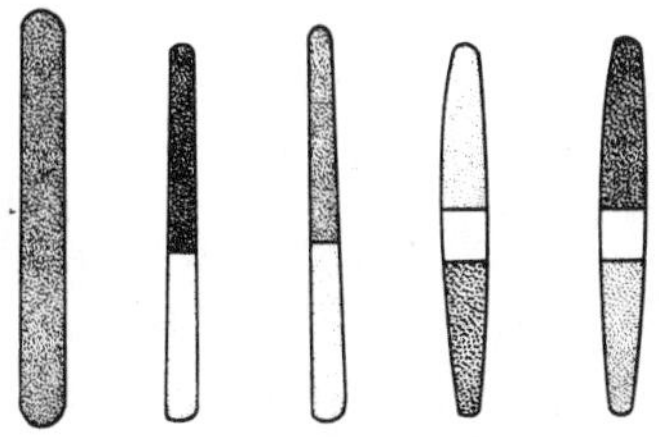

A selection of buffers

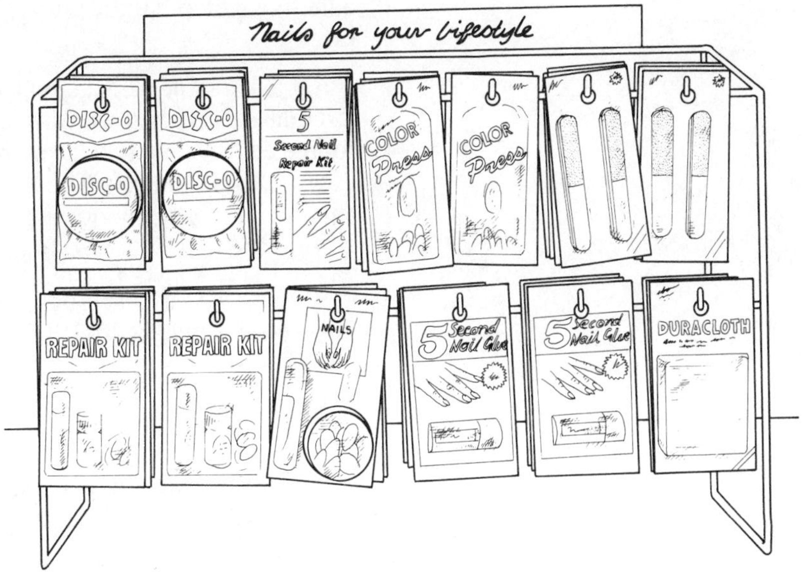

A nail bar selling a range of nail care accessories

Preparing the nails for treatment

The methods described here are typical of most of the systems currently available. Before starting treatment:

- check first that there are no contra-indications
- remove all traces of nail enamel and wipe over the hands and nails with surgical spirit
- file the nails to an even length and tidy up the cuticles if necessary. (If there is a lot of work required on the cuticles, this is best done during a full manicure the day before.)

Files and buffers

New items of manicure equipment have been developed to produce the best results with false nails and extensions. The files and buffers used for nail technology systems are produced in various thicknesses and textures. Unlike paper files, the abrasives adhere to woven cloth fibres, which means that they last longer. Filing is much faster and there are no loose filing particles. The files and buffers are usually colour coded according to their different uses.

Gel system 1: gel only

This method is often recommended for clients with brittle nails to help keep them protected as they grow to an attractive length. The gel coating hardens on the nails so that the client has to return every three or four weeks to have the small ridge created by new growth buffed away and the nails regelled. In this way a smooth nail surface is maintained and the nails do not become top heavy. A full set of gel nails applied by this method takes 30-40 minutes to complete, depending on the amount of nail repair work required.

1. Buff the nail plate with a cushioned semi-abrasive buffer. This removes any minor ridges or imperfections from the nail and helps to produce a more adherent surface. Brush away the dust that is created.
2. Apply the special primer and leave it to dry completely. This is an adhesive which has anti-fungal properties to help prevent nail disease.
3. Using a dry sable brush, apply the first amount of gel in small circular movements working over the entire nail plate from cuticle to free edge. Apply two layers by this method, then drag off the excess with the brush. The third coat should be applied like nail enamel leaving a smooth edge. Use an orange stick to tidy up around the nail.

   Some gels need to be 'cured' to set them. This is done by either the use of a special set spray or by exposing them to ultra-violet light for about two minutes.

   A light box is used to cure the four fingers of the left hand, then those of the right hand followed by the two thumbs together.
4. Apply another layer of gel and cure in the same way if required. Otherwise, wipe away the resulting sticky surface with a spirit based liquid nail cleanser.
5. Finally, buff the nails into a perfectly smooth nail shape.

Aftercare

- After four weeks the nails should be re-shaped, buffed down, primed and the gel applied and cured as previously.
- If the client wishes to have the false nails removed, buff away most of the gel and then soak the nails for 10-15 minutes in acetone, or the special remover provided. Wipe the dissolved gel away from the nail surface at five minute intervals during the soaking period.

Gel system 2: tips and gel nail extensions

This method uses the gelling system described previously with pre-formed, contoured artificial nail tips which produce natural looking nails even without nail enamel. This system allows the nail to grow out with the extension, but regelling is required every four weeks to build up the area of new nail growth so that there is a smooth and even nail surface.

1. Clean, file and buff the nails as before.
2. The tips are available in various sizes. To select correctly, measure the width and curvature of the false nails against the natural ones. The tip should sit comfortably between 1/3 and 2/3 down the length of the nail plate. It may be necessary to file the sides of the tip gently to ensure a perfect fit.
3. Apply glue to the well in the false tip and then hold it firmly in position until it has become bonded to the nail plate. This normally takes just a few seconds.
4. Cut and file the nails in to shape and loosen the sides of the false tip from the nail walls.
5. Use a buffer flat against the nail to wear down the ridge created by the false tip. When the ridge has almost disappeared, apply glue on top of the residual powder and leave it to dry. Completely smooth the ridge away with buffers, finishing with a cushioned one.
6. Apply nail tip primer, which is an adhesive with anti-fungal properties. Leave it until nearly dry.
7. Apply, cure and finish off the gel exactly as described previously point.

Aftercare

- Recommend the client to return fortnightly for a gentle buffing and manicure. Monthly appointments should be made to reshape and file away ragged edges, buff and prime the nails and reapply the gel.
- It is not usual to remove the false tip. It is normally allowed to grow out with the natural nail, being eventually filed away. If it is essential to remove the extension, buff it down and soak off the rest in special remover or acetone.

Sculptured nail extensions

This method of nail extension involves building up a false nail tip over a foil form using a liquid and powder acrylic mixture. Some systems use of a drill with an abrasive head to smooth down the hardened compound to the correct thickness and shape. Sculptured nails can also be achieved with gels.

1 Clean and prepare the nails and cuticles as before.

2 Roughen the nail surface with an abrasive buffer and then prime the nails with the fungicide supplied by the manufacturer.

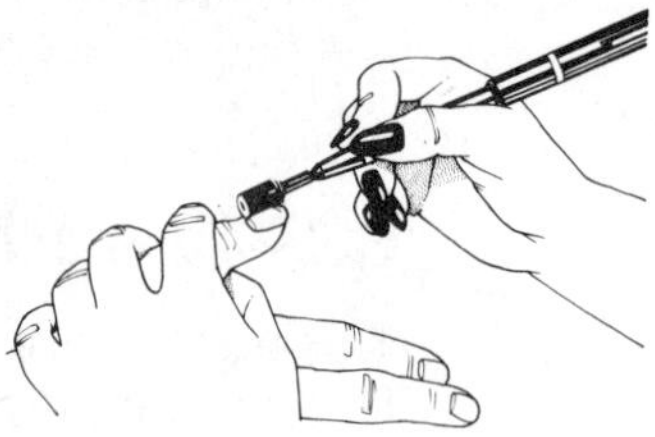

3 Fit the nail forms to the fingers, ensuring that they are aligned carefully with the edges of the cuticles. The form should not encroach onto the nail plate.

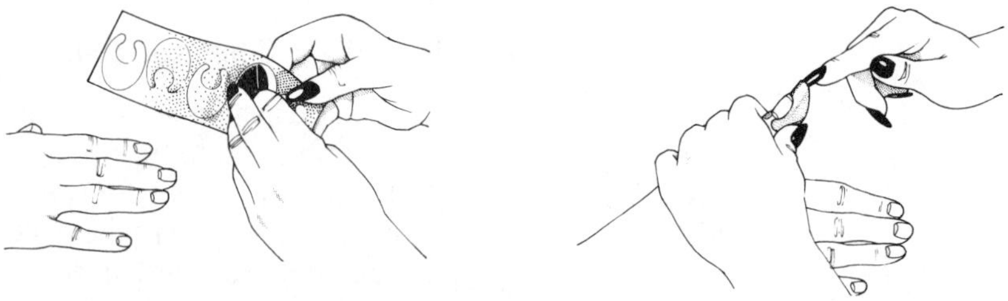

4 Mix the powder and liquid acrylic compound to a firm consistency and then gradually paint it on to the nails, working from the cuticle to the tip and beyond to create an extended nail over the nail form.

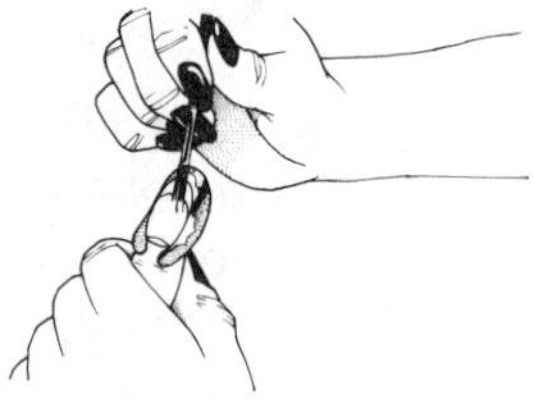

5 When the compound has set, remove the nail forms and complete the final shaping and smoothing off.

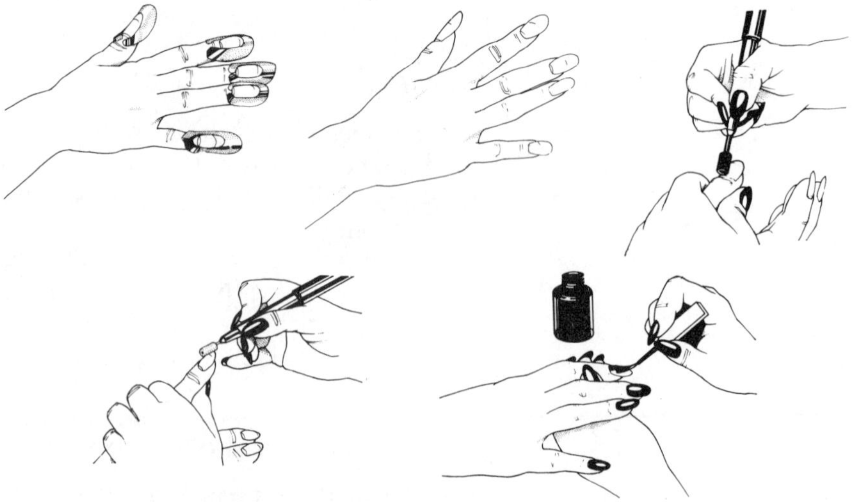

6 Some systems recommend the use of a specially formulated oil to keep the nails supple and flexible.

Nail wraps

Different types of fabric can be used with a special glue to reinforce the natural nails, or create nail extensions by securing false tips to the natural nails.

- Very fine silk is a stronger alternative to mending tissue for repairing a nail which is broken or split.
- Linen and fibreglass produce extensions to the nails which are light and strong.

Pieces of fabric are cut to the size of the nail and then eased into position over a layer of glue, taking care to avoid the cuticle. Extra layers are then built up and the resulting 'nail' is buffed smooth until it is transparent.

Semi-permanent false nails

As well as being offered in a full set, this type of nail provides a quick and effective solution for a broken nail so long as there are no signs of infection or nail bed is not exposed. The false nails are attached to the natural ones. After 10 days to 3 weeks they usually loosen sufficiently to be removed and the procedure may be repeated. This type of nail usually requires nail enamel to be worn.

1 Prepare the nails and cuticles as before.

2 Slightly roughen the surface of the natural nail with a buffer.

3 Select the false nails according to the width and curvature of the natural nails. Position them on a clean tissue in the correct order.

4 Apply glue and position false nails with their base tucked slightly under the lifted cuticle. Press the nail firmly to ensure good contact while the glue is drying. Once the nails are secure, cut and file them in to shape, bevel the edges and apply nail enamel.

A full set application is usually completed within half an hour.

Make sure that your client understands that her new nails are not indestructible! In the event of a heavy blow, they will break. This is much better than the possible damage to the nail bed which could occur if they did not break.

> *Remember*
> Strong solvents damage false nails and clients should be advised to always use acetone-free nail enamel remover.

Temporary stick-on nails

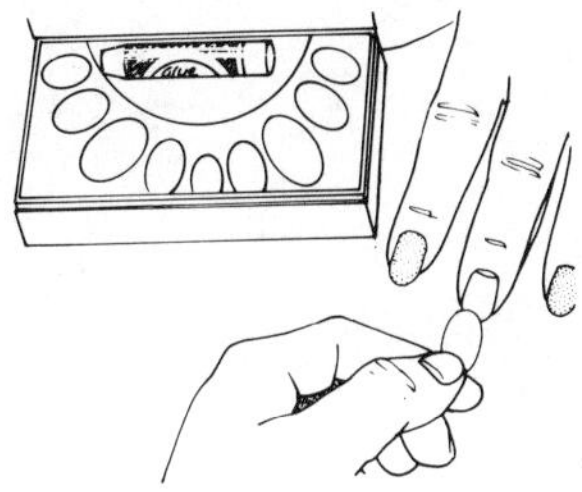

Most clients are looking for permanent effects from nail extension or false nail treatments. However, there are others for whom longer nails are not a practical choice for everyday wear. Temporary stick-on nails create a sophisticated look when nail enamel is being worn for a special event, with the advantage that they can be removed easily afterwards.

1 A full manicure may be given. It is important that the cuticles are softened well and lifted to provide a frame for the false nails.

2 Make sure that there is no moisture or grease left on the nail plate and then measure the false nails against the natural ones, matching up their width at the base.

3 The curve on some false nails may be either too shallow or too deep to fit the natural nails. This can be remedied easily by soaking them in hot water for a few minutes and bending them to the required shape while they are still soft. As the nails cool they set into the new shape. Dry the nails thoroughly before applying them.

4 Lay out the nails on a clean tissue in the order they are going to be applied. Starting with the thumbs, apply glue to the under surface of the false nail and press it on to the nail plate, making sure that the lower edge is tucked gently underneath the loosened cuticle. Keep the two surfaces in close contact while the glue dries.

5 Repeat the procedure on all the nails. Test that the false nails are secure before applying base coat and enamel in the normal way.

6 Any glue which strays on to the skin can be wiped off with a little of the special remover on a tipped orange stick.

This type of nail should not be worn for longer than a day at a time. The nails are not bonded as closely to the natural nails as with other systems and if water and other substances becoming lodged behind the false nail, the nail plate may weaken and become spongy.

Aftercare

The nails can be stored and re-used so long as all traces of glue are removed from the contact surface. Never try prising the nails off without first loosening them with the special glue solvent:

- Position the hand vertically and apply a drop of solvent behind the tip of each false nail. Wait a couple of minutes for the solvent to penetrate the glue and then gently rock the nails from side to side, gradually loosening them at the sides.
- Any remaining glue can be cleaned from the natural nails and false nails using the special solvent.

Nail technology: Multiple choice quiz

1 The hands should not be soaked in water before applying false nails because:
a) the false nails will not stick
b) the water will dilute the adhesive
c) a fungal infection may be caused
d) the natural nails will be softened.

2 Short, natural nails are coated with gel to:
a) give them gloss
b) protect them
c) smooth out ridges
d) help them grow faster.

3 Nail extensions should be applied:
a) immediately after a full manicure
b) a week after a full manicure
c) during a full manicure
d) the day after a full manicure.

4 A fungicide is contained in nail primer to:
a) prevent disease
b) help the nails to stick
c) to harden the natural nails
d) to harden the false nails.

5 Some gel nail systems use an ultra-violet light to:
a) sterilise the gel
b) strengthen the nails
c) set the nails
d) prevent disease.

6 The natural nails are buffed with an abrasive file to:
a) ensure good adhesion between the natural and false nail
b) reduce the thickness of the nails
c) reduce the length of the nails
d) remove surface dirt and stains.

7 Nail forms are used to:
a) help the client chose a nail shape
b) as a base for building up sculptured nail extensions
c) as a base for mixing up the powder compound
d) attach to the natural nails.

8 A stronger alternative to mending tissue for repairing a broken nail is:
a) cotton wool
b) calico
c) silk
d) nylon.

9 Fibreglass nails are made transparent by:
a) buffing
b) exposing to ultra-violet light
c) applying base coat
d) applying oil.

10 Temporary stick-on nails should be removed by:
a) gently easing them off with a pair of tweezers
b) soaking them in nail enamel remover before rocking them gently to loosen them
c) allowing solvent to penetrate the fixative before rocking them gently to loosen them
d) soaking the nails in hot water to soften them before removing them.

Nail technology: Self-checks

1 a) Explain the possible causes of damage to the nail plate as a result of nail extensions.
b) How would the damage affect the appearance of the nails?

2 State the advantages of using the special files and buffers which are provided for use with nail technology systems.

3 a) Explain why a client not requiring nail extensions may be recommended treatment with a gel nail system.
b) Why should the client book a follow-up appointment for four weeks after the gel nail treatment?

4 a) What is meant by 'curing' gel nails?
b) State two ways in which curing can be achieved.

5 'Clients who have been treated with tip and gel nails are contra-indicated to manicure': true or false? Explain your answer.

6 'Semi-permanent false nails are a good idea for people with badly bitten nails': true or false? Explain your answer.

7 'Temporary stick-on nails are preferable to sculptured nails for a client with an infection around the nail': true or false? Explain your answer.

8 'Nail extensions look very natural provided that coloured nail enamel is worn': true or false? Explain your answer.

Nail technology: Activities

1 Conduct a survey of the salons in your area and discover which ones offer specialised nail technology treatments.

Find out which nail systems they use and the range of services they offer.

Compare the prices of nail technology treatments offered by different salons.

2 Keep up to date with advancements in nail technology systems. Read your professional journals and visit trade exhibitions.

Gather product information and take any opportunity you can of seeing new nail systems being demonstrated.

Chapter 11

Pedicure

After working through this chapter you will be able to:

- ▶ appreciate the importance of caring for the feet
- ▶ understand the structure of the foot
- ▶ describe particular problems affecting the feet
- ▶ provide pedicure treatment
- ▶ give advice for home care.

Pedicure treatments

The feet do not generally have the attention they deserve. This is probably because, for most of the time, they are hidden in shoes and do not contribute to the overall appearance. Neglecting the feet can have quite serious consequences. Many aspects of neglect are actually forms of abuse:

- cramming the feet into shoes which bear no resemblance to the natural foot shape
- buying uncomfortable shoes with a view to breaking them in
- wearing high heels which thrust the body forward and put the natural body posture out of alignment.

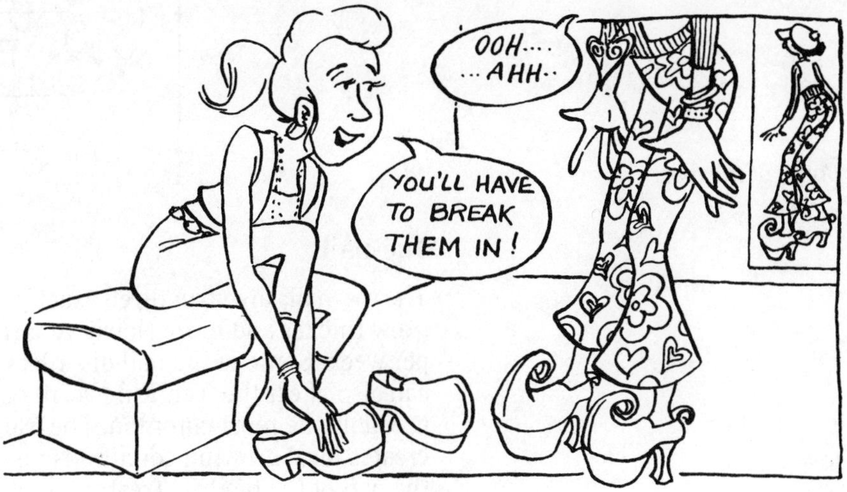

> *Remember*
> Pedicures should be promoted in the salon throughout the year and not just during the peak summer holiday months. Clients should be advised to regularly care for their feet at home, using products from the salon's retail range.

People are gradually becoming more informed about the importance of foot care, particularly those who take regular exercise and are concerned about keeping their bodies in good condition.

It is not difficult converting clients to regular pedicures once the have had their first treatment. The feet look and feel so much better afterwards.

Structure of the foot

The feet support the body and have to take a considerable strain. The main strength of the foot is in the big toe and the true centre of balance is in the ball of the foot. Damage to either affects the natural body posture. The following diagrams show how how the feet are structured to perform their very important functions.

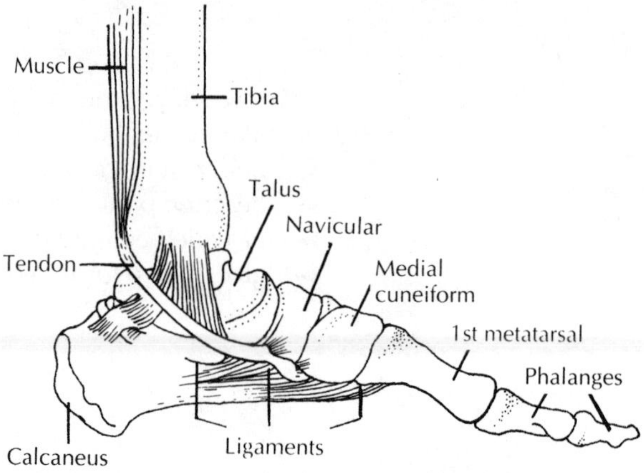

Ligaments and tendons support the arches of the foot

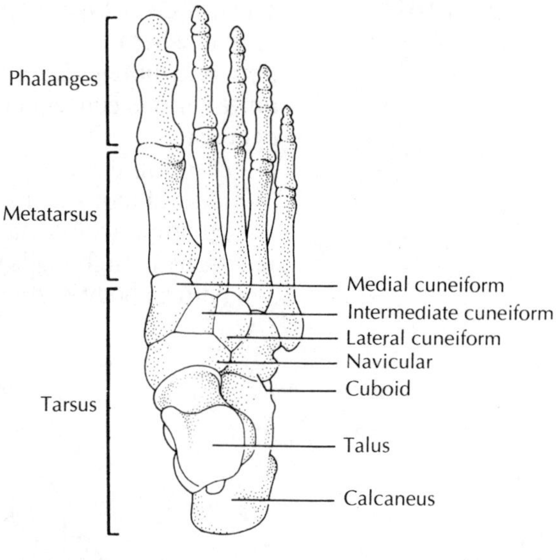

Bones of the foot

Toe-nails

The toe-nails are structured exactly the same as finger nails but they grow thicker and more slowly, at a rate of approximately 0.2–0.4 mm per week. Some of the nail disorders and diseases described previously can also affect the feet. Ringworm of the nail (*onychomycosis*) is probably the most common. The warm, moist environment of a shoe creates ideal growing conditions for the fungus, which attacks mainly the nail of the big toe. Treatment, of course, is medical. Pedicures are contra-indicated as the disease is contagious.

Common problems affecting the feet

The main damage to the feet occurs as a result of pressure, friction and congestion in footwear (which includes shoes, tights, socks and stockings). Problems arise if the toes are not able to move freely and the feet are not adequately ventilated.

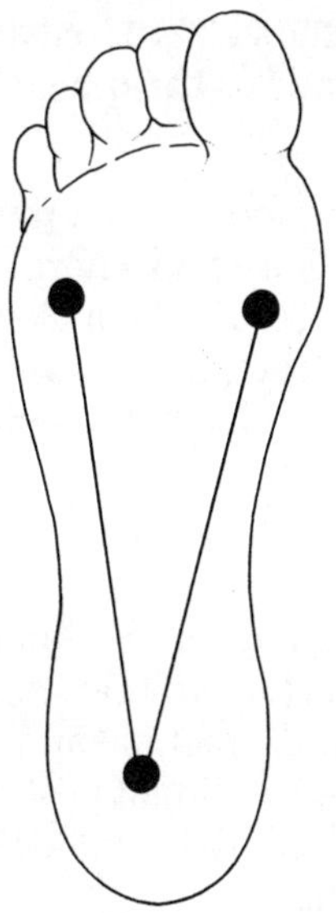

Weight-bearing points of the feet

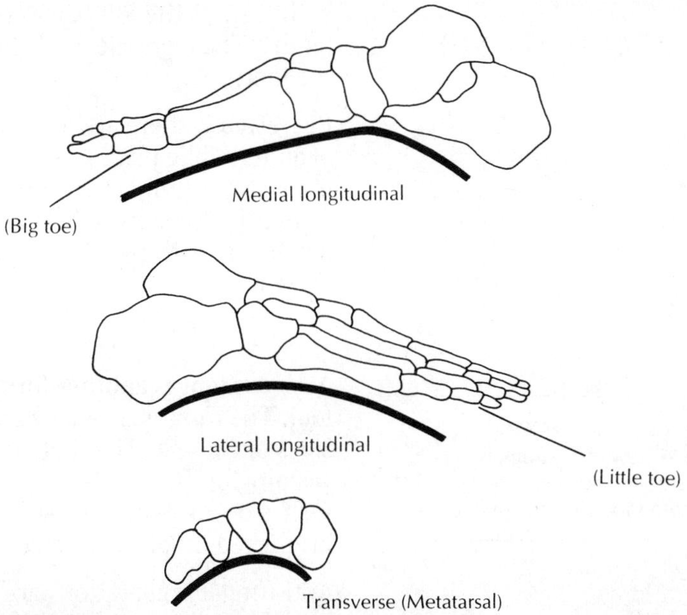

Arches of the foot

Ingrowing toe-nails

> Remember
> Always cut toe-nails straight across and never down their sides, as this forces them to grow into the skin.

Ingrowing toe-nails are very painful and occur as a result of wearing ill-fitting shoes and cutting the nails incorrectly.

If a nail cuts into the flesh, the area soon becomes infected and medical treatment is required. In serious cases the nail has to be removed surgically. Pedicure should not be given where there is pain or infection present.

Corns

> Remember
> Never let a client talk you into cutting away a corn. The treatment of corns should be left to a qualified chiropodist.

Consist of a central core surrounded by thick layers of skin. They appear frequently on the toes and soles of the feet. The skin thickens to protect against constant friction over bone. Soft corns sometimes develop between the bony points of the toes. They can become infected.

Corns are painful due to the pressure that is put on underlying nerve endings. Special plasters and pads are available which ease the pressure on the corns. Ointment can be bought from the chemist which encourages the hard skin to peel.

Calluses

> Remember
> Regular pedicures should include creaming and softening the affected skin.

These are also areas of hard skin caused by friction, but they are less painful than corns as they do not have a root. They usually occur on the sole and underneath a prominent bone. Bad posture often causes calluses. When the body's weight is not distributed evenly, excessive pressure is put on different parts of the feet.

Callus files and pumice stones are available for rubbing away patches of hard skin but, of course, they work by friction and friction causes the skin to thicken! Calluses usually clear up quite quickly once the source of pressure has been removed.

Bunion

A bunion is a harmless swelling of the joint of the big toe which is particularly common in middle-aged women; and usually affecting both feet. As the joint swells, the skin over it becomes hard, red and tender. The big toe usually becomes displaced towards the other toes of the foot.

Regrettably, there are dangers lurking for the barefoot walker, not least of all in public places where facilities have shared use and where there is a warm, humid environment. Contagious diseases can be picked up from infected skin cells left on floors, in shower trays, from towels, in fact from anything which may have previously been in contact with the disease.

Athlete's foot (Tinea pedis)

> Remember
> Athlete's foot is extremely contagious and is contra-indicated to salon treatment.

Athlete's foot is another form of ringworm which affects the skin of the foot. The fungus invades between the toes and spreads to the soles and sides of the feet. The first signs are itching, flaking, cracking and weeping of the skin between the fourth and little toe. Small blisters and rashes occur. When the soles and heels are involved, the skin develops bright red inflammation covered with white scales.

Anti-fungal preparations are available from the chemist which are usually effective within two weeks. The feet should be kept scrupulously clean, cool and dry and protected in high-risk areas such as swimming pools, changing rooms and gymnasiums.

Verrucas (Plantar warts)

Verrucas are firm and round with a rough surface. They may occur singly or in groups. If the top is scraped off, small dark spots – blood vessels supplying the wart – can be seen. Verrucas are caused by a virus and are contagious: they are picked up easily by bare feet. Because they occur commonly on the soles of the feet, the weight of the body causes them to grow inwards and become deeply embedded in the skin, which can be very painful.

Pedicure procedure

The basic manicure procedure adapts quite easily for treating the feet. Specific differences are explained in the following summary.

1 'Are you sitting comfortably?' The same basic principles of good posture apply. Seating should be adjusted so that the client's foot can be supported comfortably on the therapist's lap for treatment.

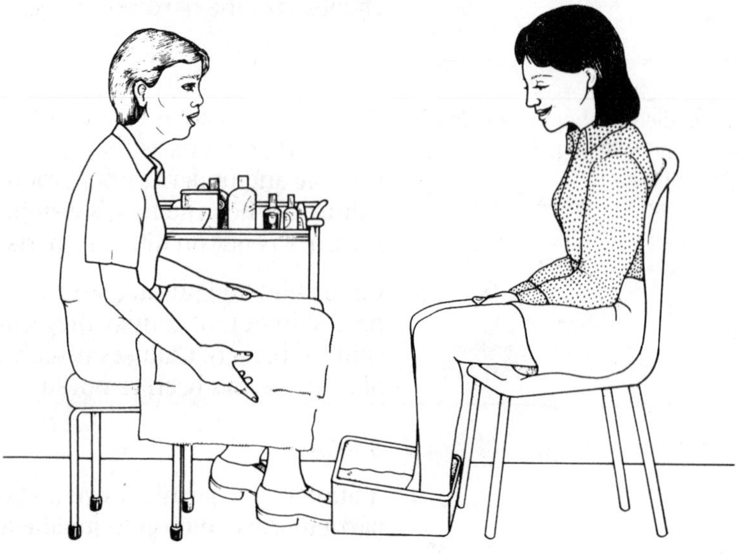

Reclining seats, foot rests and raised foot baths are available to provide extra comfort and relaxation for the client.

2 Wash hands.

3 Examine the feet and nails.

4 Soak feet in warm soapy water containing a little antiseptic.

Clients are usually grateful for the opportunity to have their feet freshened up before they are worked on by the therapist, particularly if they are tired and aching. Alternatively, if you feel that soaking the nails will make them too soft for filing, wipe over the feet with surgical spirit, which will have cleansing, cooling and antiseptic effects.

5 Choose nail enamel colour and check texture.

6 Dry both feet thoroughly and rest them on a clean towel while you replenish the soaking water in the foot bath.

7 Remove old nail enamel from both feet.

8 Where appropriate, shorten the nails with clippers.

Remember

Nail scissors have small, lightweight blades which can be damaged by using them on strong toe nails. Nail clippers are heavier duty and are designed to achieve the straight free-edge shape which is essential for avoiding ingrowing nails.

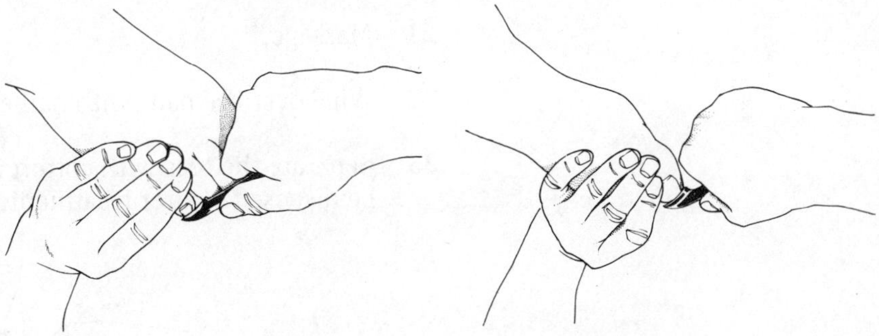

9 Foot 1: use an emery board to smoothen the free edge and achieve the final nail shape. Thick, strong nails can be bevelled slightly with an emery board to taper the shape of the free edge and complement the convex surface of the shoe.

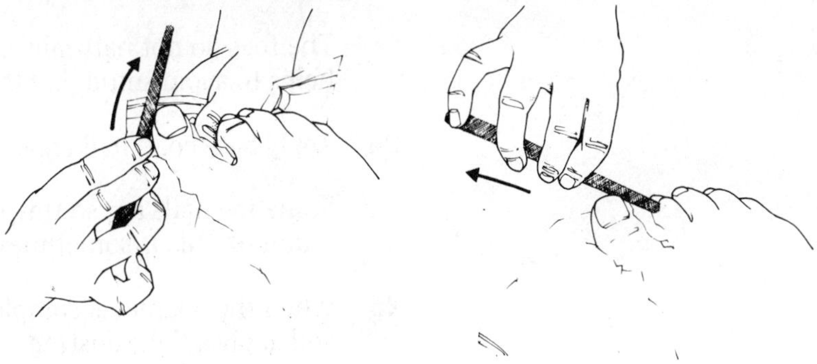

10 Use a callous file or grater where there is a build-up of hard skin. Normal sites are the heel and pads of the foot.

11 Apply cuticle cream, massage, soak.

12 Repeat stages 9-11 on Foot 2.

13 Dry Foot 1 thoroughly. Pay particular attention to the skin between the toes.

14 Apply cuticle remover. Push back, lift and clean around cuticles and free edge with a tipped orangewood stick or hoof stick.

A hoof stick is stronger than the standard orangewood stick. It has a bevelled end made of rubber. The skin at the base of the toe-nails is very sensitive and the hoof stick is considered by some to be more comfortable for pushing back the cuticles.

15 Use the cuticle knife.

16 Dry Foot 2.

17 Foot 1. Scrub nails and rinse and dry foot.

18 Repeat 14-17 on Foot 2.

19 If necessary, use cuticle nippers.

20 File away any rough edges on the nails.

21 Massage.

22 Wipe over the nails with nail enamel remover.

23 Separate the toes with cotton wool pads or rolled tissue which can be disposed of after treatment.

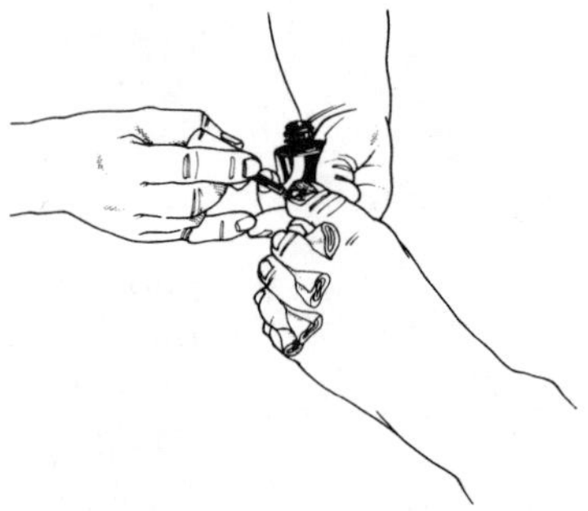

The toes do not naturally span like the fingers: separating them helps to avoid smudging the nail enamel while it is drying.

24 Apply base coat, nail enamel and top coat.

Some toe nails are so tiny that only a single stroke of enamel is required: this is sometimes done across the nail plate.

25 When the enamel is completely dry, remove the toe separators and apply a light dusting of medicated foot powder to both surfaces of the feet and between the toes.

26 Advise the client about products which may be purchased for home care use and record details of treatment.

27 Assist the client with footwear and escort from the treatment area.

Foot massage

The basic effleurage and petrissage movements used in the manicure adapt quite easily for treating the foot and lower leg, but an extra type of movement, tapotement, is usually included for working over larger muscles:

Tapotement

Tapotement covers a range of percussion movements where the hands work briskly, lightly and alternately on the body. The movements are adapted according to the shape, size and strength of underlying muscles, the amount of stimulation required and the condition of the skin.

In this massage routine, *cupping* is performed over the back of the lower leg. This improves the tone of the muscles and skin by stimulating the superficial nerves and increasing the supply of blood to the area.

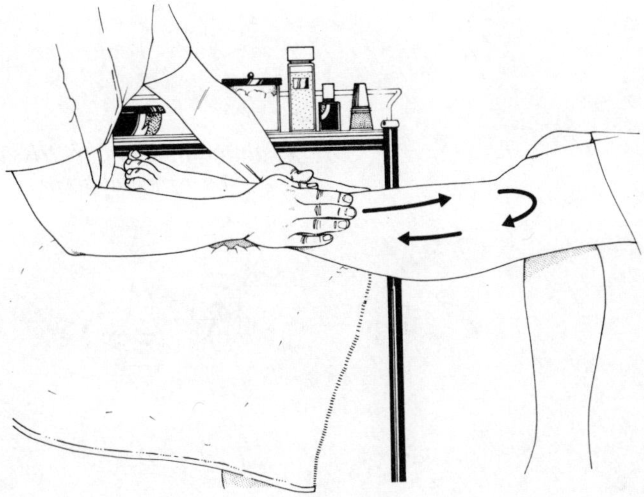

1 Massage position

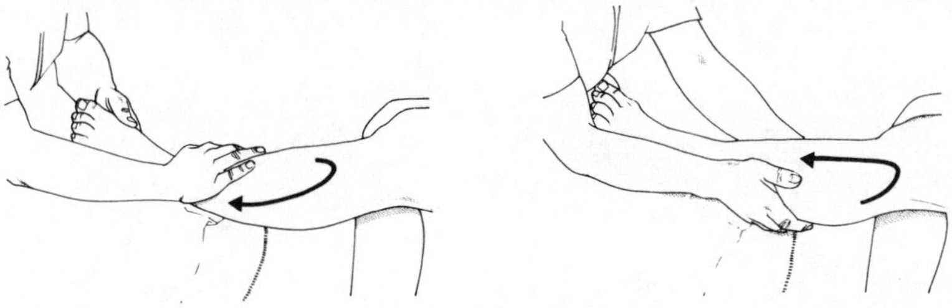

2 Stroking (effleurage) from toes to knee six times with each hand

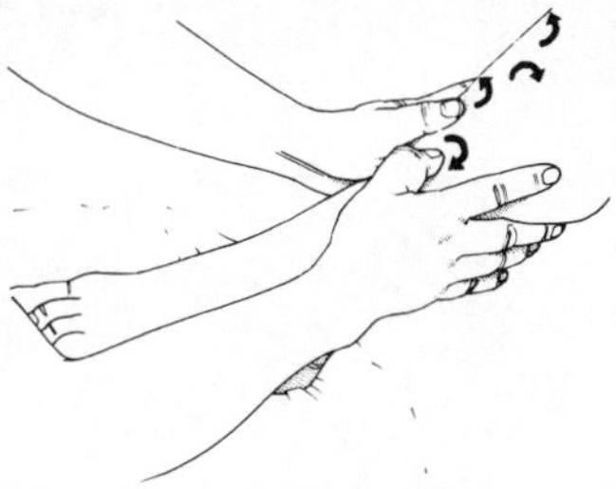

3 Thumb kneading (petrissage) to front of leg

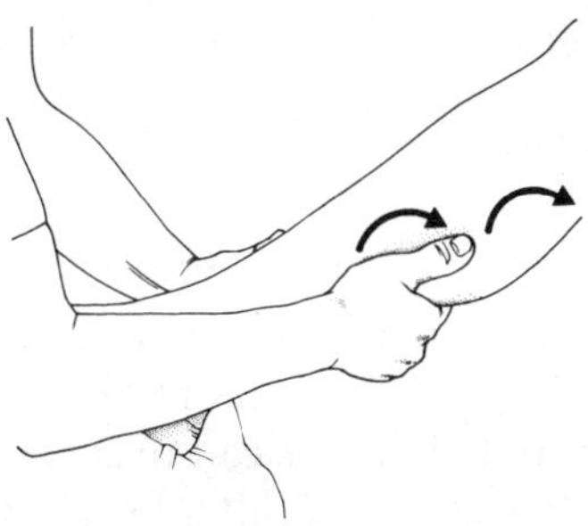

4 Palmar kneading (petrissage) to calf

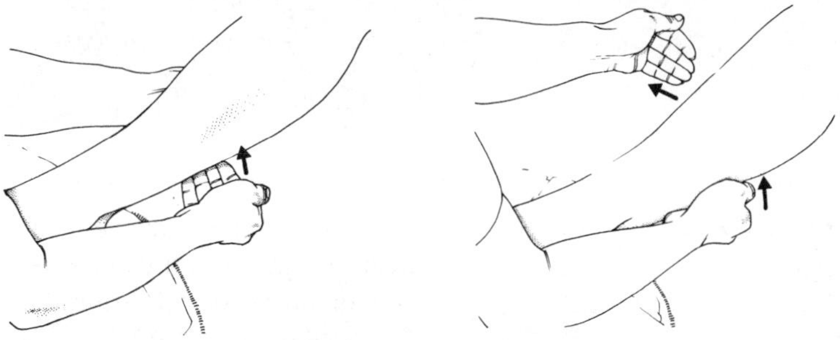

5a, b Cupping (tapotement)

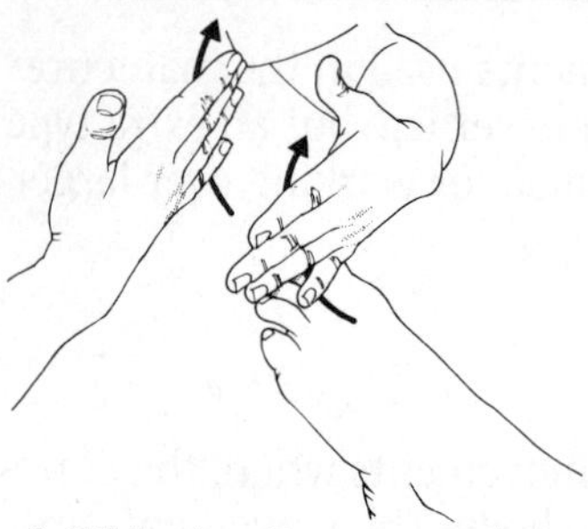

6 Whipping (tapotement)

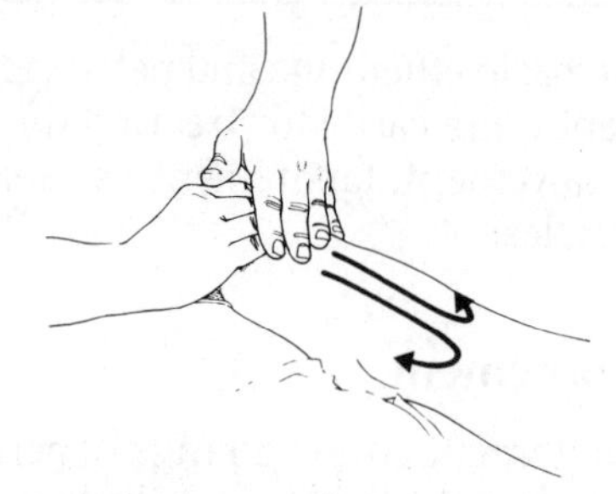

7 Stroking (effleurage) six times with each hand

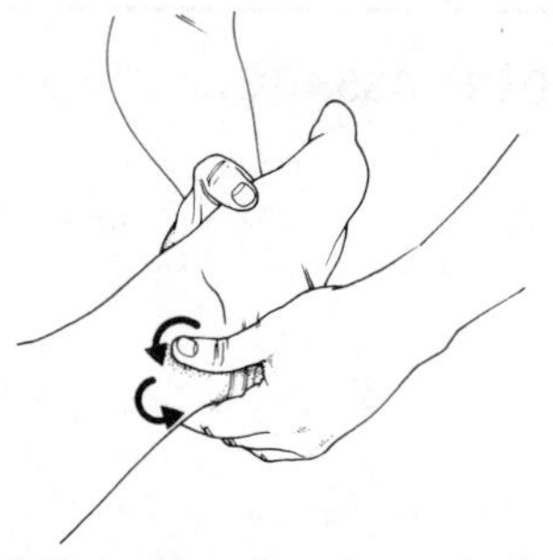

8 Kneading (petrissage) of Achilles tendon

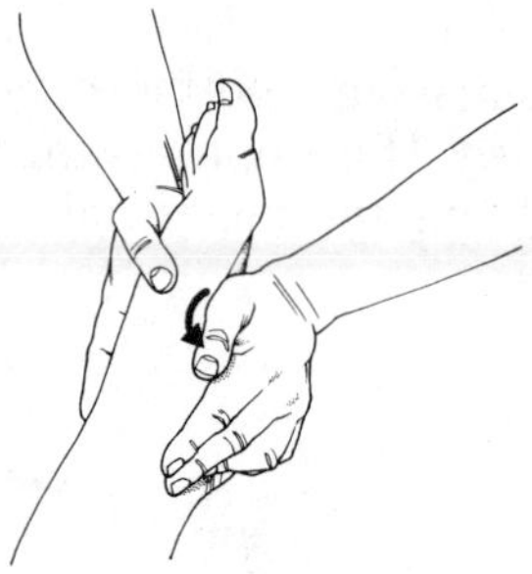

9 Palmar kneading (petrissage) over medial arch

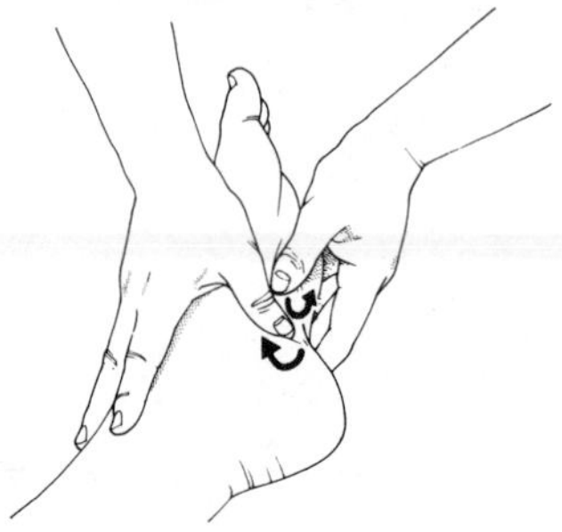

10 Thumb kneading (petrissage) on the medial arch

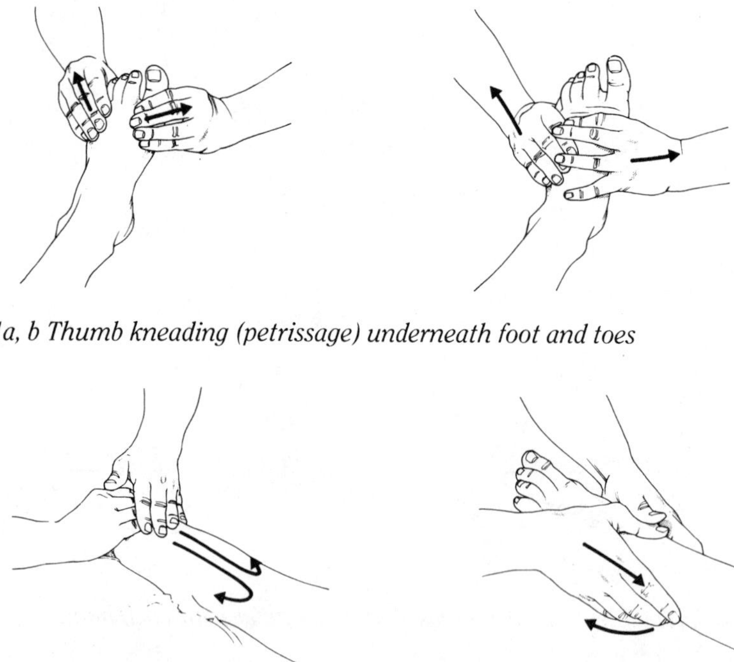

11a, b Thumb kneading (petrissage) underneath foot and toes

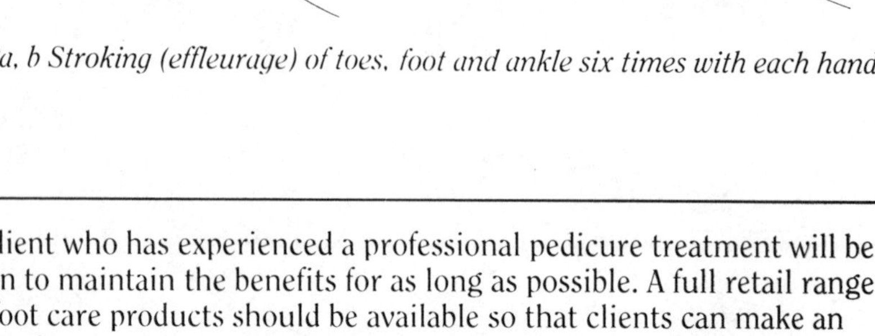

12a, b Stroking (effleurage) of toes, foot and ankle six times with each hand

Caring for the feet at home

A client who has experienced a professional pedicure treatment will be keen to maintain the benefits for as long as possible. A full retail range of foot care products should be available so that clients can make an immediate and enthusiastic start to giving the feet the attention they deserve!

The general purposes of home care treatment are to:

- keep the feet clean and dry
- prevent the build up of hard skin
- minimise the risks of infection
- avoid postural problems
- maintain an attractive appearance.

You will have explained each stage of the pedicure during the treatment, so the client should have a good idea of techniques which can be practised at home in between visits to the salon. A daily routine should be recommended, with extra tips given on the general care and maintenance of the feet.

1 The feet should be washed at least once a day, finishing with a cold rinse. Care should be taken to dry the skin well, particularly between the toes where it soon becomes warm and moist and vulnerable to infection. Scrubbing the feet briskly with a small firm brush not only helps to clean them but also stimulates the blood circulation and has an invigorating effect on the feet.

2 Dusting the feet with a foot powder after bathing and before putting on shoes helps to keep the feet dry by absorbing sweat from the skin. Foot powder is basically talc with a fungicide added to help resist diseases such as athlete's foot.

3 Excessively sweaty feet should be wiped twice a day with surgical spirit or cologne which has a cooling, astringent effect on the skin. This should be followed with a liberal dusting of foot powder.

4 Foot odours tend to be associated with sweaty feet. Sweat actually does not smell, but bacteria which are always present on the skin multiply in a sweaty environment and produce a characteristic, undesirable smell. Regular attention to keeping the feet dry and cool is the best way of tackling the problem. The feet should never be restricted in tight footwear. Shoes should be allowed to ventilate adequately between wearings. Medicated innersoles and those containing activated charcoal help to absorb odours. These are quite cheap and can be fitted into any type of footwear.

5 Deodorant and antiperspirant sprays are available, which are convenient to use during the day for cooling and refreshing the feet.

Remember

Keep a list of local chiropodists handy to whom you can refer your clients. They will appreciate your help and you may even get referrals from the professionals you have recommended.

6 Hard skin can be treated at home following the bath or shower with a pumice stone or callous file .Soften the treated area afterwards by massaging in a medicated foot cream or body lotion.

7 Tired aching feet can be revived by soaking in warm water to which has been added foot bath salts, sea salt or aromatherapy oils. The salts help by dispersing fluid in the area and reducing swelling.

8 Shoes present a healthier environment for the feet if they are allowed to ventilate properly in between being worn. If possible, shoes which have been worn all day should be aired for a day before being worn again. This advice is particularly important for synthetic shoes which are not as absorbent as leather.

Exercises for the feet

The feet spend most of their time confined and unable to exercise freely. Most people should be able to find a few minutes a day to perform these simple exercises. Try them yourself!

Foot flexing

Sit barefoot on an upright chair and cross one leg over the other. Stretch the toes downwards as far as they will go pointing towards the floor. This is called *plantar flexion*. Stretch the foot back towards you until you can feel a pull in the front of the leg. This is called *dorsi flexion*. Do the complete exercise six times then swap legs and repeat.

Foot circling

Still sitting down and with legs crossed, keep the uppermost leg as still as possible, and with the toes pointed, draw six wide circles in the air with the foot. Repeat the exercise with the other leg uppermost.

Joint stretch

Stand upright and take the body weight on one foot. Raise the heel of the other foot and bend the toe joints at right angles to the rest of the sole. Hold this position for a count of 2, then balance the foot on tiptoe for a count of 2. Return the foot to the bent position and finally to the floor. Repeat six times for each foot.

Toe toner

Stand on a thick book or step with the toes hanging over the edge. Bend the toes firmly downwards, hold for a count of 2, then pull them back strongly upwards, also for 2. Repeat the exercise ten times.

Shake and rest

Finally, stand upright and take the body weight on one foot. Lift the other foot and shake it loosely and vigorously for a few seconds. Swap legs and repeat the exercise.

Following the exercises, sit comfortably for two minutes with your legs relaxed and both feet flat on the ground.

Pedicure: Multiple choice quiz

1 The feet tend to be neglected because:
- a) people are reluctant to visit a chiropodist
- b) they can not usually be seen
- c) there is not much that can be done for them
- d there are not many products available.

2 Regular pedicures are beneficial because they:
- a) enable the client to wear fashionable shoes without hurting the feet
- b) correct the damage caused by wearing ill-fitting shoes
- c) keep the feet in good condition
- d) improve the appearance of the feet.

3 The feet are structured mainly to:
a) support body weight
b) enable walking
c) give good posture
d) grip the floor.

4 Ringworm infections of the feet are common because:
a) the fungus spreads easily from the hands
b) the feet are usually warm and moist
c) the skin of the feet is less acid
d) The fungus lives on human skin.

5 The most common cause of foot problems is:
a) heredity
b) ill-health
c) ill-fitting shoes
d) physical damage.

6 Corns are caused by:
a) a virus
b) bacteria
c) friction
d) a fungus.

7 Verrucas grow inwards because:
a) the virus lies affects the deep layers of the skin
b) the weight of the body presses down from above
c) the virus burrows through the skin
d) shoes press upwards on the feet from below.

8 Nail clippers are used to shorten the toe nails because:
a) nail scissors are curved
b) nail scissors are not strong enough
c) nail clippers are more hygienic
d) nail clippers have a straight blade.

9 A callous file should be used gently because:
a) hard skin can be painful
b) hard skin is easy to remove
c) vigorous use will cause infection
d) vigorous use will cause thickening of the skin.

10 Toe nails are shaped straight across to:
a) appear more attractive
b) avoid ingrowing toe nails
c) prevent them rubbing against the shoe
d) prevent them from bruising.

Pedicure: Self-checks

1 Over which muscle of the leg is cupping applied during the foot massage?

2 State the location of each of the three arches of the foot.

3 Name the heel bone.

4 Give two contra-indications to pedicure.

5 Why should the feet be dried thoroughly after bathing?

6 What causes foot odour?

7 Why should corns not be cut?

8 What are the benefits of exercising the feet?

9 When is the best time to promote pedicure treatments?

10 Name two retail foot care products which could be sold in the salon.

Pedicure: Activities

1 Examine the feet of your family and close friends.

Look for signs of damage by ill-fitting shoes and give appropriate advice.

Take advantage of a pair of feet on which to practise your pedicures!

2 Gather product information on specialised foot care ranges. Professional journals, wholesalers and exhibitions are good sources of information.

3 Visit a large retail chemist and see what products are available for the home treatment of athlete's foot, verrucas, corns, calluses and sweaty feet.

Make a note of their contents and an explanation of how they work.

Chapter 12

Wax depilation

After working through this chapter you will be able to:

- describe the different types and functions of hair
- identify normal and abnormal hair growth
- distinguish between depilation and epilation
- describe the structure and growth cycle of hair
- compare the benefits of wax depilation with other methods of hair removal
- advise the client about wax depilation
- apply wax depilatory treatments safely and effectively
- give appropriate home-care advice.

Treatments for superfluous hair

The skin of the face and body is virtually covered by hair. It appears either short and downy (*vellus*) or longer and coarser (*terminal*). Terminal hairs grow thickly where they are needed for extra protection:

- eyelashes: filter out dust and dirt and shade the eyes from excessive sunlight
- eyebrows: protect the eye area but also cushion the prominences of the brow bone
- scalp: prevent heat loss from the body and protect against injury to the head
- underarms/pubic area: protect against friction.

Both women and men grow terminal hairs on their legs and arms. Men also grow them on their chests and faces.

In women, the normal pattern of hair growth may change during the menopause when the balance of sex hormones is disturbed. It is not uncommon, at this time, for vellus hairs on the face to become strong and terminal, particularly above the upper lip and on the chin.

The hairs which grow on exposed areas of the body have a significant effect on overall appearance, particularly if they are dark or excessive.

Attitudes towards the presence of body hair vary between different cultures and also between individuals. In most Mediterranean countries it is considered quite normal for a woman to have dark hair growing in the moustache area. A heavy growth of hair in the underarm region is not considered to be offensive – in fact, quite the opposite!

In the United Kingdom, dark or excessive hair growth on the face and body is generally considered undesirable and the preferred look is for smooth, clear skin. Fair-skinned people usually have less hair than those with olive skins who come from Mediterranean and Middle Eastern countries; people with black skins are generally hairier than Orientals but less hairy than Caucasians.

Terminology

- Superfluous hair: excess hair which is not abnormal but may be considered socially undesirable. Superfluous hairs may be removed by depilation or epilation (see below).
- Hypertrichosis: an excessive and abnormal growth of hair. Strong, terminal hairs appear in areas usually occupied by vellus hairs.
- Hirsutism: an abnormal condition of male-pattern hair growth on a female.
- Depilation: technically, this means the removal of hair from the skin's surface and refers to methods such as shaving, clipping or using chemical depilatories.
- The term is, however, commonly used to describe all temporary methods of hair removal, including waxing.
- Epilation: this term is used to describe permanent methods of hair removal using an electrical current.
- In fact the word 'epilation' means the removal of hair completely from the skin (not just partial removal) and should also be used to describe methods such as tweezing and waxing.

Dark hairs may be bleached using a commercially prepared cream or paste. The skin should be patch-tested beforehand (at least twenty-four hours) to check for sensitivity, and the product used according to the manufacturer's instructions.

Bleaching is usually quite successful when used for lightening vellus hairs, but two treatments may be needed to strip out the reddish tones in very dark hair.

Treatments for superfluous hair: Self-checks

1 What are the main differences between terminal and vellus hairs?

2 Why do women sometimes have problems with facial hair around the time of the menopause?

3 Why is depilation not strictly the correct term for describing the removal of hair with wax?

Hair growth

The hair which shows above the skin's surface is dead. It is composed mainly of keratin, the same protein which makes up the skin and nails. Each hair grows from a narrow, tube-like depression in the skin called a hair follicle. The base of the hair follicle surrounds the hair papilla. This area has an abundant supply of blood vessels which supply nourishment to the hair. Each papilla is surrounded by hair germ cells which develop into a bulb and then grow up the follicle to form a hair. Hairs are soft at the base but gradually harden and die as they approach the surface.

> Remember
> The average lifetime of eyebrow and eyelash hairs is 4-5 months; scalp hairs may keep growing for up to seven years.

Hair stops growing when it is removed from its source of nourishment. This happens naturally during the normal cycle of hair growth and replacement. The papilla which contains blood vessels degenerates, the blood supply ceases and the hair falls out.

Eventually a new hair is formed with an active blood supply and the cycle of events leading to the growth of a new hair is repeated.

Stages of growth

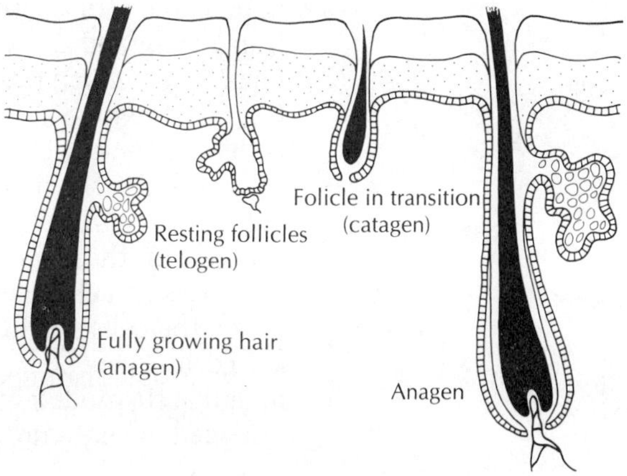

- Anagen: the active growing stage which may last from a few months up to several years. Hair germ cells reproduce at the matrix and pass upwards to form the hair bulb. They then split and change to form different layers. Hairs grow at an average rate of about 1.5 cm per month.
- Catagen A: transition stage from active to resting, which lasts between two and four weeks. The hair stops growing but there is still some activity at the papilla. The hair bulb separates from the papilla and moves slowly up the follicle.
- Telogen: this is the resting stage. It does not last long. The blood supply ceases, the hair bulb closes and the hair prepares to be shed. Meanwhile, a new replacement hair starts to grow at the base of the follicle.

The only way of stopping this cycle permanently is to destroy the structures involved with reproducing hair cells. Treatment with electrical epilation can do this.

An electrical current is passed down a fine needle to the base of the hair follicle. Depending on the type of current used, destruction takes place either by heat or chemically.

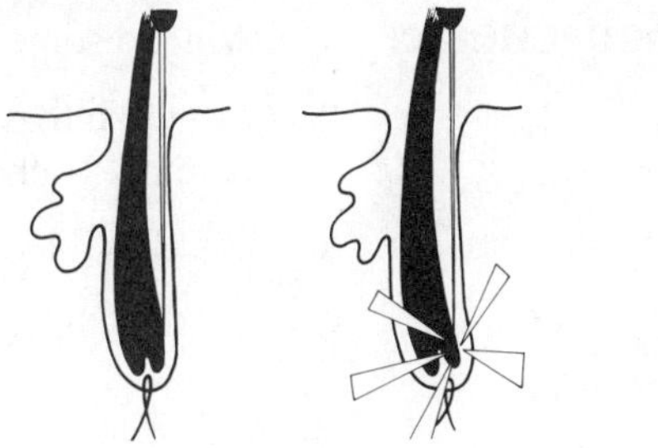

Some people cannot tolerate the feeling of the current used in electrical epilation and prefer to use other methods of dealing with superfluous hair. For others, the long-term effects of the treatment compensate for the patience required and the expense involved.

The structure of hair

A hair is made up of three layers:

- cuticle: the tough, outer protective layer of the hair. The cells are translucent and allow colour from beneath to show through. They form scales which overlap away from the skin towards the hair tip. Chemicals which are applied to lighten or tint the hairs have to penetrate the cuticle in order to work on cells in the deeper layer
- cortex: this is the main part of the hair which contains the colour pigments *melanin* (brown/black) and *pheomelanin* (yellow/red). The cells in the cortex contain bundles of fibres. The strength, thickness and elasticity of the hair is determined by the way in which the cells and fibres are held together. *Keratin* is formed in the cortex
- medulla: the middle 'core' of the hair, which is not always present. The medulla does not appear to have a function.

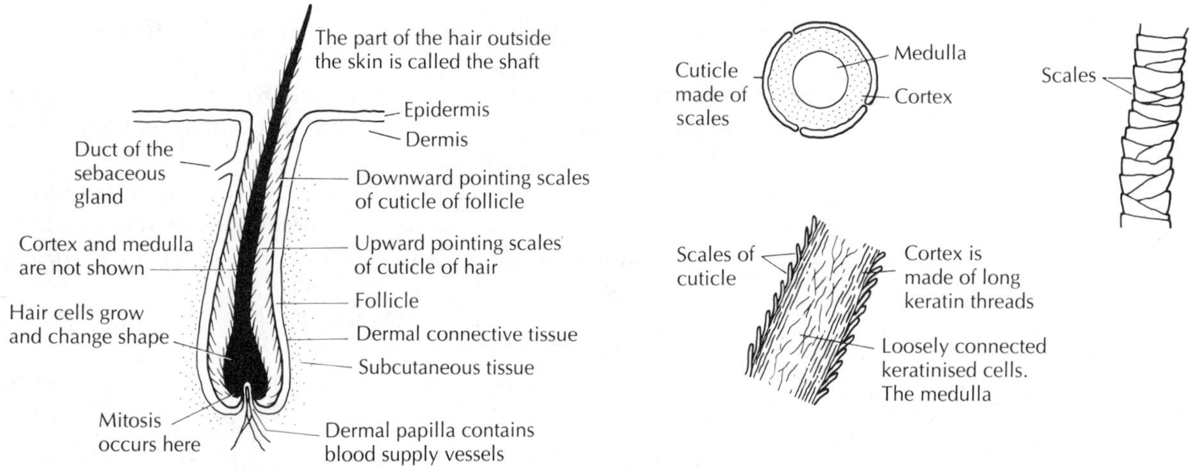

The structure of hair

Hair growth: Self-checks

1. Why do some hairs grow coarser than others?
2. Give three reasons why a client may prefer to have wax depilatory treatments rather than electrical epilation.
3. How does electrical epilation destroy hair?

Wax depilation

There are many people for whom the appearance of facial or body hair is either a nuisance or extremely embarrassing. Wax depilation provides a quick and efficient way of clearing small and large areas of unwanted hair. The treatment is very popular in the salon, particularly during the summer months when more of the body is exposed.

Waxing is a very profitable salon service:

- only small quantities of products and consumable materials are used
- running costs of equipment are low
- only a short amount of time is needed by a skilled operator
- there are opportunities for linked retail sales.

Remember
One bad experience can put the client off waxing forever. Worse still, they may decide to go to a different salon next time so that you lose their custom altogether.

During a depilatory treatment, wax is heated and applied to the skin so that it grips the hairs. When the wax is removed, the hairs are pulled out completely, leaving the skin soft and smooth.

It is obviously very important that the treatment is made quick and painless for the client. Wax depilation can be very uncomfortable if adequate care is not taken.

Wax depilatories

Hot wax depilatories

Hot wax depilatories have been available for a long time but they are less popular now than the low temperature products which have been developed more recently. Hot wax is supplied as blocks or beads. The products usually contain beeswax and resin. Soothing ingredients such as azulene may be added. Beeswax liquefies on heating and contracts around the hairs, gripping them tightly as it cools. Resin makes the wax pliable so that it can be removed from the skin in a continuous strip without cracking or breaking.

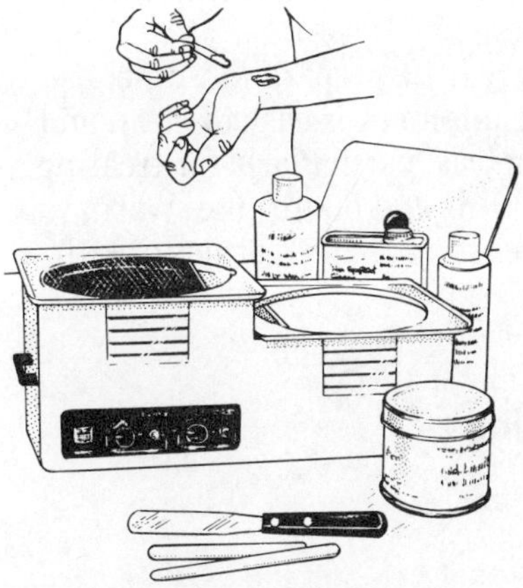

A thermostatically controlled heater maintains the wax at a working temperature of approximately 48 °C (118 °F).

Warm wax

Warm wax is usually supplied in a tin or firm plastic container. The products contain wax with a low melting point, such as paraffin wax. Synthetic resins and other organic materials are often added to improve the texture and quality of the product.

'Organic' waxes are very popular. These are based on a glucose syrup or honey. They do not set when cold but become more fluid when heated. Some warm wax products are available in cream form.

Warm wax affects the hair differently from hot wax. It creates a sticky coating on the hairs which make them adhere to a fabric or paper strip which is applied over the top. The hair is depilated when the strip is pulled away from the skin.

Remember
If your wax heater is supplied with a filter, ignore it! It is no longer considered acceptable to filter and recycle used depilatory wax. Surface skin cells, sweat and, sometimes, spots of blood become impregnated in the wax. They can not be removed by filtering.

The high temperature needed to sterilise used hot wax spoils its texture. The wax becomes brittle and unsuitable for treatment.

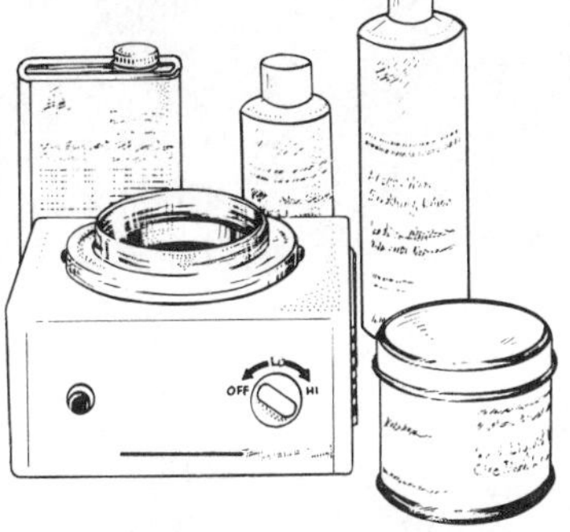

A thermostatically controlled single pan heater maintains the wax at a working temperature of approximately 43 °C (110 °F).

Some warm wax systems provide all the necessary equipment and materials in a compact, self-contained unit which takes up very little space. Pre-filled, disposable, roll-on applicators are available as an alternative to wooden spatulas. They are produced in a range of sizes for treating different areas of the body. The applicators are warmed in a special heater which maintains them at a comfortable working temperature. They are very easy to clean and maintain. The heads are detachable so that they can be washed and sterilised before being re-used.

Which treatment?

Both methods of depilatory waxing produce very good results. Hairs are removed from out of the skin, not just from off the top, and it usually takes at least four weeks for new hairs to appear.

- Hot wax: the strong, gripping action of the wax makes this method particularly effective for removing coarse deep-rooted hairs. Some therapists who have originally trained with, and become expert in, hot wax depilation prefer it to other methods for treating dark, strong hair growth.
- Warm wax: this method requires very little preparation time, the treatments are very quick and the equipment is easy to clean and maintain. Clients often prefer warm wax, particularly for treating sensitive areas like the face, under-arms and bikini-line. Warm wax treatments produce a milder skin reaction than treatments with hot wax.

Contra-indications to wax depilation

General

- Allergy to the products
- Broken skin
- Recent scar tissue
- Bruising
- Moles or warts
- Inflammation, swelling, pus
- Rashes
- Very thin or crepey skin
- Very sensitive skin
- Immediately after sunbathing or sunbed treatment

NB People with diabetes have skin which is very slow to heal. They should be treated with a low-temperature wax. Their skin should be watched closely to make sure it does not over-react to the treatment.

Specific

- Legs: varicose veins
- Underarm: mastitis
- Lip and chin: cold sores
- Eyebrows: styes, conjunctivitis

Preparing for wax depilation

1. Turn on wax heater: allow enough time for the wax to heat up and reach a comfortable working temperature before the client arrives. This usually takes at least 40 minutes for hot wax and 15

> *Remember*
> Do not forget about the wax once you have switched on the heater. Keep a check on its consistency and, if necessary, adjust the thermostat control. If depilatory wax gets too hot, it begins to smoke and give off a very pungent smell. Also, valuable treatment time is wasted waiting for the wax to cool.

> *Remember*
> Depilatory wax will make a mess if spilled on bedding, clothing, towels or floors:

minutes for warm, depending on the amount of wax and the size of the heater.

2 Prepare a trolley: you will need surgical spirit, an antiseptic skin cleanser, talcum powder, wooden spatulas, after-care lotion, cotton-wool, clean towels, tissues, tweezers and a pair of small scissors soaking in disinfectant. Fabric or paper strips will be needed for a warm wax treatment.

3 Protect the couch: use polythene sheeting followed by a soft paper sheet for the client to rest on.

4 Position the wax.: place the heater at a safe distance from the client but near enough to the couch to avoid spills or premature cooling of the wax before it is applied.

Use hot wax in an area which is well ventilated.
- be very careful when moving a container of molten wax
- make sure the heater is resting on a secure base
- keep the wax heater well way from the client
- prevent the lead of the wax heater from trailing where it could cause an accident.

5 Examine the skin and hair: do this in good light. Note contra-indications and patterns of hair growth. Hairs need to be 5–10 mm long for wax depilation.

> *Remember*
> You should wear a plastic apron to protect your overall.

6 Protect clothing: use tissues to protect the client's clothing and remove any jewellery from the area to be treated. The hair should be covered with a towel when treating the face. A client who is having a bikini-line treatment may prefer to wear disposable panties. (The client's position for this treatment is not very elegant and a modesty towel is usually appreciated!)

> *Remember*
> Don't struggle to reach awkward areas. It is much better for you to re-position the client so that you can apply and remove the wax efficiently.

7 Position the client: make sure they are comfortable and that the area to be treated is supported well.

8 Prepare the skin and hair: wipe over the skin with surgical spirit or a special pre-wax cleanser.

Trim excessively long hairs with scissors. This reduces the discomfort of hair removal.

Apply a light dusting of talc against the direction of hair growth. This lifts the hairs and helps them to become covered by the wax. It also helps prevent the wax from sticking to the skin.

9 Advise the client: explain to the client what you are going to do, how it will feel and the probable skin reaction. Warn your client particularly about:
- the likelihood of tiny red spots appearing as a result of stimulating blood to the follicles. These will disappear once the skin calms down
- the possibility of a small amount of blood appearing when hair is removed from the underarm and bikini-line areas. This is due to the coarse thick texture of the hair in these areas.

10 Test the wax: apply a little of the wax to the inside of your wrist or to the sensitive skin between the thumb and index finger. If the wax feels comfortable for you, it should feel comfortable for the client. Test a small amount of wax on the client's wrist

Applying hot wax

1. Take up some wax on the spatula and twist it round over your free hand to control the drips.
2. Apply the wax to the skin in strips, working against, with and against the direction of hair growth.
3. Use your free hand to stretch the skin so that all hairs in the area get covered by the wax.
4. Adapt the size of the strips to the area which is being treated. (The strips should be no wider than 5 cm, or they will be difficult to remove.)
5. Build up the thickness of the strips to approximately 3 mm.
6. Where possible, apply a few strips at a time, working quickly to keep the treatment flowing (see Sequence of treatment).

Removing hot wax

1. When the surface of the wax is dry but still warm, press the strip to the contours of the area.
2. Create a 'lip' by flicking up the lower edge of the strip. Support the surrounding skin while you do this.
3. Grip the lip firmly and remove the wax strip swiftly against the direction of hair growth.
4. Immediately apply pressure or rub the skin lightly but briskly to reduce the stinging effect.
5. Remove small patches of remaining wax immediately by pressing the exposed side of the warm strip over the area. It is best to fold the strip with the hairy sides together before doing this.

> *Remember*
> You should take particular care when touching the client's skin following wax depilation. This is because of the risk of slight bleeding from follicles which contained strong hairs. Make sure that you cover any cuts or breaks in the skin of your hands before the treatment, thereby protecting yourself from possible infection.

> *Remember*
> The strips must always be applied in relation to the direction of natural hair growth.

Sequence of treatment for wax depilation: guidelines for treatment

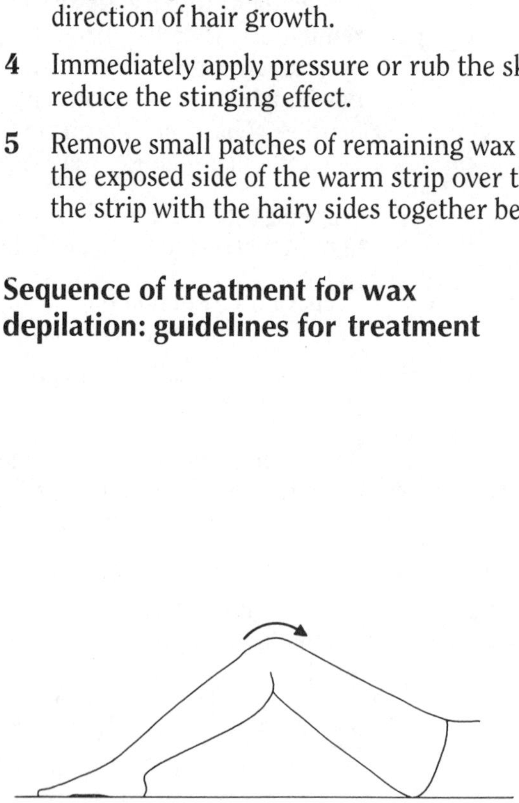

Front leg: bend the leg when waxing over the knee. Short strips are quicker and easier to work with than long ones. With experience, fewer and longer strips may be needed.

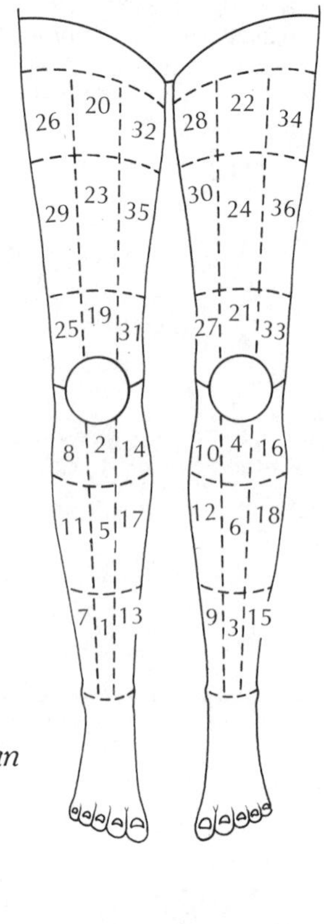

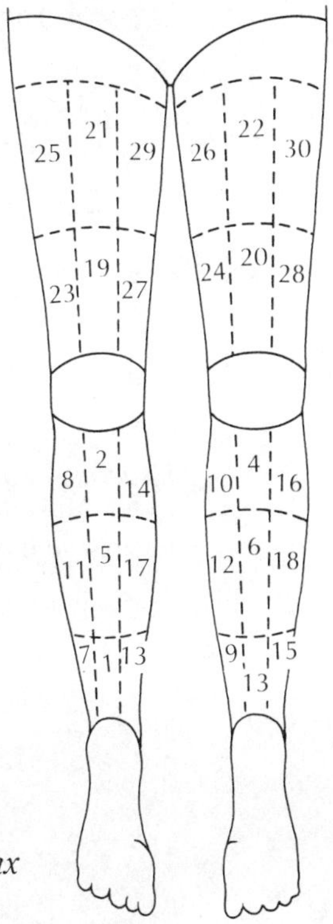

Back leg: do not apply wax over the back of the knee.

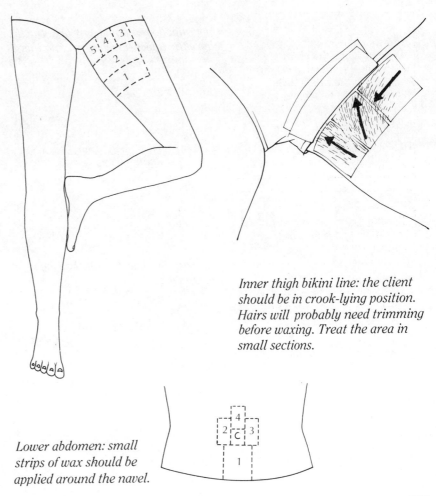

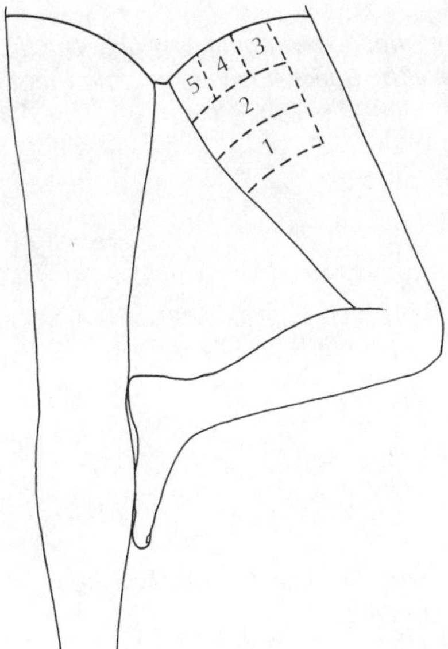

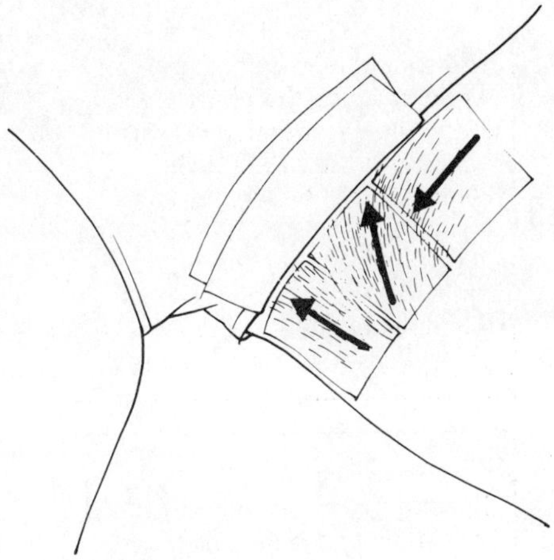

Inner thigh bikini line: the client should be in crook-lying position. Hairs will probably need trimming before waxing. Treat the area in small sections.

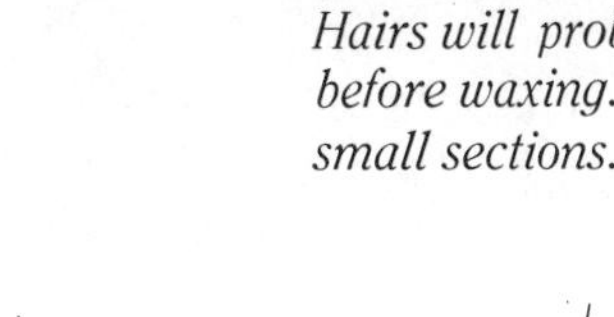

Lower abdomen: small strips of wax should be applied around the navel.

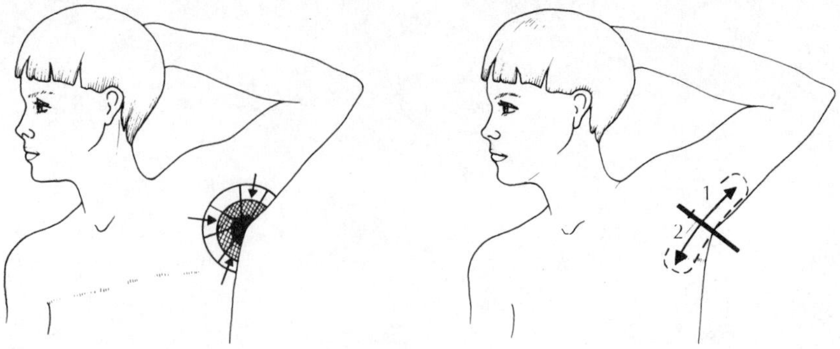

Underarm: apply wax either in small strips working from the outside, in towards the heavier growth in the centre, or in two strips, one each side of where the hairs part in the axilla.

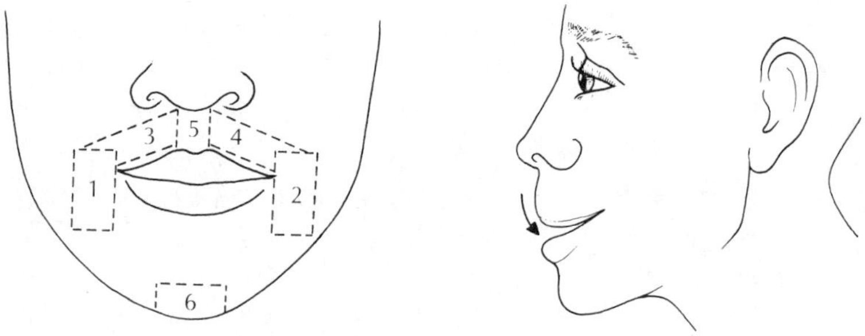

Upper lip: do not apply wax over the lip. Ask the client to stretch the skin above the upper lip when waxing there.

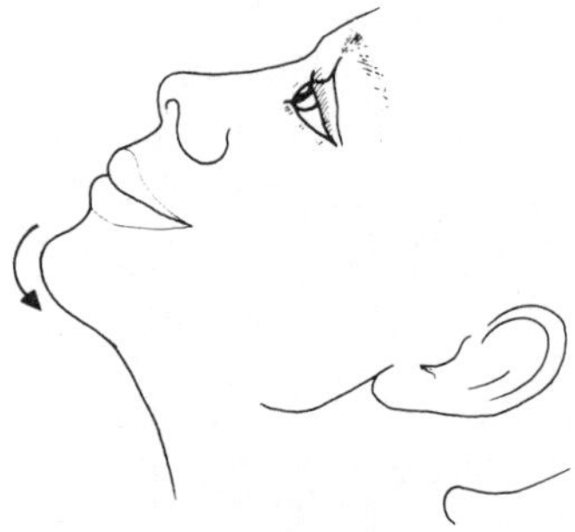

Chin: ask the client to tilt their head back so that the skin is pulled taut over the chin when waxing.

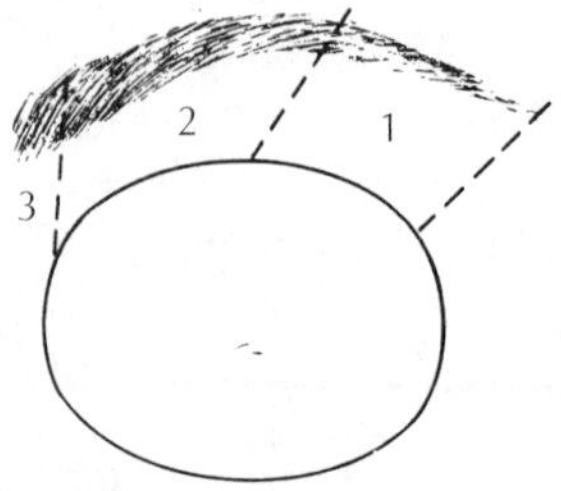

Eyebrow: pull the skin beneath the brow up and outwards before applying wax.

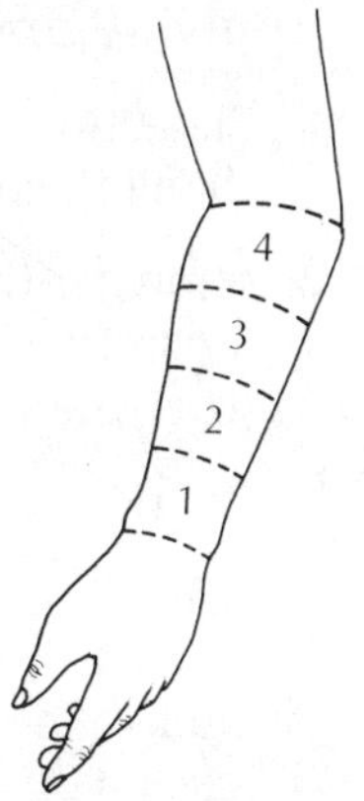

Arms

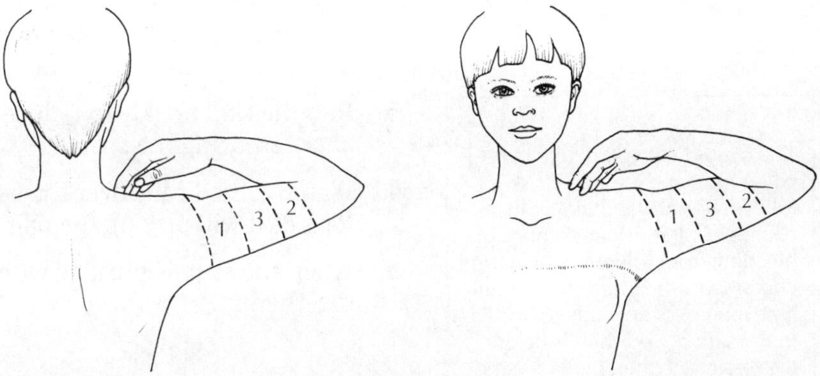

Upper arm: to treat the upper arm, ask the client to touch their shoulder and apply wax from the front or back as appropriate.

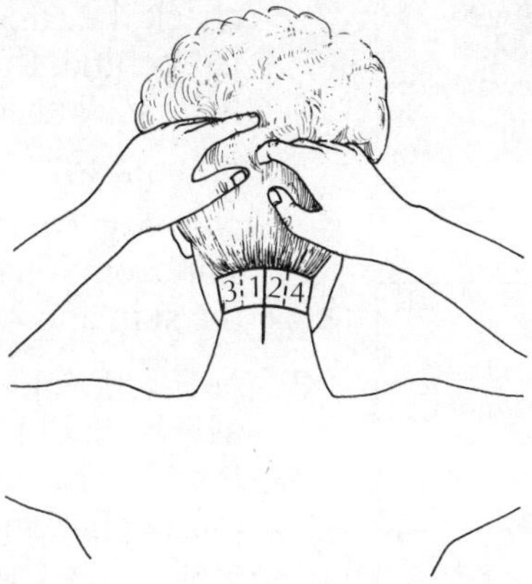

Nape of the neck: any hair longer than 1 cm should be secured out of the way.

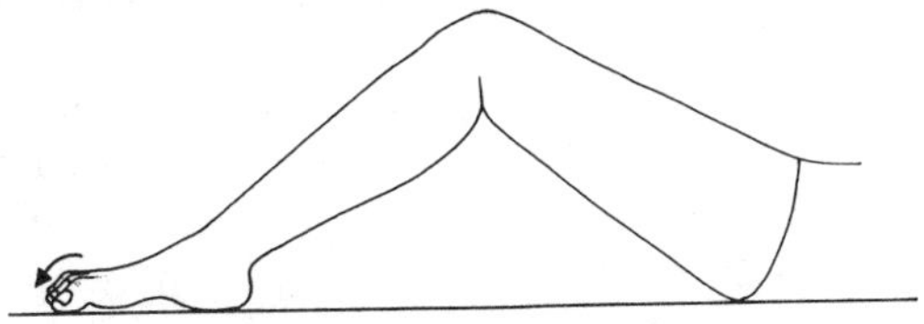

Toes: the client should bend the toes to pull the skin taut.

Applying and removing warm wax

1 Take up some wax on a spatula and twist it round over your free hand to control the drips.

2 Transfer the wax to the skin. Holding the spatula or roll-on applicator at a right angle to the skin, spread a very thin film of wax over the whole of the exposed area.

3 Work in one direction only, i.e. with the natural hair growth, supporting the skin with your free hand.

4 Press a fabric or paper strip onto the wax and smooth over it with your hand in the direction of hair growth. Make sure the strip has a clean edge for gripping.

5 Pull the strip away, quickly, from the skin against the direction of hair growth.

The strip should be pulled back parallel with the skin surface and not vertically from the skin.

6 Rub the skin briskly to reduce the stinging effect which may occur after removing the strip.

7 Work methodically over the whole area, using the same strip for as long as it will pick up the hairs.

8 When the strip is finished with, fold it up with the waxed sides together.

> *Remember*
> You should take particular care when touching the client's skin following wax depilation. This is because of the risk of slight bleeding from follicles which contained strong hairs. Make sure that you cover any cuts or breaks in the skin of your hands before the treatment, thereby protecting yourself from possible infection.

> *Remember*
> Treatment with depilatory wax also removes surface cells and grease which normally protect the skin. Do not re-apply wax for at least 48 hours if the skin appears pink and shiny.

> *Remember*
> The skin needs extra protection after a depilatory wax treatment. Empty hair follicles provide a route for bacteria.

> *Remember*
> An after-wax lotion could also be used as a hand moisturiser, body lotion or for after-sun skin care: sell it!

Completing wax depilation

1 Assess results: examine the skin. Look for remaining hairs and check the condition of the skin. If there are just one or two hairs left behind, they may be removed by tweezing. Patches of stubborn hairs may need a second application of wax.

2 Provide after-care: wipe over the skin with an antiseptic after-wax cleanser. This will remove any sticky residue and help protect the skin from infection. Apply a soothing after-wax lotion to help cool the skin and replace lost moisture.

3 Advise the client on home care: explain the special precautions which should be taken until the area has completely settled down. It takes between 24 and 48 hours for the skin to stabilise itself after wax depilation. The actual recovery time depends on the sensitivity of the skin, the amount and type of hair that has been removed and the method of treatment which has been used. Clients should be advised to take the following precautions for at least 24 hours after wax depilation and for longer if the skin still feels sensitive:
   - apply a soothing after-wax lotion or gel regularly to keep the skin soft and minimise any redness or irritation
   - have only lukewarm showers and baths
   - refrain from applying anti-perspirant, deodorant or perfumed products to the area
   - avoid applying make-up over the area
   - avoid sunbathing or having a sunbed treatment

4 Fill in record card: record details of treatment and sales.

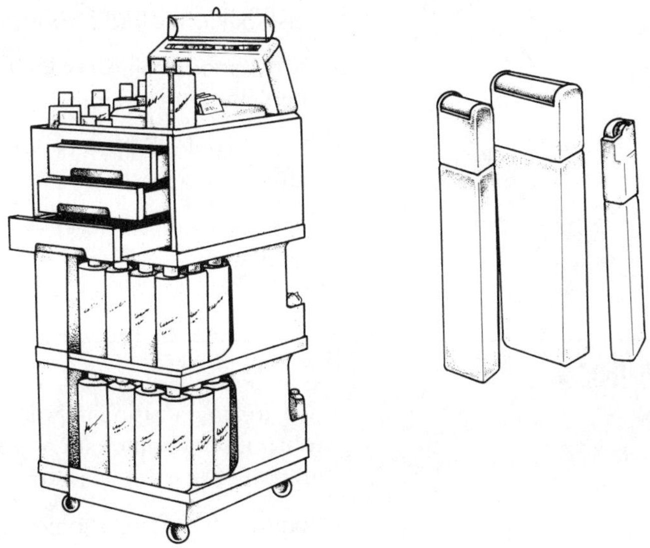

Roll-on warm wax system and applicators (not drawn to scale)

> Remember
>
> Surgical spirit is very effective for cleaning up after hot wax depilation. Wipe over the equipment while it is still warm. Wax is much more difficult to remove once it has cooled and gone hard.

5 Clear up:
- dispose of used spatulas, wax, strips and waste in a sealed plastic bag.
- remove used towels
- clean the equipment with an appropriate solvent. Some warm waxes are water-soluble and can be wiped away with a damp cloth. Others require surgical spirit or a special wax cleaner to remove them.
- detach the heads of roll-on applicators and remove wax from them with the special cleaner provided.
- finish off by wiping with surgical spirit and then soak them in a solution of disinfectant.

Wax depilation: Self-checks

1 When is a particularly good time for promoting wax depilatory treatments in the salon?

2 List four ways of minimising client discomfort when removing hair with hot wax.

3 What would happen if a resin was not included in the hot wax formulation?

4 What is the suitable working temperature for hot wax?

5 How are the ingredients of warm wax products different from hot wax?

6 Compare the action upon hair of hot wax and warm wax.

7 What is the suitable working temperature of warm wax?

8 State three advantages of using roller type applicators for applying warm wax.

9 List the contra-indications to wax depilation.

10 Why is the position of the client important when giving a wax depilatory treatment?

11 Why should a client be advised against having a sunbed treatment after wax depilation?

12 Why is the application of a soothing lotion necessary after wax depilation?

Wax depilation: Activities

1 Working with a partner, try to work out the average profit on a half-leg wax treatment using a) hot wax and b) warm wax. You will need to work out how much it costs to give the treatment and take that amount from the price that is charged to the client.

You may have to do some practical work to help you estimate the amount of wax and other consumable items needed for the treatment. When you have managed to agree on an answer, compare your salon's prices with those of other salons in the area.

2 Using the information you have gained from Activity 1, decide how you could run a special promotion for leg waxing. Consider a range of suitable alternative types on offer, for example price reduction, free gift, and then work out which one is least costly for the salon.

Design a newspaper advertisement for promoting your offer.

Waxing problems

The ones that got away!

It is very frustrating to find that some of the hairs you thought you had depilated managed to escape!

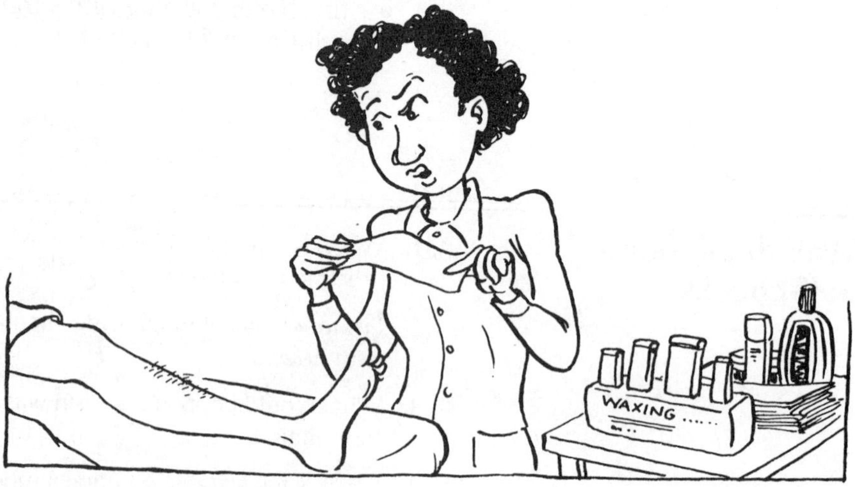

Here are some possible reasons for hairs remaining after a wax depilatory treatment:

- the hairs were too short to wax
- the warm wax was applied too thickly for the strip to grip the hairs
- the hot wax was too thick to contract tightly around the hairs
- the wax was applied and removed in the wrong direction
- the wax was removed too slowly
- the skin was not pulled taut and hairs were caught in creases.

Over-reaction

The skin normally looks slightly pink after wax epilation, even when a low temperature product has been used. Extreme redness and skin irritation suggest an over-reaction to the treatment. Possible causes of this could be:

- failing to recognise a sensitive skin and not giving a skin test before treatment
- the wax was too hot
- overlapping applications of hot wax
- applying pressure with the side of the spatula when applying warm wax
- pulling off the wax strip upwards rather than back on itself
- failing to pull the skin taut when removing the wax.

Some questions and answers

Q How long do the effects of wax depilation last?
A Usually about 4-8 weeks, but this varies between individuals. People who have very sensitive hair germ cells produce replacement hairs more quickly than others.

> Remember
> Hairs which have been cut or shaved feel thicker because they have blunt ends. After wax depilation a new replacement hair grows which has a fine, tapered end.

Q Do depilatory wax treatments make the hair grow back thicker?
A There is evidence both for and against this theory. Most clients claim that hair growth is more sparse after depilatory waxing. This is probably because the hairs are depilated at different stages of the growth cycle so the replacement hairs do not appear at the same time.

It is possible that the stimulating effects of repeated wax depilatory treatments could strengthen the follicles and increase their blood supply. This would result in replacement hairs growing back coarser and more firmly rooted.

Q Is it all right to have wax depilation in between electrical epilation treatments?
A No, definitely not. Regular depilatory wax treatments can distort the hair follicle and make subsequent treatment with electrical epilation very difficult.

Q Does depilatory waxing hurt?
A No, not if it is done properly. When the wax is removed, the feeling is similar to having a plaster pulled off. Any skin sensation soon stops once soothing after-care has been applied.

Q How long do wax treatments take?
A It depends on the amount and type of hair growth and the method of waxing used. As a guideline, the average time for a half leg-wax treatment (ankle-knee) with warm (cool) wax is 10–15 minutes. With hot wax, treatment to the same area takes nearer 30 minutes.

Other methods of hair removal

There are options available to the client for dealing with unwanted hair at home. You need to know about these so that you can give advice about the advantages of professional treatments.

> Remember
> The skin also contains keratin and must also be affected by the cream. This type of depilatory should never be used on the face. A skin test should be given before using it elsewhere on the body.

Depilatory creams

Depilatory creams contain a chemical such as calcium thioglycollate which breaks down the protein keratin and dissolves the hair so that it can be wiped away. Hair is removed from slightly below the skin's surface. They provide a very short-term solution to the problem of unwanted hair.

Clipping

Scissors are used to cut the hair at skin level. Clipping removes the tapered end of the hair and leaves it blunt. A smooth finish cannot be achieved, as a close cut is not possible with scissors.

> Remember
> Razors which are not cleaned and stored hygienically are likely to cause a skin infection.

Shaving

Shaving creates a blunt tip which replaces the natural, tapered one. This gives the effect of a thicker regrowth. If the skin is stretched while shaving, the hair is removed from just beneath the skin's surface. Razors are quick and easy to use but they produce a stubble and are not hygienic.

Plucking

Plucking is normally done with tweezers and removes one hair at a time from the hair follicle. The hair will not break so long as the skin is prepared properly and the hair is pulled out in the direction of growth. Plucking is only suitable for treating small areas, for example the eyebrows.

Threading

Threading is practised expertly by some Mediterranean and Asian communities. A piece of cotton is wrapped around the fingers and then twisted and rolled over the skin. The hair is caught up in the thread and is pulled swiftly out of the follicle. Whilst some hairs may be removed completely, it is likely that others will be broken off at the skin's surface. When performed skilfully, threading has the same effect as plucking.

Pre-waxed strips

Strips of cellophane are coated with a cold wax; the cold wax sticks to the hairs, some of which are removed when the strip is pulled off. The basic principles of treatment are the same as for warm wax, but the results are less satisfactory: for depilation to be effective, it is the hairs which need to be coated with wax, not the cellophane! The strips are easy to apply but painful to remove.

Sugaring

This technique has been practised for centuries in the Middle East. Sugar, water and lemon juice are cooked together to produce a caramel. The mixture is then poured on to a plate and rolled into little balls. The caramel balls are pressed firmly onto the skin and then pulled off sharply, taking hair with them. The effect of sugaring is similar to warm wax depilation

Abrasives

A pumice stone or abrasive glove is rubbed over the skin in circular movements and the hair is broken off at the skin's surface. The effects of abrasion on the skin are probably more useful than the effects on hair growth, provided that the skin is not damaged.

Chapter 13

Ear piercing

After working through this chapter you will be able to:

- understand the importance of hygiene and safety when piercing ears
- identify contra-indications to ear piercing
- prepare the client for ear piercing
- use ear-piercing equipment safely and effectively
- give appropriate after-care and advice to the client.

Ear piercing

Ear piercing is becoming increasingly popular in the salon. Clients know they will get a professional treatment and that standards of hygiene and safety will be high. These are essential for ensuring that the ear does not become damaged or infected. Modern ear-piercing systems allow the whole procedure to take place without any direct contact between the hands and the stud fastenings.

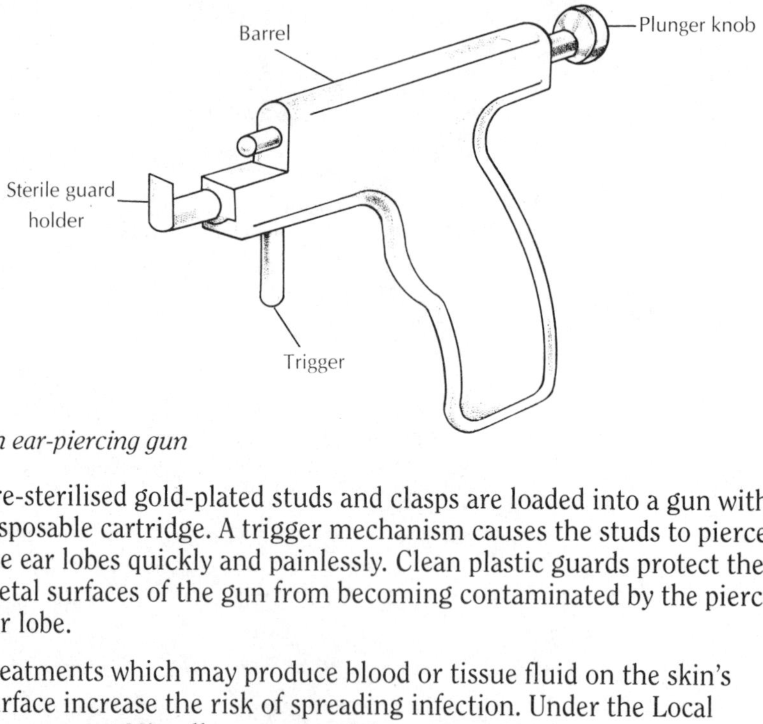

An ear-piercing gun

Pre-sterilised gold-plated studs and clasps are loaded into a gun with a disposable cartridge. A trigger mechanism causes the studs to pierce the ear lobes quickly and painlessly. Clean plastic guards protect the metal surfaces of the gun from becoming contaminated by the pierced ear lobe.

Treatments which may produce blood or tissue fluid on the skin's surface increase the risk of spreading infection. Under the Local Government Miscellaneous Provisions Act 1982, there can be very serious consequences for a salon which does not take the necessary precautions when giving these treatments. Make sure you follow the Government guidelines for ear piercing by:

- using only equipment approved by the Environmental Health Authority
- maintaining high standards of hygiene and safety
- disposing of waste correctly
- giving the correct after-care advice.

> *Remember*
> People and premises which offer ear piercing treatments must be registered with the Local Environmental Health Authority. Failure to do so may result in serious consequences.

Preparing for ear piercing

Make sure that the room is warm and well ventilated and that you will be working in a good light. You will need:

- an ear piercing gun which has been cleaned and sterilised
- a sealed blister pack containing sterile studs, guard and stud holders
- a clean marker pen
- medical swabs (impregnated with 70% isopropyl alcohol) or surgical spirit
- soothing antiseptic lotion
- towel
- a clean bowl containing cotton-wool
- closed, lined container for waste
- hair clips
- mirror
- record card (plus consent form signed by a parent if the client is under 18).

Preparing the client

It is understandable for a client to be nervous before ear piercing. You can help by appearing confident and in control.

1 Make sure the client is seated comfortably with head supported in the upright position.

2 Place a towel across the shoulders. If a stud or clasp is dropped, it will be easier to retrieve from a towel than by rummaging in the client's clothing!

3 Wash your hands.

> *Remember*
> Make sure you record that you have checked for contra-indications in case the client returns with a problem later on.

4 Examine the ears and check that there are no contra-indications. The following are contra-indications to ear piercing:
   - broken skin
   - lumps, swellings, moles, warts, scar tissue in the area to be pierced
   - any signs of infection or open wounds
   - diabetes (because of the poor healing quality of the skin)
   - epilepsy
   - infection by hepatitis or HIV
   - circulatory disorders.

5 Consult client about specific requirements and selection of studs.

> *Remember*
> The ear lobes have a very good blood supply. Bacteria which invades through pierced skin can be transported by the blood to other areas, causing a more widespread infection.

6 Cleanse the outer ear, front and back, with a medical swab or surgical spirit on cotton wool. This will remove any harmful bacteria present which could invade the pierced skin.

7 Agree the positioning of the stud with the client and mark it in an identical place on both ears. Check with the client again before piercing the skin.

Deciding where to pierce

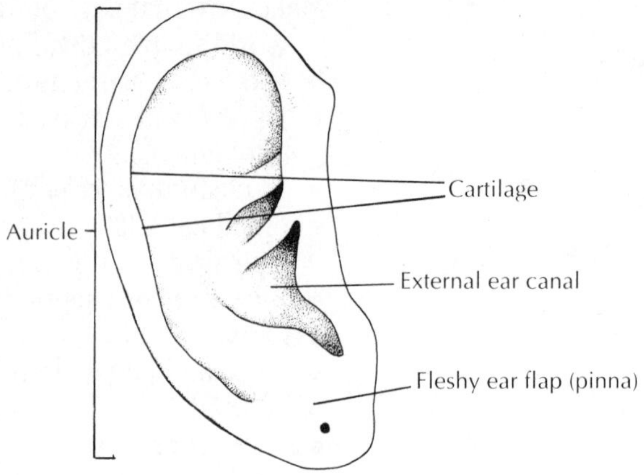

The ear should be pierced in the fleshy part of the lobe. Above this, the ear is made up of fibrous cartilage covered by firmly adherent skin.

Piercing through cartilage is very painful. If pierced too close to the edge, the ear could split. Damage to the cartilage can cause *cauliflower ear* (the ear flap appears large and deformed): this is very unpleasant. Infected cartilage is difficult to treat.

Piercing the ears

Always follow the manufacturer's instructions when loading the gun and lining up the stud and clasp with the ear markings.

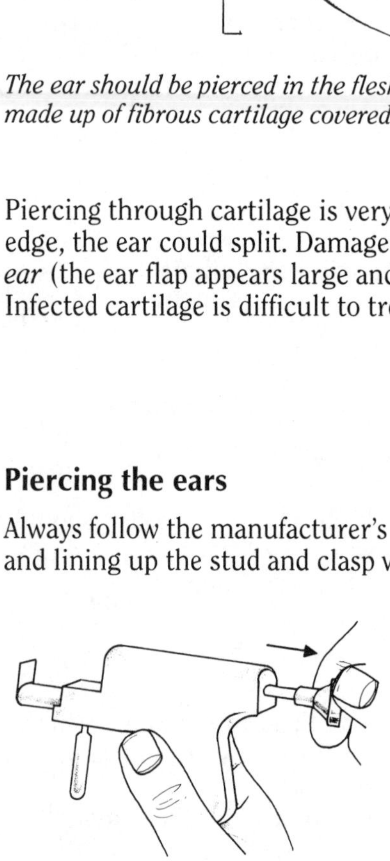

Pulling back the plunger

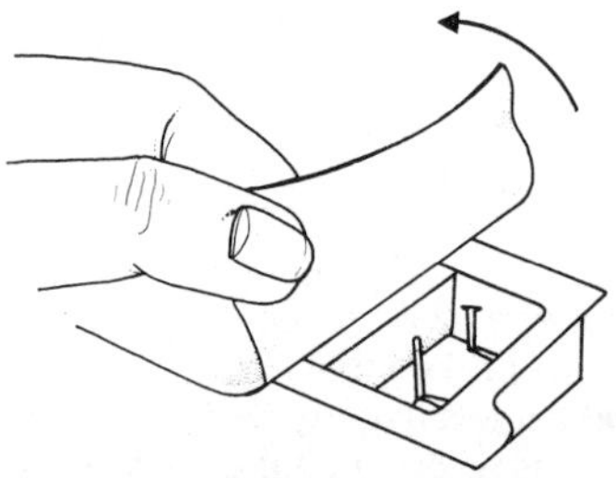

Carefully opening the blister pack

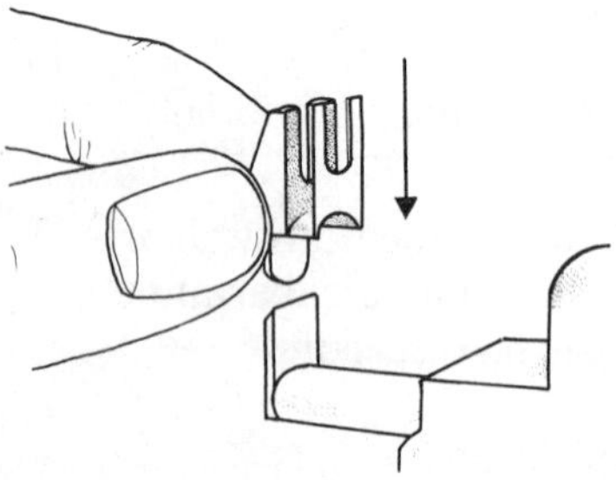

Positioning the plastic guards and loading up the gun. No touching!

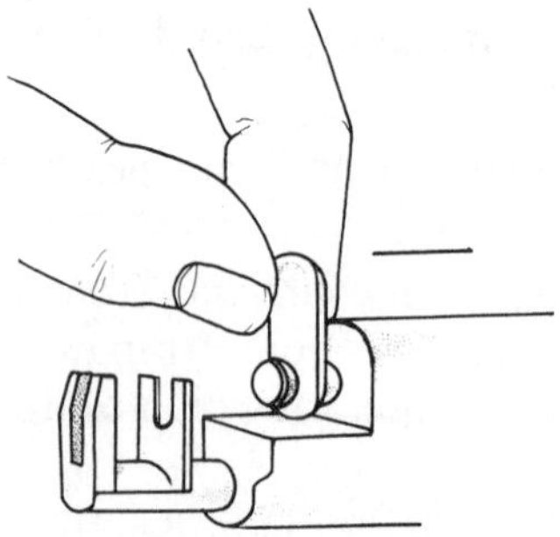

Placing the sterile stud holder in the barrel of the instrument

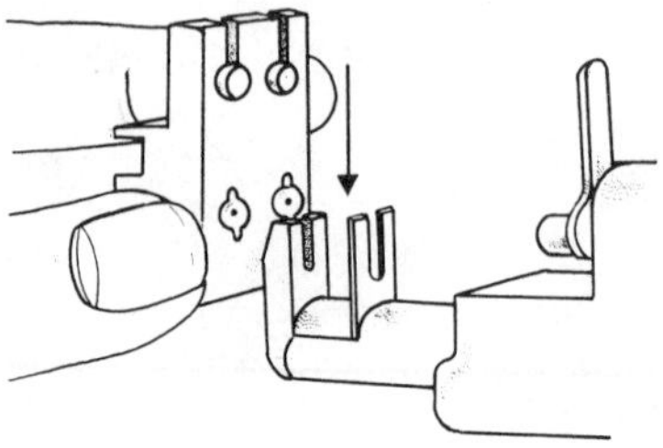

Sliding the back clasp or butterfly into the rear of the sterile guard

> Remember
> The studs and clasps are usually sealed in pairs. If a client is having only one ear pierced, the remaining stud, clasp and mounts must be discarded.
>
> Throw away all disposable holders and guards immediately after use.

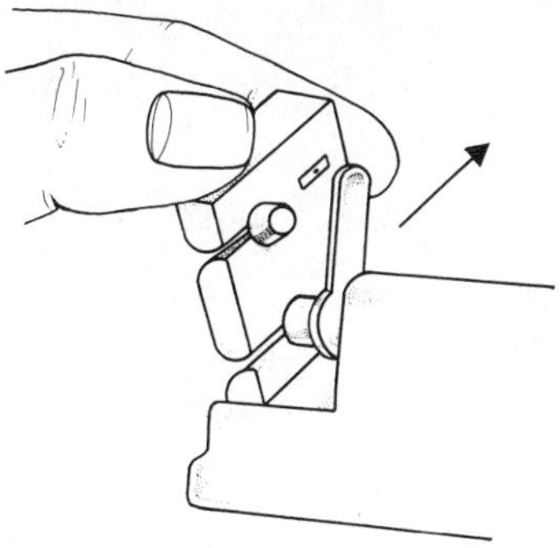

Sliding the ear stud into the sterile stud holder

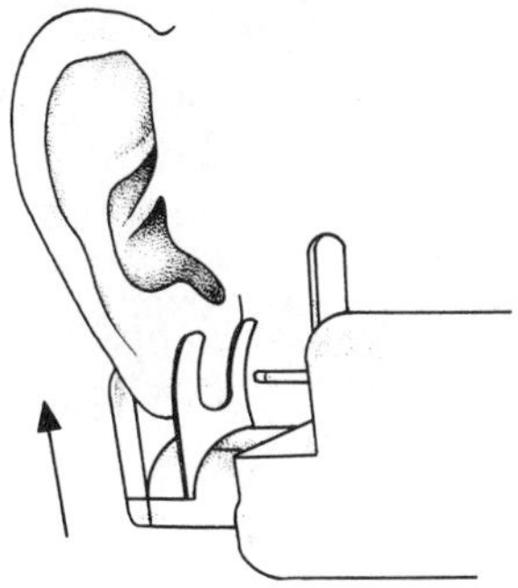

Positioning the ear lobe and lining up

> Remember
> You will need to consult your records if a client returns to you with a problem such as an infection. If the client attends the salon regularly for treatment, you may use your records to help check up on how well the skin is healing.

> Remember
> Make sure the client is advised to use the correct strength of liquid antiseptic if using a proprietary brand. Using undiluted antiseptic can irritate the skin.

> Remember
> After six weeks, the studs should be replaced with gold or silver earrings. Other types of metal may cause an infection or irritation if worn too soon after ear piercing.

Afterwards, wipe over the ear with a soothing, antiseptic lotion. Record treatment details and give the client advice for after-care.

After-care

The hole which has been formed must be kept clean and the studs kept in place for at least six weeks. After this time, healing should be complete and the studs can be replaced with earrings of the client's choice.

The client should be given the following advice for after-care.

1. To prevent infection:
   - avoid unnecessary handling of the ears and studs; don't fiddle!
   - do not replace studs with other earrings during the initial six week period
   - bathe the ear lobe twice a day with an antiseptic lotion
   - wash hands before touching ears and studs and cleanse back and front of ear lobe with surgical spirit or special after-care lotion
   - do not allow soap or shampoo to build up behind the stud or clasp. Rinse well after washing
   - cover ears when spraying perfume, antiperspirant, hairspray.
2. To prevent holes from closing:
   - do not take studs out for at least six weeks
   - turn studs at least twice daily when bathing ears with antiseptic.
3. If infection or irritation occurs:
   - rinse area regularly with warm salt water
   - contact doctor if problem becomes serious.

Ear piercing: Self-checks

1. What is the professional code of working practice with regard to ear piercing?
2. Why is there a particular risk of spreading infection when piercing ears?
3. Why is it important to protect the package containing the studs and clasps?

4 Why is a client with diabetes contra-indicated to ear piercing?

5 Why must extreme care be taken when deciding on the position of the stud?

6 For how long should the client be advised to keep the studs in place?

7 What questions would you ask a client who complained of developing sore and inflamed ears within days of having their ears pierced?

8 What advice would you give a young teenager who requested an appointment to have her ears pierced?

9 Why is it important to keep records of ear-piercing treatments?

10 Who enforces the law relating to ear-piercing treatments?

Ear piercing: Activity

Remember

A stud which fits too tightly will not turn readily in the ear and there may be problems with healing. A client with fat ear lobes should be advised of the risk of friction and irritation causing damage to the skin and underlying blood vessels.

If the client experiences discomfort, the stud should be removed and hygienic after-care procedures continued until the skin has healed.

1 Handle an ear-piercing gun before using it on a client for the first time. Practise loading the cartridges without touching the studs and clasps with your fingers. You may use the same set for repeating your practices, but on no account must you use them for actually piercing ears.

Index